PSYCHIATRIC DRUGS EXPLAINED

David Healy MD FRCPsych
Director
North Wales Department of Psychological Medicine
University of Wales
College of Medicine
Bangor
UK

SIXTH EDITION

ELSEVIER

Edinburgh London New York Oxford Philadelphia St Louis Sydney Toronto 2016

ELSEVIER

ISBN 978-0-7020-4508-0

Printed in China

Last digit is the print number: 9 8 7 6 5 4 3 2 1

PSYCHIATRIC DRUGS EXPLAINED

For Elsevier
Content Strategist: Alison Taylor
Content Development Specialist: Martin Mellor Publishing Services Ltd/Carole McMurray
Project Manager: Andrew Riley
Designer/Design Direction: Miles Hitchen

CONTENTS

PREFACE

In 1993 when the first edition of this book was written evidence based medicine (EBM) was just emerging, and prescribing by nurses in the UK and pharmacists or psychologists elsewhere was just starting to be talked about.

The biggest need in 1993 for a book like this seemed to be the need to assert the primacy of the language that people used in trying to describe what was happening to them and that those working in health care used when witnessing what was happening to people on treatment over a new biological language about lowered serotonin levels and dopamine receptor blockade.

EBM initially seemed like an ally in this effort as it was explicitly about combining the best evidence with patient and clinical values, and it put much more weight on clinical trials than on biology. EBM has however become as big a threat to the ability of two people in a clinical situation to interact in a human way as the biomythologies ever were.

Instead of a language of chemical imbalances, we now have a language of controlled trials and epidemiological data and guidelines based on these trials and the system puts more weight on these than on the merits of looking at and listening to what a person on a treatment is saying about what the treatment is doing to them. EBM is about average effects rather than what is actually happening to the person talking to me. And the pharmaceutical industry has been masters at arguing that if controlled trials haven't shown that something is happening then it's not happening and patients need to be told that their complaints are all in their mind.

From 1993, this book has been about what might be called data based medicine (DBM). When most people hear EBM they assume they are dealing with DBM when in fact they aren't. The first and key message of this book is that the person on treatment is the data. Being scientific means that we and the person or people on treatment need in a collaborative way to attempt to map the experience the person on treatment is having and perhaps after that attempt to explain it. Dismissing what is happening as coming from their mental illness is not scientific.

Many medical prescribers tell patients that they the doctors are the scientists and unless the patient has had 10 years' training in medicine their views don't count. But one of the cardinal rules of science is that a scientist is supposed to be keeping an eye out for the observations that don't fit into the current world view. She is supposed to be looking out for the Black Swans – the examples that don't fit with the observation that all swans are white. We need to encourage anyone on treatment and anyone working with someone on treatment to form Black Swan Clubs that challenge those who deny experiences – however they are explained – to be scientific.

This will not be an easy task. While the original purpose of EBM was to empower the patient, it has effectively been co-opted by pharmaceutical companies and we now have a world in which it is more and more difficult for anyone to believe the evidence of their own eyes or what they are being told by someone on treatment.

The main argument put forward against listening to the person on treatment is that we want objective knowledge and what patients have to say is often too subjective. That begs the question as to where objectivity comes from.

This book is committed to the idea that for the most part people when they report something are going to be correct and health care staff when they see something are likely to be correct also. Not always, but mostly. It was women and their hair stylists who noticed the effects of oral contraceptives on hair – not doctors.

If the person reporting what happens or the clinician reporting what they see invites others with a different point of view (a different bias) to consider the issues and they also come to the same conclusion that the drug seems to have triggered this particular problem then this is even more likely to be correct and is in this sense more objective. If several people taking drugs report the same thing and several different people not on the drug – even pharmaceutical company employees – having looked at all the issues in these people's case agree that the most likely explanation for what is happening is that treatment has triggered it then it becomes ever more likely that this is the case. This drug can cause this effect. It may not usually cause it and we may not know how it causes it in some people and not others but it causes it.

This is where objectivity comes from. Science is a group process. It doesn't depend on experts or people being free of bias. It's about replicating something in front of us. The 'biased' person can help by pointing to details we may not have taken into account. The expert can help but not when it comes to novel effects when by definition no-one is an expert. The expert can be more helpful later in accounting for the effects.

Compared with the opportunities to investigate all angles of individual cases and to weigh different factors, controlled trials are simply mechanical exercises that depend on the observations of clinicians and patients in the first instance. Rating scales are no substitute for the ability to talk in detail to a person. Trials that depend on scales and adhere to rigid protocols are blunt instruments that are not designed to look at the fine grain of behaviour. Objectivity does not come from a mechanical exercise like this. To err is human, to really foul things up needs a controlled trial.

I am not contrasting the Art of Medicine here with the Science found in trials. The Science of Medicine lies in being able to explore experiences with an individual patient and in attempting to account for their experience. Trials, and in particular those linked to industry, are perhaps better seen as the Artifice of Medicine.

Fifty years ago a mother presenting to a doctor or hospital with a newborn infant saying that something was wrong was not believed, especially if the tests showed nothing wrong. Now all the books say believe the mother even if the tests show nothing wrong.

When things go wrong, someone taking a psychotropic drug today is in a similar position to mothers 50 years ago. The challenge to us all is to change this. The challenge to non-medical prescribers will be to do better than doctors.

INTRODUCTION

CHAPTER CONTENTS

There are typically three parties to the act of taking any psychotropic drug: the taker, the prescriber and the company that produces and markets the drug. All three are bound up by the history of our attitudes to psychological problems, to psychotropic drug taking and to the processes of industrialisation that take place both within the pharmaceutical industry and within medicine. All three are also shaped by changing attitudes in society at large, one of which involves an increasing awareness of the rights of individuals, included in which is a right to information about treatments they may be given.

These forces have conspired in recent years to bring about the production of handbooks about drugs that cover their mode of action, their potential benefits and their possible side effects. However, such handbooks consist mostly of lists of drugs with bold statements of reputed modes of action and comprehensive lists of side effects. These give little flavour of how the drugs concerned may interfere with individual functioning or impinge on individual well-being.

One of the aims of this book, in contrast to these others, is to produce a text that makes the issues live. To this end, there is a lot of detail about the history of different drugs. On the question of what the various drugs do, both current thinking and current confusions are outlined. Too much certainty is, I believe, the enemy of both progress and science. And apparent academic certainty tends to invalidate the perceptions of a drug taker – who is actually one of the individuals best placed to contribute to the further development of psychopharmacology.

I also include an attempt to assess the influence of the pharmaceutical industry on the perceptions of both clinicians and patients.

More importantly, rather than simply give a list of benefits and side effects, I attempt to give a fuller description of what the experience of the side effects may be like and how these impinge on normal living. To try to put some flesh on the bare bones of a list of side effects means that I have compromised between being comprehensive and being significant. Readers should be aware that this book does not include every known side effect. It does not include precise figures as to the frequency of each side effect. It does not include all known interactions with other compounds. What it does include are the reactions and interactions that occur regularly, and the book attempts to give some feel for how important or otherwise these are.

What emerges, nevertheless, is a list of side effects that, in many respects, is rather fearsome – to add to a set of motives on the part of both prescribers and the pharmaceutical industry that are often venal. Many of my colleagues wonder whether taking this course of action is advisable. I have a number of reasons for thinking it is.

CONSUMERS AND COMPLIANCE

The final arbiter of whether psychotropic medication is useful or not is the taker. The taking of any psychiatric drug involves a trade-off between the benefits the drug confers and the risks it entails. Until recently, prescribers have been accustomed to making this trade-off for those for whom they prescribe. In general medicine, where respiratory or cardiac function is concerned, this is often the only possible course of action. But where psychotropic drugs are concerned, this is not the only option and – arguably – it is not the best option.

In psychiatry, prescribers often moan about non-compliance with the regimens they prescribe. In the absence of any systematic work on why the takers of the drugs we prescribe are non-compliant, the vacuum tends to be filled with a vague view that patient recalcitrance amounts almost to a culpable or moral failing. It seems that we rarely stop to appreciate that anyone worth their salt is going to think seriously about continuing treatments with medications that may obliterate their sex life, make them suicidal or generally make them feel worse than they were before they began treatment. There have always been prescribers sensitive to issues like this, but there have also been far too many of us who, when faced with complaints about the medications we prescribe, have tended almost reflexly to increase the dose of what has been prescribed or to add some antidote to counteract the side effects of the first prescription, rather than to listen carefully to the substance of the complaint.

We are taking a tremendous burden on ourselves in proceeding this way. But, more importantly, in doing so we neglect the services of a group of potential mental health workers whose services come for free – our patients. Fully informing the client of the nature of the compounds, of their potential benefits and equally of their limitations and side effects, and of the available alternatives, at the very least has the merit of deflecting legal criticism. More importantly, however, it has the potential benefit of enlisting the takers of psychotropic drugs in the enterprise of handling their own condition, regarding which they may often be uniquely sensitive.

INDIVIDUAL END-POINTS

The reason for this last claim is that, where drugs are concerned, one person's cure may be another's poison. My first awareness of this came from a very simple practical exercise, almost 30 years ago in medical school. A group of 10 of us were given a beta-blocker to take. This should slow the heart rate, and it did – for nine of us – but one of the group had a marked increase in heart rate. This suggested that she was 'wired up' differently to the rest of us.

A few years later the lesson was brought home again in a study in which clonidine was given to some colleagues. Clonidine lowers the concentration of noradrenaline in the bloodstream, and in the group as a whole it clearly did so, but in 20% of those investigated it produced an increase.

In the central nervous system, where there is a multiplicity of receptors for each drug to act on, and where all of us have different proportions of each of these, the likelihood of a uniform response to any one drug is rather low. A diversity of responses, rather than uniformity, should be expected. Nevertheless, in practice prescribers tend to operate as though uniform responses were the norm. It is emerging that in some cases this inflexibility may be fatal. Where psychological problems are concerned, however, we traditionally have had the escape route of blaming the undesirable behaviour of our patients – such as their killing themselves because the drugs we prescribe make them feel worse – on the neurosis or irrationality that brought them for treatment in the first instance. This avenue of escape – blaming the patient – is one we should be reluctant to adopt.

PHARMACOPSYCHOLOGY

There is another reason for taking this approach, which is that the takers of psychotropic drugs are potentially engaged in a scientific experiment every time they consume a prescribed medication. By treating psychotropic drugs just like any other group of drugs, most books manage to obscure the scientific drama involved.

At the end of the 19th century, when the first psychoactive agents became available, Emil Kraepelin coined a name for the study of the effects of these drugs on psychological functioning: pharmacopsychology. The current term is psychopharmacology. The difference between these two terms indicates a major shift in the thinking that has taken place over the course of the past 100 years, a shift that to some extent needs to be reversed today to restore balance to the field.

Psychopharmacology today is science concerned with discovering the receptors that psychoactive drugs bind to, the levels they achieve in the brain and the benefits that these drugs offer to hospital services or general practitioners in reducing the disruption caused by psychological problems, or the frequency of attendance of individuals with mental health problems.

Pharmacopsychology, in contrast, as conceived by Kraepelin, was a discipline that would concern itself with exploring the construction of the psyche by means of the use of drugs. Every taking of a psychoactive drug, from tea and coffee to alcohol or barbiturates, Kraepelin believed, could potentially reveal something about the way psychological operations function or about how the constituent parts of the psyche are put together.

This remains a legitimate scientific programme today. It has been suspended over the past 50 years, largely because of our reluctance to take at face value the verbal reports of individuals who take the drugs we prescribe.

This reluctance has been engendered, in part, by behaviourist theories of psychology, which generally ignore any so-called internal mental events. It has been reinforced by the psychoanalytical approaches to psychological disorder, which broadly propose that there is no point in paying much heed to the obvious or face-value meanings of what individuals with psychological problems may say, as there would be no problem if their statements could be taken at face value. Finally, this reluctance has been supplemented by psychopharmacologists who, in trying to unravel the mysteries of the mechanisms of action of psychoactive compounds and of brain functioning, have in general paid little heed to the statements of the takers of these drugs, and have focused instead on the drugs as probes of physiological status.

However, even a biologically reductionist programme could have benefited significantly from paying more heed to the statements of psychotropic drug takers. For example, I believe, there would never have been a dopamine hypothesis of schizophrenia if the statements of individuals who took neuroleptics had been taken into account (see Chapter 2).

What seems to be needed today is the re-creation of a science of pharmacopsychology. Such a science would work closely with the takers of psychotropic drugs to determine what changes they experience on the compounds they take, in an effort to work back from those experiences to an understanding of how the mind works.

The person on treatment

1

CHAPTER CONTENTS

You are on a drug or working with someone who says they are having an unusual experience on a new drug – topiramate. Everything seems to be changing size in front of their eyes or speeding up and slowing down – it's almost like Alice in Wonderland. Could the drug be causing the problem? It's not in the textbooks. You Google it – nothing shows. Do you say you don't know?

The next step may be to go to a doctor – who says 'this is psychosis, we need to add another drug – an antipsychotic'. This doesn't feel right to you – but how do you challenge a doctor?

The first step is to believe the person. This might be easier if it is you experiencing the problem. If you have genital numbness and no libido and you are not functioning sexually, even though the drug has been stopped for months, it may be clear to you the drug has caused the problem. You may be confident about this even if your doctor or others insist that the problem is caused by a mood disorder or that something like this could not be caused by a drug stopped so long ago.

You need to distinguish between what is happening and what anyone thinks the cause might be. The next step is to get a really good description. It may be important for instance to distinguish when taking a selective serotonin re-uptake inhibitor (SSRI) between turning blue from the waist up versus turning blue from the waist down.

Frequently books will say just because something happened after going on a drug doesn't mean the drug has caused it; but, whilst true, the first rule of cause and effect is that an effect needs to happen after its cause. If something happens shortly after going on a drug, particularly if this is something unusual that can't easily be otherwise explained, the drug is likely to be the cause. If we weren't able to learn about poisons in this way, humanity would be extinct by now.

Healthcare workers desperately want to improve the lives of the person that they're helping, and this blinds prescribers to the fact that the magic of medicine is one that involves bringing good out of the use of a poison, just as the art of surgery involves bringing good out a mutilation. And just as a mutilation can go wrong, so too can a poison.

The human body was not designed to be poisoned. It can withstand insults in the short term but when drugs are given in the longer term, close monitoring is needed to keep track of what is actually happening. The clinical trials done on most drugs last a few weeks, and we do not have good information about the longer term effects of most of the drugs referred to in this book. There are many discoveries still to be made.

The next point is never to underestimate the capabilities of a motivated patient. If something goes wrong for them, even if they have no background in health care and dropped out of school early, chances are they will have done their research on the issue and have consulted with friends and Google. A motivated person can do extraordinary things. Chances are they will have done many of these things before they raise the issue with their doctor.

As will become clear later, clinical trials are not a good tool to establish what a drug is doing (Chapter 27). When trying to work out if a drug can cause a problem, the basic tool is to observe what is happening and then, if possible, stop the drug to see what happens and, if there is an opportunity, restart the drug to see what happens then.

CHRISTMAS TREE LIGHT BULB TEST

In the days when Christmas tree lights used real bulbs rather than light emitting diodes (LEDs), the lights were taken down from the attic once a year, and typically on plugging them in they didn't work. The trick was to go around to each bulb and unscrew it until unscrewing the dud bulb that was breaking the circuit led to the lights coming on. Screwing it in back again would cause the lights to go off.

These are the principles of challenge, de-challenge and re-challenge. They are 100% causal (see Figure 1.1).

So for our person with Alice in Wonderland syndrome described above, if the problem clears up on stopping topiramate and comes back on restarting it, the topiramate causes Alice in Wonderland syndrome.

We may not know how topiramate causes this problem, but we do know for certain that it is causing this person this problem and that it has the potential to cause the same problem for others. We don't know from individual cases how often it causes this problem, and controlled trials don't tell us this either.

If it's not possible to stop taking a drug and restart it, a further possibility is to vary the dose. If reducing the dose helps and increasing the dose aggravates this, it is also good evidence that the drug is causing the problem. Dose–response curves are causal. It is possible to get a drug approved by the regulators simply based on demonstrating a dose–response curve.

It is helpful to be able to explain the effects biologically but not necessary. This may help in particular for enduring problems (legacy effects – see Chapter 23) where stopping a drug doesn't lead to the problem clearing up. In this case, a really good description of the problem may make it easier for someone who knows the relevant biology to work out what might be going on.

Trigger Algorithm

1 Are there previous reports of this reaction in the manufacturer's literature, FDA database, or RxISK database?

Score 1 if previous reports, Score 3 if PRR* = 2–3, Score 5 if PRR* > 3 No = –1, DK = 0

↓

2 When did you start the drug? When did the problem start?

If the event came after starting Drug, Score 3; If there before the Drug, Score –1 DK = 0

↓

3 Did the problem start or get worse after a dose increase?

If started/got worse after dose increase, Score 3; If no change with Dose, Score 0 DK = 0

↓

4 Did you lower the dose? Did the problem clear up?

If improved on lowering the dose, Score 2; If didn't improve on lowering Score 0 DK = 0

↓

5 Did you stop the drug? Did the problem clear up?

If cleared on stopping the drug Score 2; If didn't clear on stopping Score 0 DK = 0

↓

6 Did you try any other treatment as an antidote? Did the problem clear up?

If cleared with antidote, Score 2; If didn't clear with antidote, Score 0 DK = 0

↓

7 Did you restart the drug? Did the problem reappear?

If the problem got worse, Score 3; If not, Score = 0 DK = 0

↓

8 Have you ever had this reaction before on another drug of the same type?

If you had on the same type of drug, Score 2; If you had on another type of drug Score 1 DK = 0

↓

9 Have you ever had this happen to you before when not on a drug?

If you had Score –1; If not Score 1 DK = 0

↓

10 Could anything else be causing this problem?

If it could, Score –1; If it couldn't, Score 1 DK = 0

↓

11 Have you ever been told you are a poor metabolizer of drugs and need lower doses, or do you have a history of sensitivity to drugs?

If you have, Score 1; If not Score 0 DK = 0

↓

12 Could you have taken too high a dose?

If you could, Score 1; If not Score 0 DK = 0

↓

13 Does a prescriber or a pharmacist see a link?

If they do, Score 2; If not Score –2 DK = 0

↓

14 If a name has been put on your condition, is it rare off drugs?

If it is very Rare, Score 5; If Rare, Score 3; If common Score 0 DK = 0

Total Score
9+ points to a link – bring to your prescriber/pharmacist
5–8 points to a likely link – bring to your prescriber/pharmacist
0–4 needs information or input from your prescriber/pharmacist
PRR, Proportional Reporting Ratio.

FIGURE 1.1 Trigger algorithm. For more information on PRR and Trigger Algorithm, see http://www.RxISK.org

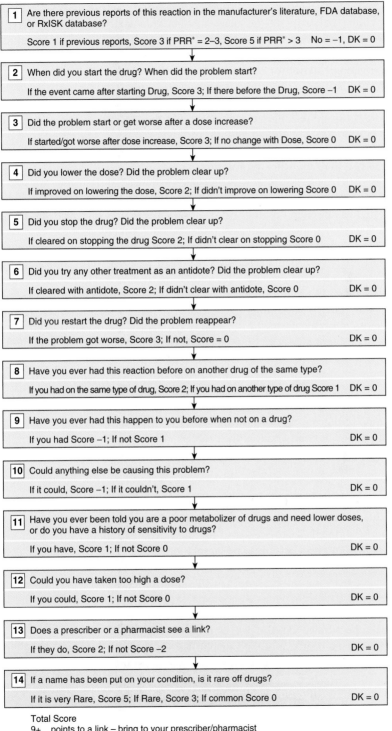

One biological tool is an antidote. For example, if a drug makes you restless and coffee makes the restlessness worse but alcohol dramatically relieves it, this is an indication that the original drug causes restlessness. An antidote that more specifically reverses the effect of the original drug offers even more convincing evidence for causality.

A further way to confirm that a drug is causing a problem is to see if there are reports of the same problem elsewhere and, in particular, if there are reports from quite different regions or different countries. For example, this can be done by consulting reports of adverse events submitted to the US Food and Drug Administration (FDA). (There are a number of sites such as RxISK.org that offer this information.)

Sites such as RxISK offer raw data and proportional reporting rates (PRR). A higher PRR means that reports of this problem on this drug are happening at a higher rate than on other drugs or other problems on this drug. Usually a PRR greater than 2.0 indicates a link, but this isn't always the case, and a PRR less than 1.0 can occur when there is a strong link to treatment.

Alice in Wonderland syndrome has been reported with topiramate, the asthma drug Montelukast, Oseltamivir (Tamiflu) for viral illnesses, and metoprolol, a beta-blocker, with very high PRR values in each case.

There are two key points to remember. First, we seem to think numbers are more objective than words. They aren't. Words come before numbers. To solve a problem means getting the words right first – the numbers will follow.

Second, it is even more important to stress that it is not super-scientists who find out whether drugs cause events or not. For example, it is women on oral contraceptives who notice changes in their hair, or their hairdressers, who make discoveries. The people who make discoveries are often people with no background in healthcare, who find themselves drinking more after being put on an SSRI and that the problem clears up once the drug is stopped, who put two and two together and discover that the drug has caused the problem. The super-scientist may work out how the drug does this – but it is ordinary people inadvertently doing science that establish the 'something' the drug is doing.

The role of those of us not on the drug is to offer support, confirm the validity of people's experiences if not their explanation and support them in trying to explore what might be happening.

In doing this we may be helped by prescribers but will often run into more disbelief than we might expect in this quarter. Not every prescriber when faced with a clash between a convincing account from a patient and the supposed evidence (ghostwritten with lack of access to the data) is able to envisage the possibility that the patient might be right.

Prescribers can be inhibited further by the fact that they have been genuinely attempting to help and are in denial that they may have caused problems.

Ultimately, they and we need to bear in mind that there is likely more to be learnt about psychiatric drugs than we now know. Every prescription is an exploration.

SECTION 1
MANAGEMENT OF THE PSYCHOSES

SECTION CONTENTS

The antipsychotics

2

CHAPTER CONTENTS

INTRODUCTION

Traditionally, the major psychiatric illnesses have been divided in three – schizophrenia, manic-depressive psychosis and a third group including the paranoid or delusional disorders and acute and transient or atypical psychoses. The appearances of diagnostic precision are misleading, however, as all of these disorders in practice are managed with antipsychotics.[1] The concept of schizophrenia has looked like it might fragment for some time with developments in pharmacogenetics and neuroimaging, but there have been few substantive developments in the last twenty years, except for changes driven by marketing for instance, from diagnoses of schizophrenia to bipolar disorder.

The antipsychotics were initially called neuroleptics or major tranqulisers. Chlorpromazine and haloperidol were amongst the first-generation neuroleptics. Clozapine and a series of 'atypical' antipsychotics are now the most commonly prescribed.

Table 2.1 lists first- and second-generation antipsychotic drugs.

The antipsychotics, however, are also used for conditions such as obsessive-compulsive disorder, a range of severe anxiety states and even as hypnotics. Accordingly, there will also be references to the use of these drugs in the

Table 2.1 ***The antipsychotics***

Drug name	UK trade name	US trade name
First-generation		
Chlorpromazine	Largactil	Thorazine
Flupenthixol	Fluanxol/Depixol	n/a
Zuclopenthixol	Clopixol	n/a
Perphenazine	Fentazin	Trilafon
Trifluoperazine	Stelazine	Stelazine
Pericyazine	Neulactil	Neulactil
Sulpiride	Sulpitil/Dolmatil/ Sulparex	n/a
Haloperidol	Serenace/Haldol/Dozic	Haldol
Tetrabenazine	Xenazine	
Molindone	n/a	Moban/Lidone
Second-generation		
Amisulpride	Solian	n/a
Aripiprazole	Abilify	Abilify
Asenapine	Saphris	Saphris
Clozapine	Clozaril	Clozaril
Iloperidone	Fanapt	Fanapt
Lurasidone	Latuda	Latuda
Olanzapine	Zyprexa	Zyprexa
Paliperidone	Invega	Invega
Quetiapine	Seroquel	Seroquel
Risperidone	Risperdal	Risperdal
Ziprasidone	n/a	Geodon
Zotepine	Zoleptil	n/a

n/a, Not applicable.

chapters on the management of both mood disorders and anxiety. There is also a place for both benzodiazepines and stimulants in the management of schizophrenia or other severe psychotic disturbances, which will be outlined later.

There has been controversy over whether the antipsychotics led to the emptying of the mental hospitals or whether this was happening prior to their introduction. This is not an issue that can be easily answered. There were and almost certainly are people whose lives have been transformed for the better by these drugs, but the availability of the drugs does something else – it engenders confidence and a willingness to take risks. The existence of this group of drugs provides a safety net, which has meant that some people have been talked to or discharged home who previously would have been left to vegetate in back wards. It is in fact often not possible to tease apart contributions made by a drug, the interaction with staff or a discharge. No drug is ever given in isolation, and the talking that goes with drug administration and the context in which it is given may be of critical importance.[1]

An example may highlight the issues. In the 1960s and 1970s, there was a vogue for token economy programmes in many hospitals. Schemes were put in place whereby in return for 'good' behaviours patients would receive tokens, which they could then use to buy cigarettes or other benefits. It seemed to work. But did it do so because of the principles of learning theory involved, because it forced patients and nursing staff to spend more time talking to each other, or because it offered patients some more control of their lives in heavily regulated wards? Today there is an interest in cognitive approaches for hallucinations and delusions – but do these work because of something new or because they encourage us to spend more time with patients?

The interaction between two human beings may be incredibly potent. The giving and taking of psychotropic drugs should be part of and should facilitate such interactions rather than substitute for them.

HISTORY OF THE ANTIPSYCHOTICS

Chlorpromazine, the first of the antipsychotics, was synthesised in 1950. Its use for nervous disorders led to the synthesis of the antidepressants, the anxiolytics and most other drugs now used for nervous problems. Despite this enormous effect on all our lives, no Nobel Prize was ever given for its discovery – owing to a bitter controversy over who discovered it. This controversy is relevant to the question of what these drugs do.[1]

Chlorpromazine was made as a centrally acting antihistamine. In the course of its use as part of an anaesthetic cocktail in 1952, Henri Laborit, a surgeon, described a striking change in subjects who had taken it – they were not sedated in the usual way with anaesthetic agents, but rather appeared to become indifferent to what was going on around them. This effect was visible within minutes of having had the drug – in normal subjects.

In 1952, Jean Delay and Pierre Deniker reported that chlorpromazine was of benefit in controlling states of manic and psychotic agitation. There was no suggestion initially that chlorpromazine was in any way specific to schizophrenia – in fact quite the contrary. In the mid-1950s, chlorpromazine was reported as being useful for almost every psychiatric condition, except for chronic schizophrenia. The new drug was also useful for nausea, vomiting and itching (hence its European trade name Largactil – Large Action).

The battle lines were drawn between Laborit and Delay and Deniker as to who made the discovery. Taking sides in this dispute depends on whether you see the antipsychotics as being in some way curative of psychotic illness or as producing a useful anti-agitation effect in anyone who takes them whether or not they have a psychological problem.

Within a few years of their use, it became clear that the new group of drugs produced extrapyramidal side effects, most notably Parkinsonism. As further compounds came on stream, it seemed that only those that produced extrapyramidal effects brought about benefits in the psychoses. This led to two things. First, the drugs as a group came to be called neuroleptics by Delay, a term that literally means 'nerve seizing'. This insight led to the dopamine hypothesis of schizophrenia. The second effect was that for 30 years little effort was put into finding antipsychotics that would not produce extrapyramidal effects – atypical antipsychotics as such agents are now called. It was only with the rediscovery of clozapine – a drug with much fewer extrapyramidal effects – that the picture changed.

ARE ANTIPSYCHOTICS ANTISCHIZOPHRENIC?

The evidence that the antipsychotics are antischizophrenic comes from a series of studies which have shown that subjects who take them after discharge from hospital are much less likely to be readmitted than those who do not.[2] This kind of evidence was reinforced by the dopamine hypothesis of schizophrenia, which stated that all antipsychotics block the dopamine system in the brain, and as they are beneficial in schizophrenia, therefore there must be something wrong with the dopamine system in the brains of individuals with schizophrenia.

Decades were spent trying to test the dopamine hypothesis and to develop new drugs that were active on the dopamine system. There have been two consequences of this. One has been that many researchers have had a vested interest in believing that antipsychotics are antischizophrenic. In addition, given the 'known' abnormalities in the dopamine system in schizophrenia, the fact that the drugs work on the dopamine system seems to mean that they are antischizophrenic.

For those who take the approach that antipsychotics correct the core disturbance in schizophrenia, the response to patients not getting better has been to give more of the drugs and the idea that an individual might not take their drugs is viewed very seriously. In addition, for some clinicians the idea of paying heed to what those taking the drugs have to say about whether the drug is helpful or not seems irrelevant – after all, these drugs cure an illness that causes loss of insight.

In contrast, the view taken here is that antipsychotics are not specifically antischizophrenic. In daily practice, many who are agitated are prescribed an antipsychotic, whether or not they have schizophrenia. Whether or not the person has schizophrenia, it makes sense to pay heed to whether they say the drug they are on is suiting them or not.

There is also evidence from a number of studies that patients who use these drugs 'cleverly', that is who take the drugs when they feel themselves 'slipping', but who may even discontinue when they feel better again, are no more likely to be readmitted to hospital than patients who take the drugs continuously.[3,4] The evidence from these trials, however, is compromised by the fact that antipsychotics can cause dependence, and this may produce problems on discontinuation, even in people who do not have chronic illnesses.

Further evidence in favour of the notion that antipsychotics dampen agitation rather than cure schizophrenia comes from three sources. First, whilst antipsychotics help patients get out of hospital, they self-evidently do not cure schizophrenia. Second, brain imaging studies have revealed that the dopamine system in the brain of individuals with schizophrenia is normal.[5] Finally, the reports from individuals who take these drugs point to anti-agitation effects rather than to cures.

What of the evidence that these drugs work on the dopamine system? If the drugs are useful and work through the dopamine system, this can also be taken to indicate that whatever is wrong in schizophrenia cannot be wrong with the dopamine system. A good analogy would be with the use of aspirin in arthritis. Aspirin works on the prostaglandin system. The fact that aspirin is helpful (not curative) in arthritis indicates that despite whatever is wrong in this condition, there is nothing wrong with the prostaglandin system. In the case of the antipsychotics, this raises the question of what do they do that is comparable to the anti-inflammatory effects of aspirin, and the answer, when discovered, was that they 'tranquilise'.

HOW ANTIPSYCHOTICS WORK

During the 1960s it was shown that brain cells work by releasing neurotransmitters. There are now over 100 known neurotransmitters. These act by binding to a receptor protein on a target cell. Most drugs that act on the brain do so by attaching themselves to these receptors, either blocking or enhancing the action of the neurotransmitter that naturally binds there.

Most neurotransmitters have up to six or seven different receptors to which they bind. Ordinarily drugs will bind to one or two of these, but not all, so that some, but not all, actions of that particular neurotransmitter are enhanced or blocked. However, the same medications will also bind to the receptors of other neurotransmitter systems. Thus, whilst antipsychotics primarily act on the dopamine system, they also act on the noradrenaline, serotonin, acetylcholine and other systems. These drugs are Cocktail Compounds rather than Magic Bullets that select and hit one target.

DOPAMINE

Dopamine was discovered by Arvid Carlsson in the late 1950s. It was subsequently shown that Parkinson's disease involves a loss of dopamine-containing nerve cells and that the disease could be treated with the dopamine precursor, L-dopa, or with dopamine agonists. The antipsychotics all bind to and block the dopamine-2 receptor – they are D2 antagonists.

What does blocking D2 receptors do? In very low doses, it reduces stereotyped behaviour. This lays the basis for the use of these drugs in Tourette's syndrome or Huntington's chorea, where sufferers have stereotyped utterances and gestures that interrupt normal speech and behaviour. Many individuals in the throes of a psychosis display repetitive thinking and actions, and, indeed, agitation may make us all stereotyped to some extent.

Perhaps linked to this action, dopamine blockade produces a feeling of indifference, a sense of being shielded from stress – a 'who cares' feeling that many people find immensely useful. It is for this reason that the antipsychotics have also been called major tranquilisers. However, the tranquilisation they produce is not like the wave of calm relaxation that lorazepam, diazepam or alcohol produce. Subjectively, the experience is more a case of finding oneself not getting worked up rather than finding oneself relaxed. From the outside, it can look more like immobilisation or non-reaction than relaxation or sedation, and it was this non-reaction in someone who remained awake that led to the word tranquiliser.

SEROTONIN

In addition to binding to D2 receptors, almost all antipsychotics act on the serotonin system, binding in particular to serotonin S2 receptors (see Chapter 11). Despite the fact that LSD and other hallucinogens act through the S2 receptor and chlorpromazine blocks the effects of LSD, so powerful did the 'neuroleptic' idea and the dopamine hypothesis become that for years pharmaceutical companies tried to produce compounds that would bind only to dopamine receptors. The purest compounds of this sort, sulpiride and amisulpiride, appear to be good, but somewhat less potent, antipsychotics. Perhaps surprisingly, given their selective action on dopamine, sulpiride and amisulpiride have fewer than average extrapyramidal side effects.

In the late 1980s, clozapine, a drug first produced in 1958, was rediscovered, and with it came the recognition that a drug could be 'antipsychotic' without triggering extrapyramidal syndromes and without binding potently to the D2 receptor. The trend up until then had been to produce compounds with increasing specificity for one receptor. Clozapine seemed a step back into the past – it was a 'dirty' drug that bound to many receptors. Its binding to S2 receptors was particularly striking. This has led a number of companies to bring out compounds that bind to both D2 and S2 receptors, hoping to find another clozapine. S2 antagonists block the hallucinogenic effects of LSD. They can also be anxiolytic and sleep enhancing, but when used alone, S2 antagonists have not proven useful in the treatment of psychosis.

At present it no longer seems clear that the route to finding the best antipsychotic lies in finding the right receptor to bind to. An alternative comes from a long-standing view of psychosis that has seen psychosis in terms of a defective filter that permits the psyche to be bombarded with too much stimulation. Perhaps 'dirty' drugs help by damping down more components of the filter system than do cleaner compounds.

Yet another possibility is that there is a spectrum of antipsychotics from the sedative dirty drugs like clozapine at one end to non-sedative selective agents like amisulpiride at the other and that some of us will suit drugs from one end of the spectrum whilst others will do better with an agent from the other end. In other words, there is no best drug, just a best drug for me.

A 'WHO CARES' FEELING

In the 1950s, before the idea that the antipsychotics were antischizophrenic took hold, there were attempts to pinpoint what it is these drugs do – what state of mind they bring about. In general, the verdict was that they produce a feeling of detachment – of being less bothered by what had formerly been bothering.

When these drugs are working properly, takers report beneficial effects on their ability to focus or concentrate on things. Subjects may find themselves more alert mentally, more able to focus on tasks that need doing, less in a daydream, and less distracted by internal dialogues, strange thoughts or intrusive imagery. The voices, thoughts or obsessions may be described as being still present but as having receded from centre stage. At least part of the person's mind has been left free to get on with other thoughts.

However, for the past two decades, under the influence of the notion that antipsychotics are antischizophrenic, interest in these drugs has focused almost exclusively on the fact that their use seems to get people out of hospital. There has been little interest in the changes the drugs bring about to get people out of hospital, and as a consequence, despite 60 years of use, it is difficult to be precise about the beneficial effects of antipsychotics. The unfortunate consequence of this is that we do not routinely tell people what we expect an antipsychotic to do that is helpful and then ask them to let us know whether the treatment is doing what it is supposed to do.

Reducing tension may be a good thing that may make some people better, but not others. At present when someone fails to respond, our almost reflex response is to increase the dose of the drug, but this will not be of any benefit if the drug is already working in the sense of relieving tension. In such cases, something else is called for: either a completely different type of drug, perhaps an antidepressant, or a behavioural or cognitive intervention.

Everyone who takes an antipsychotic is affected by them whether or not they have a mental illness. In affecting everyone in much the same way, antipsychotics resemble tea, coffee, nicotine or alcohol. Just like tea and coffee, they act within a few minutes, and the effect usually lasts for 4–6 hours. For this reason, just like tea or coffee, they are often given several times a day.

Broadly speaking, more of an antipsychotic gives more of a 'who cares' feeling up to a certain level, just as more coffee gives a more stimulating effect up to a certain level. However, beyond the point at which marked extrapyramidal effects kick in, more of an antipsychotic may start to make you feel worse just as too much coffee can. Like tea, coffee or aspirin, antipsychotics do not cure an illness – except for the delirious states which they effectively do cure. On the other hand, just as aspirin may help a range of conditions from headaches to fevers and arthritis, so also the antipsychotics if used properly may be very helpful for a number of different nervous conditions and non-nervous states including vomiting, itching and coughing.

ANTIPSYCHOTICS AND POSITIVE SYMPTOMS OF PSYCHOSIS

Antipsychotics are almost invariably given to individuals who have hallucinations or who have what others consider unrealistic beliefs (delusions). These symptoms are called the positive symptoms of schizophrenia in contrast to states of social withdrawal and apathy, which are termed negative symptoms. To observers, it often appears that the voices or delusions seem to lose their grip, and the person seems less likely to act on them after some days or weeks on the drugs. It is this 'clearing up' that has led to the impression that antipsychotics are antischizophrenic. More often than not, however, questioning reveals that the hallucinations or delusions have not entirely disappeared. It is more usual that takers of antipsychotics will still have their voices or some of their ideas, but they are less worried by them.

Where the management of voices and delusions is concerned, a number of points should be borne in mind. One is that many so-called normal people hear voices or have what may seem very strange beliefs. It is not a foregone conclusion that voices need to be removed or odd beliefs need to be corrected. A great deal hinges on how distressing these phenomena are to the person who has them or how much they are intruding on the lives of others. Many a lonely person is comforted by the exchanges they have with their voices.

Another point is that there are now a variety of cognitive and behavioural methods for handling voices.[6,7] The present status of such techniques is that they may prove beneficial against a background of judicious drug treatment, but they are not an alternative to drug treatment. There is one group of patients, however, whose voices often do not seem to clear despite what may be heroic medication regimes – patients with voices linked to prior abuse or trauma. In such cases, a non-drug input seems essential.

ANTIPSYCHOTICS AND NEGATIVE SCHIZOPHRENIA

The second-generation antipsychotics were sold on the back of being better for the negative features of schizophrenia than the first generation. These negative features are apathy and social withdrawal, as well as poverty of thought, action and speech.

The new drugs have receptor profiles very much like chlorpromazine. Historically it is clear that chlorpromazine was reported as waking people up from psychoses and from negativity. It got them talking in a way they had not been talking before and made them more active than they were before. The early trial evidence in fact suggested that chlorpromazine was better for these features of the illness than it was for the positive symptoms of psychosis. It is now also clear from the most recent trials that the older agents are as good as the newer ones in terms of getting people well and better in terms of their side-effect profiles.[8,9]

The common experience of both mental health workers and patients changing onto newer agents during the late 1990s, however, was that the new drugs improved quality of life, re-motivated patients, and were much more likely to be taken than the older agents. Why the mismatch between the research and the clinical evidence? The answer to this almost certainly lies in the fact that clinically patients were switched in the 1990s from poisonous doses of older compounds to more appropriate doses of newer compounds. The improvements are real, but these improvements have little to do with the new agents being better than the older ones. Lower doses of the older agents would have produced similar benefits. The other side of this message is too high a dose of any of these agents can produce many of the negative features of schizophrenia – demotivation, agitation and withdrawal (see Chapter 3).

CLOZAPINE AND SECOND-GENERATION ANTIPSYCHOTICS

Clozapine was launched on the US and UK markets in the late 1980s, with claims that it constituted a radical breakthrough in the treatment of schizophrenia. Its cost at that point was 20–40 times greater than that of the older antipsychotics.

Clozapine, however, was not then a new drug.[1] In clinical trials in Europe during the 1960s, and later in China, it was found to be at least as good as, but no better than, other antipsychotics. In the course of clozapine's early use, a number of problems were noted. It could cause a fatal neuroleptic malignant syndrome. These problems led some early triallists to recommend it be abandoned, and for this reason it was never licensed in Japan. Clozapine also leads to a series of metabolic problems including diabetes and cardiac problems. The problem that caused the greatest concern was agranulocytosis – a loss of white blood cells, which in some cases was fatal. This led to its withdrawal from use.

Clozapine differed from other antipsychotics in two striking ways. First, it did not produce standard extrapyramidal problems, and this led to its designation as an atypical neuroleptic or antipsychotic. Second, it did not seem to cause tardive dyskinesia, but instead could lead to improvements in tardive dyskinesia. From the mid-1970s to the early 1990s, tardive dyskinesia was the greatest problem linked to the use of the antipsychotics (Chapter 3). When clozapine was re-introduced, however, it was for treatment-resistant psychoses rather than for tardive dyskinesia.

The re-introduction of clozapine came following trials in which it appeared that around 30 percent of individuals who were unresponsive to older antipsychotics showed some improvement on clozapine. One argument was that this improvement might stem from the fact that clozapine acts more potently on some other brain system than traditional antipsychotics, producing more effective 'filtering' or alternatively adding something of an antidepressant effect.

Another explanation for this benefit might be that clozapine binds less effectively to dopamine receptors than do other antipsychotics, and accordingly it is less capable of producing D2 'poisoning' than other antipsychotics. In the clinical trials that led to its re-introduction it was compared to poisonous doses of older agents. If the poor response of some individuals to conventional antipsychotics results from the development of side effects such as akathisia (see Chapter 3), then individuals sensitive to these effects might be expected to improve once the 'poisoning' ceases. Whatever the reason, clozapine clearly helps some people where other antipsychotics do not, although, not surprisingly, given the current climate neither patients nor their clinicians are able to put in words just what it is that clozapine does that helps them.

In the wake of clozapine, a generation of antipsychotics emerged, all marketed as atypicals supposedly providing the benefits of clozapine without the risks. Of these all are in fact typical antipsychotics in the sense that they produce extrapyramidal problems in a dose-dependent way. The term atypical is a marketing term that is scientifically meaningless.

Olanzapine along with clozapine produces more weight gain than any other antipsychotic, and both drugs raise blood lipid and sugar levels leading to diabetes and metabolic syndromes. All antipsychotics do this to some extent, although the newer drugs appear to have a greater likelihood of cardiac and metabolic complications than some of the older agents. There are therefore considerable hazards to these new drugs.

Clozapine's reputation may stem from a historical accident. Had haloperidol been removed because of some problem leaving clozapine and similar agents to dominate the market, the reintroduction of haloperidol years later would have been accompanied by stories of miraculous cures on extraordinarily low doses in patients resistant to clozapine-type antipsychotics.

This scenario suggests that the available antipsychotics fall along a spectrum with perphenazine, flupenthixol and risperidone at one end offering typical neuroleptic effects and clozapine and chlorpromazine at the other end offering more sedative effects, with some patients responding to agents from one end of the spectrum and others responding to agents from the opposite end. Whatever the truth of the matter, there is no room for complacency in that the life expectancy of patients with schizophrenia is falling relative to the rest of the population despite all the advances we claim to be making.

A NOTE ON BIOMYTHOLOGIES

One of the marketing advantages drug treatments have is that companies can appeal to biological mechanisms of action and, in doing so, create a scientific illusion. In the case of the antipsychotics, atypicality was the buzz term through the 1990s. The current illusion centres on the supposed dopamine system stabilising effects of aripiprazole stemming from its profile as a partial dopamine agonist. This supposedly means that it is 'gentler' than other agents. Aripiprazole is a partial agonist, but this drug causes more marked akathisia than most other antipsychotics and seems just as risky if not more so than other agents. Both mental-health professionals and takers are better advised to pay more heed to what a drug actually does to people than to what they are told it may be doing in the body.

Another current biomythology is that antipsychotics are neuroprotective and that treatment needs to start as early as possible to minimise the neurotoxic effects of a psychosis. Antipsychotics can be brain damaging in the very obvious sense of causing tardive dyskinesia, and they are life shortening. They need to be used with caution and can probably be only used wisely when the patient and others involved in their care have an input into what is happening.

ANTIPSYCHOTIC DOSES

From the 1960s through to the mid-1990s, the antipsychotics were delivered in ever-higher doses, culminating in megadose regimes. There were three reasons for this: the dopamine hypothesis of schizophrenia, an ongoing need for sedation and as a means of behaviour control.

If dopamine is abnormal in schizophrenia and if the antipsychotics act on this system and patients fail to get well, one reason seemed to be that the drug might not be getting into the brain. Clinicians tried to overcome this by increasing doses.

Up until 1952, the only ways to help patients who were highly disturbed and in need of 'controlling' for their own sake were isolation, physical restraint or sedation. The drugs most commonly used for sedation were the barbiturates. However, the barbiturates put patients to sleep, and it is not possible to 'work' with sleeping patients. Moreover, barbiturate overdoses can be fatal. Against this background, the antipsychotics were a major step forwards. They calm agitation without producing sleep.

With the advent of the antipsychotics, the barbiturates fell out of use, but the need for sedation remained. The antipsychotics were increasingly used for this purpose, but these drugs are not good sedatives, and so extremely large doses had to be used. Many of the problems caused by antipsychotics stem from high doses used for this purpose.

This issue came to a head in the 1990s with recognition that efforts to sedate difficult patients with antipsychotics given by intramuscular routes whilst the patient is being restrained may be fatal. This led intensive care units to develop protocols for the management of emergency sedation.[10] There is a trend towards using benzodiazepines, and in particular lorazepam, as the first line of treatment in such instances. The more sedative atypical antipsychotics are unsuitable for this purpose given their cardiovascular effects.

Whilst not truly sedative, in high doses antipsychotics do control behaviour. They do this by literally immobilising a person. In situations of difficulty, they are often used for the purpose of immobilising someone who poses a risk to themselves or others. In an emergency, this use is defensible. However, emergencies seem to occur with greater frequency under certain staff. There is a political dimension to this question. Without the use of antipsychotics in high doses, arguably given the staff–patient ratios that may be obtained on occasions in some psychiatric wards, such units would become unmanageable.

In such situations the use of immobilising doses of antipsychotics for acutely disturbed patients seems to have a 'chemical cosh' quality to it. Some takers will have had the experience of these drugs being used to 'control' them in this manner, rather than to help them; it is against this background that problems with compliance may need to be judged.

For some combination of these reasons the doses of antipsychotics during the 1970s, 1980s and 1990s rose to poisonous levels. Haloperidol narcosis was common – this involves the administration of haloperidol 10 mg intravenously hourly (equivalent to olanzapine 30 mg parenterally hourly), as was flupenthixol 2000 mg per day (risperidone 2000 mg per day). It was routine practice in some hospitals to begin all new patients, even elderly women, on haloperidol 10 mg four times a day. In contrast the evidence base for these drugs from the start pointed to much lower doses being optimal.[10–12]

FIRST-GENERATION ANTIPSYCHOTIC DOSAGES

Chlorpromazine was originally used in doses between 200 and 400 mg per day, and haloperidol in doses from 1 to 7 mg per day. At 500 mg of chlorpromazine, clear extrapyramidal problems are the norm. Until the 1990s, however, chlorpromazine was administered in doses up to 5 g per day with 100–200 mg haloperidol per day being regularly used. Clinical trial evidence now clearly indicates that more than 500 mg chlorpromazine or 10 mg haloperidol per day is unlikely to be helpful.[14–16] Given patience and an attitude that does not rely totally on drug treatment to bring about benefits, lower doses will produce the best outcomes at a reduced cost in side effects. Higher doses in fact risk making the clinical picture worse by causing demotivation and dysphoria.

Some people will tolerate much higher doses without significant problems. Doses higher than these however should ordinarily only be used if the taker finds them clearly helpful or if the taker needs to be controlled for their own good – in cases of manic excitement for instance. Particular care needs to be taken in patients who may have been abused and seem prepared to do anything to get rid of intrusive voices.

If 300–400 mg chlorpromazine, 5–10 mg haloperidol or perphenazine 16–24 mg per day fails to help, the options are to add some other non-drug treatment or a different type of drug. Benzodiazepines may be helpful[17] especially in the presence of catatonic features.[18] An alternative may be to change from an antipsychotic at the sedative end of the spectrum to one at the neuroleptic end or vice versa. A key issue is to ask the person whether the treatment is helping them or not or whether a newly introduced treatment is more or less helpful than the previous treatment and, if so, why.

A consequence of the use of high-dose antipsychotic regimes has been that mental-health workers have become deskilled when it comes to the management of disruptive or awkward behaviour by non-pharmacological means. It has been all too convenient to resort to a chemical cosh, particularly in situations of under-staffing, rather than to attempt to sort out an underlying grievance or to devise a behavioural contract to contain unhelpful behaviour.

SECOND-GENERATION ANTIPSYCHOTIC DOSAGES

The second-generation antipsychotics came on stream after the mania for megadoses of antipsychotics had passed. As a result, they are more likely to be prescribed in doses in line with the clinical trial evidence of what works best. This means, in general, that 1–6 mg of risperidone will be used, 10–20 mg of olanzapine, and 400–600 mg of clozapine and quetiapine.

For a long time, nursing or medical staff happy with a prescription of risperidone 2–4 mg per day thought doses of haloperidol 2–4 mg per day were too low, even though the trial evidence and receptor-binding data suggest that these are equivalent.

BOX 2.1 Equivalent doses of antipsychotic drugs

Chlorpromazine 100 mg	=	haloperidol 1–2 mg
	=	flupenthixol 1–2 mg
	=	perphenazine 4–8 mg
	=	amisulpride 200 mg
	=	quetiapine 200 mg
	=	olanzapine 5 mg
	=	clozapine 200 mg

Whilst there has been a general and welcome lowering of doses in recent years, the allopathic compulsion (mission to cure) that led to megadoses of first-generation antipsychotics has not gone away. Today, it expresses itself in drug cocktails. In the face of a patient failing to respond, staff want to do something. Instead of raising the dose of the original compound, they now add in others, in particular mood-stabilisers (Chapter 7).

DOSAGE EQUIVALENCE

The dose of an antipsychotic that is needed generally hinges on its potency at binding to D2 receptors. The more potent at binding, the lower the dose needed clinically. Thus 1–2 mg of haloperidol is equivalent to 100 mg chlorpromazine, but these drugs have more than one effect, so equivalence is something of a hit and miss affair.[19] Box 2.1 therefore gives approximate equivalents of the most commonly prescribed antipsychotics.

FLEXIBLE THERAPY

Antipsychotic therapy should aim at producing an effect that the taker identifies as being useful. Therapy should also involve helping the patient to identify signs of stress or possible triggers to the worsening of a schizophrenic, manic or other psychotic disorder. At such times, the optimal use of antipsychotics would be to take them 'cleverly' – to assist coping. 'Clever' self-prescribing would also involve reducing the dose, or possibly discontinuing the drug, at times when there is less stress or an illness has become more manageable or in acute and transient psychoses that clear completely between episodes. The aim of prescribing should be to produce an antipsychotic effect at the lowest possible dose: one that does not bring about side effects and therefore does not require the additional prescription of antidotes.

Adding the different side effects of each drug to the biological differences between subjects who take the drugs means that some people will find a particular drug, such as perphenazine or risperidone, produces a helpful sense of security or indifference to outside pressure. Others will find the same drug, in the same dose, uncomfortable. Those who dislike one antipsychotic, however, will often find another perfectly acceptable.

Whether a particular antipsychotic is the right one or not is something the taker can often tell after the first day – sometimes after the first dose. The evidence is that those who, from the start, like what they get do well – those who do not like the effects of the drug they are put on do not do as well.[20] This suggests that test dosing and a willingness to switch between antipsychotics until the right one is found for each individual should be standard practice. It is not standard practice.

Whatever their various side effects, antipsychotics should not make someone feel much worse. If they do, then too high a dose or the wrong drug is being prescribed. It seems that many patients when they feel worse do not think that it could be the effects of the drug: 'My doctor wouldn't have prescribed something that could make me feel worse' (Chapter 25).

In the case of the antipsychotics, confusion is particularly likely as increased restlessness could be caused either by a worsening of the illness or by the drugs. Demotivation can be caused by the illness, by the drugs or by life. Agitation can arise as a result of experiences caused by the illness or in reaction to feeling strait-jacketed by the drug.

Within therapy settings there is a default towards blaming the disease rather than the drug. If behaviour worsens or agitation increases, doctors and nurses almost always push for an increase in the drugs on the basis that the patient has become more 'psychotic'. In contrast, the approach outlined here would encourage individuals to trust their own instincts and speak out. Ideally, if the problem could possibly be the result of treatment, speaking out should lead to the dose being reduced or the drug being changed or halted, but this rarely happens (see Chapter 25).

FOR HOW LONG SHOULD TREATMENT CONTINUE?

It has been common in the past for people once started on an antipsychotic to be prescribed them virtually permanently. If the approaches outlined here were adopted, many individuals would not be on these drugs continuously for these lengths of time. The best reason for continuing a treatment indefinitely is if a particular individual finds the drugs helpful – not just simply because mental-health staff think they should continue.

There is a further group of patients who should not continue with treatment – those with acute and transient or atypical psychoses. Roughly 20% of admissions for psychoses fall into these groups. In this case, whilst the disorder may recur in the future, the current attack is likely to clear up completely in anything from a few days to half a year. Staying on treatment longer than is needed risks producing a dependence that will make it impossible to stop treatment later. How can we know if the problem has cleared up? The simplest way is to ask the person. For people with an enduring psychosis, the voices or ideas will be still there in the background, whereas in the case of an acute and transient psychosis, the voices or confusion will have gone completely.

The question of dependence on and withdrawal from antipsychotics was clearly recognised in the 1960s, but for 30 years afterwards the possibility was discounted. The current situation is that up to a third of those on antipsychotics will feel dramatically worse if they try to discontinue – even from doses as low as 1 mg of risperidone or 2.5 mg olanzapine per day taken for several months.[21]

For the past 20 years rapid relapse on discontinuing treatment has been cited as evidence that antipsychotics are antischizophrenic. However, there are other reasons why discontinuing antipsychotics may make someone feel worse. One is that these drugs can cause a nervousness, restlessness or agitation that may only become manifest when attempts are made to reduce doses (see Chapter 3). This is commonly misinterpreted as a worsening of mental state, and patients are told to restart their drugs. Both patients and their relatives are likely to be told that this problem could not be caused by withdrawal from treatment as antipsychotics are non-addictive. This is misleading. Antipsychotics can produce dependence and withdrawal. Up to a half of those taking an antipsychotic may expect to have a variety of problems from motor disturbances to nausea, stress sensitivity, pain or problems with temperature regulation upon halting treatment. The problem seems to be greater for women than for men (see Chapter 23).

The risks of withdrawal and relapse are highest in those who stop treatment abruptly and probably in those who are stopping from higher dose levels. Discontinuing treatment should therefore involve a gradual taper of dose rather than abrupt cessation. Decisions about discontinuation should probably also take into account the nature of the problems that might arise should the individual relapse and the hostility of the environment in which the individual will have to cope without their drug shield.[22]

DEPOT ANTIPSYCHOTICS

A depot is an intramuscular injection, which lasts in the system for 2–4 weeks. In the USA these preparations are called LAIs – long-acting injectables. The different preparations are shown in Table 2.2.

For some people depot antipsychotics are convenient. They offer round-the-clock protection without the bother of having to remember to take pills.

However, there is another aspect to depots. A great number of people who are prescribed antipsychotics do not take them. The single greatest determinant of compliance is the quality of the relationship between the taker and their carers.[23] Another reason must lie in the sometimes unpleasant side effects of ongoing treatment. This is particularly likely to be the case in clinics where prescribing has been insensitive – the dosages too high, the drugs continued for too long. Far from blaming the drugs or themselves, though, mental-health personnel often see the problem in terms of the patient's unreliability or lack of insight. The patient is blamed.

This non-compliance led to the introduction of depots. It is quite common to find individuals diagnosed as having schizophrenia or manic depression kept on depots for decades. All too often 'community care' seems to reduce to the control of individuals in the community by means of depot antipsychotics. If the dose is too high, a patient may be immobilised in an apartment, unable to get out and live – convenient perhaps for some but not the goal of treatment.

Finally, one of the unusual features of depot prescription is that their prescription may not lead to a discontinuation of the prescription of oral antipsychotics. Many people are prescribed both concurrently. The rationale for this may owe more to the neuroses of prescribers than anything else.

Table 2.2 *Depot antipsychotics*		
Drug name	**UK trade name**	**US trade name**
Flupenthixol	Depixol	n/a
Fluphenazine	Modecate	Prolixin
Haloperidol	Haldol	Haldol
Olanzapine	ZypAdhera	Zyprexa Relprevv
Paliperidone	Xeplion	Invega Sustenna
Zuclopenthixol	Clopixol	n/a
Risperidone	Risperdal Consta	Risperdal Consta

n/a, Not applicable.

ANTIEMETICS

Many individuals who have never considered they had a psychological problem, let alone a psychosis, will have had 'antipsychotics' when given metoclopramide, prochlorperazine or promethazine to control travel sickness or to stop vomiting.

These drugs all bind to dopamine receptors in the brain. They can all be used for antipsychotic purposes. In the doses given for nausea, little may be apparent other than an antiemetic effect, although even at these doses extrapyramidal side effects may occur. Conversely chlorpromazine, sulpiride and haloperidol may all be used effectively to counter vomiting.

ANTIPSYCHOTICS AND PSYCHOTHERAPY

Drug therapies and psychotherapy tend to be cast as opponents when caring for someone who is ill should make them complementary. Those who give drugs are seen as believing that the illness is a biological one and that talking makes little sense whilst those who practise psychotherapy view the drugs at best as a necessary evil.

In fact, early research from the 1960s indicates that there may be beneficial effects from group therapy in which patients help one another to express what the problems of therapy are and see the consequences of failures to take medications. Until the late 1960s, the dominant view was that the drugs, rather than curing people, opened them up to a point where other approaches from therapy to work or social groups might then provide further benefits.

The divide between pharmacotherapeutic and psychotherapeutic approaches leads to problems for anyone who wants to take any non-drug approach towards psychoses. An insensitive dose of an antipsychotic will lead to a demotivation or restlessness that will make any psychotherapeutic approach from behavioural manoeuvres through to cognitive interventions all but impossible. On the other hand reducing the dose of treatment can provide opportunities for therapy in that the patient, finding it was really the drugs rather than some aliens or other sinister forces that were producing a range of difficulties, may be more open to having other beliefs challenged.[24]

SIGNIFICANT INTERACTIONS

ALCOHOL

There are reports that drinking alcohol may make the emergence of antipsychotic-induced akathisia and dystonia more likely (see Chapter 3). This is probably incorrect. Alcohol may even reduce the nervousness and restlessness that some antipsychotics can cause. However, sedative antipsychotics combined with alcohol are liable to produce even more sedation than would ordinarily be the case. Both antipsychotics and alcohol raise the risk of diabetes, and their combination can be expected to increase that risk further.

LITHIUM

The combination of antipsychotics and lithium is used widely and, in general, appears to be safe, although there is a slightly increased risk of neuroleptic malignant syndrome or lithium encephalopathy and of cardiac rhythm disturbances (see Chapter 7).

BARBITURATES AND BENZODIAZEPINES

Any sedatives may interact with sedative antipsychotics such as quetiapine to produce what may be a disproportionate sedation. Interactions are much less marked with non-sedative antipsychotics.

ANALGESICS AND ORAL CONTRACEPTIVES

Sedative antipsychotics may also potentiate the sedative effects of centrally acting analgesics such as pethidine, codeine or morphine. Perhaps more importantly, many analgesics, especially opioids, can produce many of the same extrapyramidal effects as the antipsychotics – haloperidol was originally derived from pethidine. As with analgesics, oral contraceptives can produce a number of extrapyramidal side effects, and the combination of contraceptives and antipsychotics may make these problems more likely.

ANTIDEPRESSANTS, ANTICONVULSANTS AND ANTIHISTAMINES

Concurrent administration of antipsychotics and either antidepressants or anticonvulsants may result in rises in the plasma concentrations of both groups of drugs. It also seems more likely to lead to weight gain. The combination of selective serotonin reuptake inhibitor (SSRI) antidepressants and antipsychotics appears to increase the likelihood of extrapyramidal side effects. Many antipsychotics and antidepressants were derived from antihistamines in the first instance, and a number of antihistamines share properties in common with both the antipsychotics and antidepressants so that combining these apparently different drug groups can lead to an unexpected increase in side effects.

SPECIAL CONDITIONS

PREGNANCY

The effects of antipsychotics on an unborn foetus are not established, probably because the patients originally given these drugs were unlikely to get pregnant. But it now seems that all psychotropic drugs produce problems in pregnancy, and as the use of the antipsychotics spreads for bipolar disorder, problems are likely to emerge if only because both new and old compounds produce diabetes and metabolic problems that are likely to increase risk.

BREASTFEEDING

All antipsychotics except clozapine and quetiapine increase the amount of breast milk, making it uncomfortably superabundant in some instances. They also enter breast milk, although in lower doses than found in the mother's plasma, potentially causing side effects to the baby. It is probably, therefore, advisable to avoid breastfeeding whilst taking these drugs.

DRIVING

The antipsychotics are particularly problematic for driving in that they cause users to dis-engage; this shows as lack of concentration and attention. See also chapters on antidepressant side effects (Chapter 5) and benzodiazepines (Chapter 10).

OTHERS

Caution should be taken in cases of known prostatic disease, glaucoma, Parkinson's disease, thyroid problems, diabetes and cardiac problems.

MORTALITY: YOUNG AND OLD

Chlorinating promazine was designed to interfere with as many biological systems as possible in order to counteract the effects of stress. The resulting chlorpromazine affected cholinergic, histaminergic, serotonergic, adrenergic and almost all other known systems, leading to a host of cardiovascular and other effects in addition to its central 'who cares' effect. For the following 40 years, research aimed at stripping out the side effects on other systems and leaving the main neuroleptic effect. This produced a series of drugs from perphenazine to sulpiride that were remarkably safe in the short term for a range of conditions and across a wide range of doses. The controversies surrounding these drugs had more to do with the way they were administered than with their intrinsic safety.

It is not clear that the intrinsic safety of recent agents, which are a throwback to chlorpromazine, matches that of the older agents. These newer drugs have a variety of metabolic and cardiovascular effects that even in acute usage can pose problems. Increasing awareness of this has led also to a growing concern that longer-term use of the antipsychotics is linked to increased rates of mortality. This becomes especially clear in elderly populations, where the antipsychotics now come with warnings of increased mortality linked to cardiorespiratory and vascular events. This may be due to the side effects of the drugs but may also stem from the effects of the drugs on dopamine, which has a regulatory role in respiratory and cardiac systems.

It is now clear that anyone put on these drugs chronically is at increased risk of mortality and that the risk goes up in proportion to the dose of drug and the number of drugs used.[25–27] The single greatest problem is linked to triggering suicidal reactions in young people during the first year of treatment.[28]

These drugs are therefore immensely useful – when used properly. Proper use depends greatly on a close cooperation between taker and prescriber. The takers need to learn what the right antipsychotic can do for them and how best to use them. Both prescribers and takers need to recognise the limitations of these drugs – what they do not do. A failure to recognise the limitations of antipsychotics has led in the past, and still leads, to the prescription of doses that may make mental states worse and increase mortality.

In general, paradoxically the drugs may appear most useful for conditions in which they may offer a limited benefit – the acute and transient psychoses. They are most likely to be given chronically in conditions where they offer no benefit and may in fact increase mortality – chronic schizophrenia. It is in the midrange of conditions, those enduring psychoses in which the subject can identify a benefit of treatment, that the best trade-off is likely to be and where some benefit warrants taking some risks.

Antipsychotic side effects and their management

3

CHAPTER CONTENTS

INTRODUCTION

The antipsychotics all bind to dopamine receptors, but almost all of them bind to other receptors as well. People also differ. The combination of these two principles means that the side effects of an antipsychotic may differ from one individual to another.

The side effects listed here are fearsome. However, for the most part, they are reversible by reducing the dose, changing the drug, halting it or using the right antidote.

Treatment, however, may involve a trade-off. In practice many of us are prepared to tolerate the interference with daily living that some of the side effects listed may cause, in exchange for peace of mind. The reason for listing is not to deter prescribers from prescribing or takers from taking, but to involve takers and carers in making the trade-off rather than having it imposed insensitively on them and to give prescribers some feel for the nature of that trade-off.

Dissatisfaction about the balance between the benefits and side effects of treatment should not lead to unilateral action, except in an emergency, but it should lead to a process of negotiating a position acceptable to the taker and their family. Negotiation may involve showing this list of side effects to a relative, who perhaps believes that these drugs are curative and that, therefore, the taker should take them regardless. Negotiation might also reveal the need to change prescriber.

Another reason to list problems is this. For the most part, the side effects listed here will clearly seem like side effects. There are, however, a number of effects brought on by the drugs that may seem more like a worsening of the illness than side effects. It is important that takers are able to discriminate between drug-induced effects and the illness. All too often both takers and prescribers can mistake some of the problems caused by treatment for features of illness.

Although primarily referring to antidepressants, Rebekah Beddoe's *Dying for a Cure*[29] illustrates wonderfully how easy it is in the mental-health domain for a therapy to become the problem rather than the cure. Another book that brings the benefits and drawbacks to therapy to life is John Watkins' *Medicating Schizophrenia.*[30] One of the most powerful of books in all of medicine covers this area – the heartbreaking *Dear Luise* by Dorrit Cato Christensen.[31]

DOPAMINE SYSTEM EFFECTS AND SIDE EFFECTS

All antipsychotics reduce dopamine activity in the brain. As this is what they are designed to do, in one sense the dopamine system effects are not side effects, but when they occur to a greater extent than is desirable, they become side effects. These effects are in general called extrapyramidal effects. There is agreement now that treatment should avoid causing dopamine-related side effects. However, this has not always been the orthodox view. From 1955 to 1995 or so, clinicians aimed to produce dopaminergic side effects in the belief that it was only when such effects were apparent that the treatment was likely to produce its benefits.

The effects listed in 1–3 below are likely to be immediately apparent. They all form part of a Parkinsonism that follows from blocking dopamine. Parkinson's disease involves lowered dopamine, but the antipsychotics do not cause Parkinson's disease. Once they are stopped, the state clears up. *Ivan*[32] is a book about having Parkinson's disease that gives a good 'feel' for the problems Parkinsonism can cause.

The most important dopamine-related effects are 4–6 listed below. The best clinical descriptions of both Parkinsonian and other extrapyramidal problems are in a book by David Cunningham-Owens.[33]

1. STIFFNESS/LACK OF MOVEMENT: AKINESIA

This is the central feature of Parkinson's disease. When caused by antipsychotics, in a mild form it is felt as a slowing of spontaneous movements – this may not be unpleasant. In a more severe form, the feeling may be one of being restricted, even strait-jacketed, which can be distressing.

This slowing may produce clumsiness. If severe, it can lead to someone just sitting motionless in the one place like a zombie. The person may be wide-awake but not moving much, not even smiling. This happens because antipsychotics slow all movements, even down to facial expressions. There may, for instance, be noticeable delays between questions being asked and answers being offered.

Even one dose can make anyone look like a 'schizophrenic'.[34,35] A certain amount of the stigma now linked to mental illness is almost certainly tied up in obvious effects of this type that antipsychotics can produce, and this can compromise efforts to reduce stigma.

If the dopamine system is blocked to the point that an individual has a lot of parkinsonian side effects, the person may find themselves drooling, which happens when the muscles of the face and mouth get slower to react to saliva build up which therefore dribbles out. This can be put right by reducing the dose, but it is an unpleasant and unnecessary experience.

Another problem is that when the person starts to walk they may find themselves leaning forwards or to one side. They may also find it difficult to start moving or, once having started, they may find it difficult to stop. These effects can all be put right by lowering the dose, changing to a different drug or using an antidote (see below).

2. ABNORMAL MOVEMENTS: DYSKINESIAS

Abnormal movements are one of the most noticeable features of Parkinson's. The pill-rolling tremor of the hand that this illness produces is perhaps the commonest of these. When caused by antipsychotics, this tremor will be experienced as anything from a hardly noticeable fine tremor to a clear shake that makes coordination difficult, causing someone, for example, to be unable to drink tea without spilling it. This can seriously interfere with social life. Tremors can also be caused by antidepressants, lithium, valproate, caffeine and bronchodilators, and other drugs, and combinations of these drugs with an antipsychotic may need to be reviewed.

The commonest set of abnormal movements affects the hands or arms, but the legs may also be involved. This shows itself as an inability to keep one's legs still when sitting down. The muscles of the mouth and face may also be involved, giving a repetitive pouting of the lips and protrusion of the tongue. The jaw may be affected, leading to tooth-grinding and dental problems. The entire body may also writhe or shake.

One of the least recognised set of dyskinesias involves the respiratory muscles. When the movements of these muscles become discoordinated, the result is breathlessness, wheezing or shortness of breath. This may be persistent or episodic – happening only at night for instance. Commonly, what is happening may be misinterpreted as asthma or as an anxiety attack, and the treatments given may make the problem worse.

3. ABNORMAL MUSCLE TONE: DYSTONIA

The term dystonia means that a muscle has gone into spasm. Typically spasm happens abruptly. Virtually any muscle may be affected, but the muscles of the eyes, mouth and jaw are the most commonly affected.

The most dramatic spasm involves the eyeballs, which may roll up in the head so that only the whites of the eye can be seen, in what is called an oculogyric crisis. The person affected can see almost nothing. The first time this happens, the individual concerned and anyone else watching may be very alarmed. The spasm will usually wear off inside an hour. It can also be quickly reversed by an anticholinergic antidote (see below). This is relatively rare.

When the mouth or larynx is affected, there can be difficulties speaking distinctly or difficulties in eating or drinking. These conditions are readily reversed on discontinuing treatment or with an antidote, but there have been reports of serious complications. Dystonias of the larynx may also lead to a change in voice so that the person sounds hoarse. Other problems include trismus or lockjaw and clenching of the jaw, especially at night, which can lead to dental problems.

Spasms are the obvious form of dystonia, but the commonest way dystonia is experienced is in the less obvious form of pain. These pains can affect the jaw, throat, facial muscles or the limbs or trunk. The pain may lead to a mistaken diagnosis of facial pain or an atypical pain syndrome. Treatment should involve changing the drug rather than painkillers.

4. TARDIVE DYSKINESIA: LATE-ONSET DYSKINESIA

Tardive dyskinesia refers to a set of abnormal movements of the face and mouth. This dyskinesia may only appear several months after the drug has been started, or after it has been stopped, and its late onset led to the term tardive. It involves lip-smacking, protrusion of the tongue and chewing movements, and it may extend to writhing movements of the trunk and limbs.

Anything between 5% and 20% of people who take antipsychotics chronically and in high doses may be affected. The problem is commoner in women than men, in older rather than younger people, with higher doses of drugs rather than lower doses, and with some antipsychotics rather than others. Children also seem vulnerable, as does anyone with a cognitive impairment or brain injury. Clozapine and quetiapine are much less likely to cause a problem, but other newer agents may cause it as often as older agents. Whilst dose-dependent, the problem can happen after relatively low doses given for weeks rather than years, and milder versions may be seen in people who have never had an antipsychotic, suggesting that in some individuals there may be a vulnerability to this kind of problem.

Unlike other abnormal movements, tardive dyskinesia lasts for years after the drug has been discontinued. As these movements involve the face, they are obvious and socially embarrassing. There are, at present, good antidotes for most of the other side effects but not for tardive dyskinesia. One option now is to switch anyone who has this problem to quetiapine or clozapine, as both have been demonstrated to suppress dyskinesia. Some cases may respond to cholinesterase inhibitors (see Chapter 18). A further option is to put the person back on a drug they may have been taken off or to increase the dose of the drug they are on.

The occurrence of tardive dyskinesia led to legal actions in the United States, and these stopped the production of new antipsychotics through the 1970s and 1980s.[1] The re-emergence of clozapine owes a lot to the fact that it does not cause this problem and may even clear it up. There is a belief that newer agents are less likely to cause tardive dyskinesia, but this is probably wrong. Tardive dyskinesia is dose dependent, and probably appeared more often with older agents because they were used in higher doses.

5. RESTLESSNESS, NERVOUSNESS, AGITATION, TURMOIL: AKATHISIA

Akathisia may be the most serious side effect of antipsychotics. This is a complex, unpleasant, emotional state that often leads to visible restlessness. Throughout the 1970s and 1980s, visible restlessness was all that most people meant when they used the word akathisia, referring literally to an inability to sit still. However, there may be no obvious restlessness. The problem may be only subjectively apparent, in which case an individual may feel anything from being mildly twitchy to being unable to stay still or to feeling like leaping out of their skin. It may be difficult to decide from the outside whether this is normal fidgetiness or akathisia.

The best word from the sufferer's point of view to describe what is happening is probably mental turmoil. Restlessness does not convey all that may be involved. The first descriptions of this problem were in normal people taking reserpine for blood pressure problems. This led to quotes like the following: 'increased tenseness, restlessness, insomnia and a feeling of being very uncomfortable', 'the first few doses frequently made them anxious and apprehensive … they reported increased feelings of strangeness, verbalised by statements such as "I don't feel like myself" … or "I'm afraid of some of the unusual impulses that I have"'. Also, take the case of CJ, who on the first day of treatment reacted with marked anxiety and weeping, and on the second day 'felt so terrible with such marked panic at night that the medication was cancelled'.[36,37]

The phenomenon therefore includes the emergence of strange and unusual impulses, often of an aggressive nature. Dysphoria is a much better word for what is at the heart of akathisia than restlessness. Turmoil is probably the best everyday word. Akathisia is an emotional rather than a motor disorder. If it were a motor disorder, it would be classified under the dyskinesias.

One study of healthy volunteers taking haloperidol done by King and colleagues found that up to 50% taking doses as low as 4 mg may feel uncomfortable, ill at ease with themselves and unable to settle. Some volunteers found it almost impossible to remain in the room but at the same time found it very difficult to explain what was wrong.[38] Many psychiatrists who have tried antipsychotics have experienced this, and a number have said it was close to the worst experience of their lives. We have found similar results to the King study, with the extra twist that discomfort and irritability were still clearly present in some of our volunteers up to a week later.[34,35,39] Others have found similar effects.[40,41]

It is important to bear akathisia in mind when faced with 'difficult' behaviour on the part of some people when they come into hospital. Patients who develop akathisia may be seen as getting more ill, and as a result they may be put on more treatment. Alternatively the individual affected may feel he has to get out of hospital quickly, and if he is not obviously deluded, ward staff may consider that they have little option but to let him leave. People leaving hospital in circumstances like this, or developing problems like this at home, are probably at high risk of suicide. Accordingly, reports of increased irritability or impulsivity from anyone taking an antipsychotic should be taken seriously. They are often not taken as seriously as they should be because antipsychotics are expected to reduce irritability and impulsivity, not increase it.

Whether in healthy volunteers or patients, akathisia sometimes responds to an anticholinergic antidote or to propranolol. One of the most effective agents, however, appears to be red wine. This is a problem, therefore, that may literally drive a patient to drink. In other cases, halting the medication completely may be the only way to alleviate the problem. In a proportion of subjects who have been on antipsychotics for a long time, it may take several months after discontinuation of the drug for the akathisia to wear off. High-potency (low-dose) antipsychotics such as haloperidol, risperidone, olanzapine or aripiprazole seem particularly likely to cause this problem. Low-potency (high-dose) treatments like chlorpromazine, quetiapine or clozapine are less likely to do so.

Akathisia may present from the first few hours of treatment, or it may only emerge weeks or months later as the drug builds up in the system. This form of tardive akathisia is a hazard with depot antipsychotics. Akathisia may also emerge only during attempts to discontinue antipsychotics, when it may incorrectly lead both takers and prescribers to think that the taker's mental problems are getting worse.

Having been neglected for 50 years, the risks linked to akathisia have come to the fore recently. Part of the risk lies in the fact that the person suffering may not realise the problem is caused by their treatment. They may feel as though their nerves have got worse. If the akathisia involves an unbearable worsening, it may lead frantic people to contemplate anything – even suicide – to bring it to an end. A milder form of akathisia may initially be interpreted as a worsening of the illness despite treatment, and this in turn may lead slowly to hopelessness and a conclusion that suicide is the only way out.

There is a high incidence of suicide in young patients with schizophrenia or psychosis who have recently been diagnosed and put on drug treatment.[28,42] This has been interpreted as a fatalistic reaction on the part of intelligent sufferers, who, appalled at the prospect of what lies in front of them, opt to bring their suffering to an end as quickly as possible. This may account for some cases of suicide, but a successful or attempted suicide is more likely to follow the development of akathisia. Unfortunately, the first exposure to treatment, without warning as to what can happen and how the problem can be put right, leads takers to misattribute what is happening to a worsening of their mental state. Suicide was rare in patients with chronic psychoses before the advent of the antipsychotics and now may be up to twenty times commoner.[48] (See below.)

6. LACK OF INTEREST: DEMOTIVATION

Antipsychotics produce a state of indifference, and the problem here is that long-term use or too high a dose may leave a user apathetic, listless and indifferent to everything. Parkinson's disease is in some respects a profound state of indifference. Before drug treatment of Parkinson's disease with L-dopa, it was often observed that people might simply sit on a chair for days on end, seemingly unable to move. However, a fire alarm might produce rapid fluent movement, indicating that in part what was lacking was not the ability to move but sufficient motivation to do so.

It is known that people who take antipsychotics are significantly less likely to relapse and to have to be re-admitted to hospital. However, studies also suggest that they may be also less likely to get married or involved in significant relationships, to find themselves jobs, or to get on with their lives compared with individuals who have the same illness but who do not take continuous antipsychotics.[2]

Another finding is that all emotions may be blunted, rather than just certain emotions that have been troubling. Many takers complain that all feelings, from joy to anger, are dulled. Not all people have this side effect. Broadly speaking, it depends on the dose being taken, although some people will be clearly affected at very modest doses.

As this is a psychological rather than a physical side effect of antipsychotics, it is in many ways far more important than the other side effects mentioned. It can be pernicious in that the person may become indifferent to being indifferent. It is also important because there are few antidotes for it other than halting the drugs, although stimulants can sometimes be used.

It may, in addition, be very difficult to distinguish drug-induced demotivation from psychotic or depressive demotivation, or life itself. Trying to tease out what is happening may require great skill and cooperation between the taker of the drug and the prescriber. All too often, the appearance of apathy and listlessness results in individuals, who are taking antipsychotics, being inappropriately prescribed an antidepressant. Antidepressants do not help this condition.

One of the things most commonly mentioned by people reducing antipsychotics is a return of interest in things, along with finding that they have more 'get up and go' and that simple things are no longer impossibly difficult. This can lead to problems if an unwary individual throws themselves into things and gets stressed or overloaded as a consequence. It can also be somewhat frightening as feelings such as anger, temper outbursts or a more vivid appreciation of the sexuality of others may re-emerge in all their potential awkwardness.

7. HORMONAL CHANGES

All antipsychotics, except clozapine and quetiapine, increase the level of the hormone prolactin through D2 receptor binding. As the name suggests, this hormone is central to lactation. As a consequence, taking an antipsychotic in some cases can lead to women who are already lactating having a much more profuse supply of milk. It can lead to women who are not lactating starting to lactate. It can also lead to a large increase in breast size.

Increased prolactin can also lead some men to have a mild degree of breast swelling. This is reversible and usually disappears quickly once the drug is halted. In some instances men may produce small amounts of milk. This is best managed by changing the drug, but it can also be managed by adding bromocriptine, which suppresses prolactin production.

In part because of their effect on prolactin, the antipsychotics are also liable to cause disturbances in menstrual regularity and may even lead to menses ceasing altogether. This can lead to a belief that one is infertile and to unprotected sexual intercourse, but pregnancy is still possible in these circumstances. Given that this situation may be brought on by the use of an antipsychotic in low doses for anxiety, it perhaps brings home what is often forgotten, that is that every prescription involves a trade-off between a benefit and a risk.

There are a number of other effects of antipsychotics on sexual functioning that are not caused by their effects on prolactin – these are outlined below and in Section 8. On the positive side, antipsychotics may lead to a decrease in the intensity of period pains.

8. OTHER DOPAMINE-RELATED SIDE EFFECTS

There are many aspects of parkinsonian states that are still poorly understood and often unrecognised. One of these is that Parkinson's disease is sometimes accompanied by painful sensory symptoms. Other features include change in the oiliness of the skin or hair. Similar changes may also occur with antipsychotics. The risk is that complaints of this type will be dismissed as impossible. The general effect of all these changes is to produce a great deal of what is now seen as a 'schizophrenic look'. Effects like this may also produce subtle changes in smell that can have real interpersonal effects.

NON-DOPAMINE SIDE EFFECTS

Dopamine-related side effects may be found with all antipsychotics, but they are more common with some antipsychotics than with others. They are least common with clozapine. However, a number of other side effects are more likely to occur with clozapine and related drugs, and yet other side effects are common to all antipsychotics, but unrelated to dopamine.

1. WEIGHT GAIN

This is the commonest side effect of antipsychotics at standard doses. The only treatment that does not cause it is tetrabenazine. The reason for this weight gain is uncertain. It may stem from a reduction in activity because of demotivation with no compensatory reduction in appetite. It may stem in part from an increase in thirst antipsychotics cause, which leads takers to high-calorie drinks. However, there also appears to be some stimulation of appetite and/or a reduction in metabolic rate that stems directly from the drug. Not all antipsychotics are the same on this issue. Blocking S2 receptors appears to make weight gain more likely, as do actions on the histamine system. Many of these drugs increase concentrations of the hormone leptin, which is linked to weight gain. Broadly speaking, olanzapine and clozapine cause the most marked weight gain, sometimes a 20 kg weight gain, whilst almost all other agents also cause at least some weight gain.

This 'cosmetic' consequence of treatment was initially considered trivial by prescribers, who believed that the dopamine-related side effects were likely to be of much greater concern to patients. However, surveys of people generally indicate that weight gain is their most important concern, and when prescribers are asked what would worry them most if they had to take treatment, weight gain also comes out as the most important side effect.

This may lead to dieting or to instructions from a general practitioner to lose weight. Dieting alone is rarely successful in these cases, and the failure to lose weight may lead to frustration and guilt if it is not realised that the drugs are responsible.

Many seem to think that weight gain is in some way the fault of the taker, who should adjust their lifestyle. A better bet is to switch antipsychotic, or where possible lower the dose or stop treatment.

2. METABOLIC SYNDROMES

Some of the agents responsible for the most weight gain, especially olanzapine and clozapine, also increase blood sugar and lipid levels and cause diabetes. The combination of weight gain, raised lipid levels and diabetes is commonly referred to as metabolic syndrome and is thought to place individuals at high risk of later cardiovascular complications. For this reason, regular general health screens are now seen as important for anyone on an antipsychotic.

3. DIABETES

In addition to causing more weight gain than other agents, olanzapine and clozapine in particular but other antipsychotics to some extent can cause diabetes. This seems to be an effect of treatment that is independent of weight gain. Exactly how it is produced is still uncertain, but both molecules share structural features in common. The studies designed to investigate this do not exonerate other antipsychotics, but at present the problem seems most clear with olanzapine, quetiapine and clozapine. The rate of onset of diabetes in patients on antipsychotics is double the expected rate for the population at large. The insulin resistance these drugs cause has also been linked to a range of problems, such as polycystic ovaries.

4. SYMPATHETIC SYSTEM EFFECTS

Many antipsychotics including chlorpromazine, clozapine, olanzapine and quetiapine also bind to receptors in the sympathetic system, producing sedation and a lowering of blood pressure. All these treatments should be started in lower doses and titrated up for this reason.

The drop in blood pressure on antipsychotics is ordinarily not marked. In most cases, the only awareness that an individual will have of blood pressure changes will be a slight exaggeration of the tendency we all have to feel faint when we leap up from a chair or jump out of bed. However, in some cases the drop in pressure may be substantial leading to fainting or falling, with bruising or cuts and even fractures. Problems of this sort if suspected are good grounds for changing treatment.

The combined effects of sedation and a marked lowering of blood pressure make chlorpromazine, quetiapine, olanzapine or clozapine hazardous when given acutely in situations where the level of observation is low. Even on psychiatric wards with adequate staff levels, patients may be at risk of damaging falls or accidents. Elderly individuals in residential homes may run an equivalent risk from much lower doses.

An action on the sympathetic system may also lead to palpitations or what may be thought to be panic attacks – when the taker is aware of their heart beating quickly or irregularly. This is usually not serious, although it may very alarming. However, whilst usually mild, this effect indicates that these drugs have a knock-on effect on the cardiovascular system, making precipitate administration of large amounts of these drugs hazardous.

Another effect in men, which may in part be mediated through the sympathetic system, may be an inability to sustain an erection (see Section 8). This, as with the other symptoms above, is reversed once the drug is halted.

Finally, sympathetic system effects may produce difficulties passing water and constipation. This may range from an uncomfortable fullness of the bladder, to difficulties in passing water – being slower to start and longer to stop – to complete urinary retention. In the past this was described as an anticholinergic effect of these drugs, but it is now clear that it is sympathetic in origin. Whilst this problem may be worse in older men with prostate problems, it can happen even to young women.

Related to this, sympathetic system effects can lead to marked and painful constipation. This is something doctors are likely to discount as insignificant. However, both constipation and urinary retention can have marked effects on our mental states as the vigilance systems in our brain are wired to pay more heed to internal threats than to external threats.

5. ANTICHOLINERGIC EFFECTS

Olanzapine and chlorpromazine also have prominent anticholinergic effects, as do a number of other antipsychotics. The commonest consequence of this is a dry mouth. In some cases this may be quite severe. There may also be a nasal drying, which some people find uncomfortable.

Anticholinergic effects may also lead to blurred vision, and therefore any apparent worsening of eyesight should not lead the person to seek an eye test until the drugs have been discontinued.

Ordinarily, antipsychotics are given to people to reduce agitation, suppress delusional beliefs and to abolish hallucinations. However, in some cases, particularly in the elderly, the anticholinergic effects of chlorpromazine, for instance, may cause agitation, confusion and hallucinations.

Mild anticholinergic side effects usually wear off with time. If they are marked enough to make someone clearly uncomfortable and do not clear up after a few days, the drug should be changed or discontinued.

6. THIRST: COMPULSIVE DRINKING

Up to 20% of individuals on long-term antipsychotics drink excessive volumes of fluid in the form of water, high-calorie soft drinks, or tea and coffee. It is not clear whether this is caused by the dry mouth some antipsychotics can induce or whether the drugs also cause repetitive drinking apart from this.

Excess drinking may cause problems if allied to cigarette smoking. Many individuals on chronic antipsychotics smoke more than the average. One reason may be that smoking provides something to do in an otherwise boring day. Smoking may also ameliorate some of the side effects of antipsychotics. Combined with excess drinking, this can cause a problem in that nicotine can reduce the volume of urine produced and lead to water intoxication with convulsions and disorientation.

7. SEDATION AND AROUSAL

Although not nearly as sedating as the barbiturates, the sedative effects of antipsychotics mediated through the sympathetic and the histaminergic systems may be extremely useful in some cases, particularly to help sleep. In other cases the taker may prefer to have a non-sedating antipsychotic or marked sedation may interfere with activities such as driving a car.

Given the widespread belief that antipsychotics generally are sedative, the effects of these drugs on levels of arousal are contradictory and sometimes surprising. When given in low doses, it may be necessary to restrict the prescription of antipsychotics to the morning as, if given in the evening, they may interfere with sleep.

Even when given in somewhat larger doses at night, antipsychotics may sedate yet give a very unsatisfying sleep. A common report of people who discontinue these drugs is that they sleep more soundly when not taking them.

These effects vary from individual to individual and from drug to drug. The very same dose of an antipsychotic given to one individual in the evening may lead to sleeplessness, whereas another person may be sedated by it. Olanzapine, quetiapine, clozapine, chlorpromazine and levomepromazine are more sedative than other antipsychotics.

8. SEXUAL SIDE EFFECTS

Until recently the limited surveys that had been undertaken indicated that sexual side effects may occur in up to 50% of individuals on treatment, but even this now seems an underestimate.

The most commonly reported side effects in men are an inability to sustain erections or a delay in or inability to ejaculate. These effects may occur in up to 50% of men taking antipsychotics but most probably relate to dosage so that at lower doses they are less likely to be present. The opposite effect of involuntary and sustained erections (priapism) has also been reported, on most antipsychotics, as have involuntary ejaculations.

Also very common is a decrease in libido (sex drive). This is probably part and parcel of a general demotivation syndrome (see above). A change in the quality of orgasms has been reported, although exactly what kind of change has not been clearly specified.

In women, there can be decreased libido, change in the quality of orgasm and anorgasmia, but in general there is less awareness of what the impact of antipsychotics is on female sexual functioning (see Section 8).[43]

9. SKIN RASHES

All drugs may cause skin rashes of one sort or another. These are commonly allergic reactions. In the case of a marked reaction, the drug should be stopped. The rash will usually clear up in 24–48 hours. A different antipsychotic should then be taken, if one is still needed.

Chlorpromazine can also cause a photosensitivity that makes takers more likely to burn when exposed to sunlight for any length of time. If this happens, the drug should usually be stopped. It can also cause an uncomfortable itchiness, probably linked to a jaundice it uniquely triggers, which may start some weeks after the drug has been started and clears up when treatment is discontinued.

10. AGGRESSION AND IMPATIENCE

Antipsychotics are so often given to control aggression that for many mental-health staff it is difficult to believe that they could also cause aggression. One way that this can happen is through the production of akathisia. A common report from takers is that they feel more impatient, irritable and liable to fly off the handle. Whether all of this can be put down to akathisia is not clear. Whatever the cause, whilst there are no trials showing that antipsychotics cause aggression or impatience, drug companies clearly believe this can happen and have listed it as a side effect on the data sheet of most of these drugs. There is also good evidence from antidepressant trials that drug-induced akathisia may lead to violence and assault.[44]

11. NEUROLEPTIC MALIGNANT SYNDROME

Neuroleptic malignant syndrome (NMS) is a state where individuals, usually shortly after being put on neuroleptics, become stiff, feverish and out of touch. This condition may be fatal if not detected quickly. NMS is closely related to catatonia, which also comes in fatal or malignant forms.

Severe forms of NMS are uncommon. Milder forms may occur and resolve spontaneously. The severe forms are most likely to happen in individuals on higher doses of antipsychotics combined with other drugs and if the individual develops an additional low-grade infection or other physical problem. This type of reaction is commoner in older individuals, perhaps because they are prone to other physical conditions.

Treatment until recently involved discontinuing all drugs and intensive care unit monitoring for dehydration. There has been a recent revolution with current recommendations that lorazepam in doses of up to 15–20 mg per day be used as the first line of treatment. If this fails, electroconvulsive therapy produces rapid responses in most cases.

12. CATATONIA

Catatonia is a state in which perception and volition are cut off from movement.[45] It is closely related to NMS. Movements may become stereotyped and perseverative. The person may be non-communicative and may look like they are responding to visual or auditory stimuli, when in fact they aren't. The usual response is to view the state as psychotic and increase the dose of antipsychotic when in fact it is being caused by the antipsychotic, and the best treatment is reducing or stopping the antipsychotic and giving a high dose of a benzodiazepine.

13. CARDIOVASCULAR CONDITIONS

Beyond the acute effects of antipsychotics on blood pressure noted above, there are effects on the cardiovascular system that are the subject of growing scrutiny. The headline effect some of these drugs cause is a lengthening of the Q-T interval on electrocardiograph tracings. The first drug to cause concern in this area was thioridazine. A second was pimozide, and a third was sertindole. All can lead to a lengthening of the Q-T interval in the heart, potentially causing arrhythmias. These three and others have been discontinued or greatly restricted as a result.

It is now clear that almost all antipsychotics and antidepressants have similar effects. One problem with this is that no one is clear on what is a safe level of Q-T interval lengthening, neither are they absolutely clear on whether there are lifestyle or other physical factors that can make Q-T changes more problematic. There is a real risk of someone ending up on several different drugs all of which cause a little Q-T lengthening, none of which are dangerous in their own right, but where the combination of treatments and other physical factors is lethal.[46]

In addition to this well-documented problem, there are others. Clozapine and some other drugs in the group appear to cause a myocarditis (an inflammation of the heart muscle) that can be fatal. This is most likely to happen in the first few weeks of treatment. Clozapine has also been linked to cardiomyopathy (an excessive growth of cardiac muscle), which has its onset after months or years of treatment when it shows up as heart failure. Whilst most takers of clozapine will have none of these problems, it is clear that there should be a greater level of routine cardiac screening in anyone taking an antipsychotic than has been customary up until now.

In addition to the above, antipsychotics are associated with a six-fold increase in the risk of clots (thrombosis), which is particularly likely to be a hazard in those who are older or who are immobilised for one reason or another, or in those on contraceptives or other treatments that increase the risk of thrombosis.

Finally, both dopamine agonists used to treat Parkinson's disease and dopamine antagonists can cause cardiorespiratory failure through their effects on dopamine, which has a role in regulating breathing and cardiac function. This may be a particular hazard in the elderly.

14. EPILEPSY

All antipsychotics may trigger epileptic convulsions in susceptible individuals. This ranges from rare with haloperidol to more common with clozapine.

15. SUICIDE

In recent years, clozapine has been promoted as a treatment particularly suited to patients who are suicidal. The evidence that clozapine has benefits in this area is minimal.

In clinical trials submitted to regulators, olanzapine and risperidone have been linked to more completed suicides than other drugs. Lilly, the makers of olanzapine, have refused to reveal the data on the number of suicidal acts that occurred in their clinical trials.

The clinical wisdom on this issue has been that suicide happens in patients with schizophrenia or psychoses because of insight on a future devastated by illness. Whilst this might be right in some cases, it is almost certainly wrong in most cases. Suicide was rare in schizophrenia before chlorpromazine, which suggests that many people are reacting adversely to the treatment they are put on.[28] Another factor pointing to the drug is that the suicide rate during the first year of treatment is much higher than at any other time. There may be a host of factors linked to suicide such as patients ending up in isolated circumstances or abusing alcohol or street drugs, but the treatment they are given is the one thing both patients and their carers can readily change. This should mean that we take very seriously the need to ensure that anyone on an antipsychotic is on the right drug for them and in the right dose.

16. WITHDRAWAL EFFECTS

These are dealt with in greater detail in Chapter 23. They include a wide range of neurological problems and other disturbances. Any of the problems mentioned above can appear in the withdrawal phase, including dyskinesias, dystonias manifested as pain or spasms, akathisia, irritability, aggression, suicidality or tardive dyskinesia. There may be stress intolerance, appetite problems, pain all over the body even on brushing one's hair and a labile emotional state that might seem like depression to others.

17. SURPRISE EFFECTS

Another unusual problem on clozapine is bed-wetting. This may occur in up to one in five patients. This rather unusual side effect has been inserted for two reasons – one is to warn people that it may happen. A second reason is to draw attention to the fact that many unusual side effects may happen on a drug – some of which will not appear in any textbook and some of which may be unknown to the professionals involved in an individual's care. It is important to create an atmosphere that facilitates the reporting of problems, particularly ones that seem unlikely to stem from treatment. It is also important to maintain an open mind as to whether problems that are reported may indeed stem from treatment. At the very least, they are being reported because the person is having problems with some aspect of being treated.

Another surprising problem that may not look like a side effect of antipsychotic treatment is toothlessness. In fact, patients treated with antipsychotics are much more likely to lose their teeth than is normal. This may be because some of those treated end up homeless and in situations where it is difficult to look after their physical health and it is this that leads to toothlessness, but there are good grounds to think that antipsychotics and antidepressants might also contribute to toothlessness by causing dyskinesias and dystonias of the jaw.

MANAGEMENT OF SIDE EFFECTS

A number of different drugs are used to manage some of the side effects of the antipsychotics. These include anticholinergics, benzodiazepines, propranolol, psychostimulants and tetrabenazine.

ANTICHOLINERGICS

The anticholinergic group of drugs (Table 3.1) is often used to alleviate the motor side effects of the antipsychotics. These drugs antagonise the action of the neurotransmitter acetylcholine (ACh) at one of its receptors, the

Table 3.1 ***Anticholinergic drugs***

Generic drug name	UK trade name	US trade name
Trihexyphenidyl (benzhexol)	Artane/Broflex	Artane
Benztropine	n/a	Cogentin
Orphenadrine	Disipal/Biorphen	Disipal
Procyclidine	Kemadrin/Arpicolin	Kemadrin
Biperiden	Akineton	Akineton

n/a, Not applicable.

muscarinic receptor. The French physician Jean Martin Charcot was the first to use an anticholinergic drug, atropine, in the form of Belladonna, to treat Parkinson's disease in the 1880s, leading to the use of anticholinergic drugs ever since for parkinsonian problems, although they have largely been superseded now by the use of L-dopa and dopamine agonists. However, before L-dopa came on stream, the recognition that most antipsychotics cause parkinsonian symptoms led to the anticholinergics being used routinely to alleviate these side effects.

L-dopa and dopamine agonists have not replaced the anticholinergic drugs for this purpose because of concerns that dopamine agonists such as L-dopa might make schizophrenia worse. The evidence for this is not good, and there is a good deal of evidence to suggest that stimulants can reverse some of the parkinsonian problems of the antipsychotics. There may be a place for testing out other new antiparkinsonian treatments also.

From the 1970s onwards, the anticholinergic drugs were almost certainly used too routinely.[47] It became common practice to co-prescribe an anticholinergic agent with an antipsychotic from the start, even before side effects had appeared. The rationale for this was a belief that the emergence of side effects might compromise an individual's willingness to continue with medication. However, in many cases an early prescription of an anticholinergic will have meant that hospital staff or a general practitioner was not called out of hours by a distressed patient, who might otherwise have been alarmed by a dystonic reaction or other side effect. In the past, when much larger doses of antipsychotics were prescribed, the occurrence of parkinsonian side effects were all but inevitable, and the co-prescription of anticholinergic agents could be defended on this basis. Today, with the emphasis on much lower antipsychotic doses, the routine prescription of anticholinergic agents is less defensible, particularly as these agents bring their own problems and risks. The common side effects are shown in Box 3.1.

In many texts, this list of side effects will still include urinary difficulties, with a feeling of uncomfortable bladder fullness and possible retention.

BOX 3.1 Common side effects of anticholinergics

- Dry mouth
- Constipation
- Dizziness
- Blurred vision and a possible onset of glaucoma in susceptible individuals
- Theoretically, difficulties with having an erection might be expected, but in practice this does not seem to be a problem.
- An anterograde amnesia, so that subjects appear not to take in and retain things that happen whilst on these drugs. Similar problems are produced by alcohol and benzodiazepines so that elderly subjects, in particular, taking both anticholinergic agents and a benzodiazepine may have marked impairments of memory – enough to lead to worries about dementia.
- Dissociative reactions (see Chapter 5). These may include acute confusion and disorientation.

Whilst anticholinergics likely can give some urinary retention, these difficulties are usually caused by sympathetic system effects.

There is some evidence that the concurrent taking of anticholinergics may increase the risk for two of the most serious complications of antipsychotic therapy – tardive dyskinesia and NMS.

The stiffness, tremor and acute muscular spasm brought about by antipsychotics will often respond to anticholinergics – often with dramatic speed. In some instances, akathisia may also respond, but many cases of akathisia and most dyskinesias, in particular tardive dyskinesia, do not respond.

It seems increasingly reasonable to suggest that antipsychotics should be prescribed in such a way that side effects do not emerge; that is, low doses should be prescribed from the start, and there should be a willingness to change antipsychotics to find one that does not cause side effects. If such an approach is taken, there should be a considerable reduction in the amount of anticholinergics needed. One of the saddest things in clinical practice is to have a patient thank me for the marvellous tranquillisers they have been put on – only to realise that they are referring to their anticholinergic antidote.

There is a further intriguing possibility. For the past three decades the anticholinergic effects of antidepressants have been portrayed as a bad thing. However, any trials carried out for anticholinergic agent use in depression point strongly to the fact that this action may be antidepressant. This is not surprising because the anticholinergics are euphoriant.

STIMULANTS

Stimulants can be useful in treating antipsychotic side effects. For years they were avoided in anyone with psychosis in the belief that they might worsen the psychosis. With the demise of the dopamine hypothesis of schizophrenia, the way is open to renewing the investigation of the usefulness of these drugs and other dopamine agonists. This group is dealt with further in Section 4. Stimulants can be particularly useful for antipsychotic-induced demotivation.

BENZODIAZEPINES

A number of cases of akathisia respond to benzodiazepines, as does NMS and some dystonias. At present lorazepam is assuming a status in many units not unlike that formerly occupied by the anticholinergics: it is almost routinely prescribed in the early phases of treatment. This use is possibly excessive, but it may be coincidentally blocking the emergence of NMS or catatonic features in some patients.

BETA-BLOCKERS AND ANTIHISTAMINES

These are occasionally given for akathisia.[48,49]

TETRABENAZINE

Tetrabenazine is a derivative of reserpine that acts presynaptically. This has a number of consequences. First, whilst it also causes dyskinesias, dystonias and akathisia, many of the chronic drug-induced dyskinesias or dystonias caused by other antipsychotics improve on tetrabenazine – and this is the most common reason for its use. However, tetrabenazine is also an antipsychotic, and one that is not linked to weight gain. In patients for whom weight gain is a particular problem, tetrabenazine is an option to consider.

REFERENCES

1. Healy D. The creation of psychopharmacology. Cambridge, MA: Harvard University Press; 2002.
2. Johnstone EC, Crow TJ, Frith CD, et al. The Northwick Park 'functional' psychosis study: diagnosis and treatment. Lancet 1988;ii:119–25.
3. Healy D. Schizophrenia: basic, reactive, release and defect processes. Hum Psychopharm 1990;4(5):101–21.
4. Harrow M, Jobe T. Does long-term treatment of schizophrenia with antipsychotic medication facilitate recovery? Schizophr Bull 2013;39:962–5.
5. Healy D. D1 and D2 and D3. Br J Psychiatry 1991;159:319–24.
6. Chadwick PJ, Lowe CF. Measurement and modification of delusional beliefs. Br J Clin Psychol 1990;26:257–65.
7. Romme MAJ, Escher S. Accepting voices. London: MIND Publications; 1994.
8. Lieberman JA, Stroup TS, McEvoy JP, et al. Effective of antipsychotic drugs in patients with chronic schizophrenia. N Engl J Med 2005;353:1209–23.
9. Jones PB, Barnes TE, Davies L, et al. Cost utility of the latest antipsychotic drugs in schizophrenia study (CUTLASS 1). Arch Gen Psychiatry 2006;63:1079–87.
10. Pilowsky LS, Ring H, Shine PJ, et al. Rapid tranquillisation. Br J Psychiatry 1992;160:831–5.
11. Baldessarini RJ, Cohen BM, Teicher MH. Significance of antipsychotic doses and plasma levels in the pharmacological management of the psychoses. Arch Gen Psychiatry 1988;45:79–91.
12. Jusic N, Lader M. Post-mortem antipsychotic drug concentrations and unexplained deaths. Br J Psychiatry 1994;165:787–91.
13. Thompson C. The use of high-dose antipsychotic medication. Br J Psychiatry 1994;164:448–58.
14. Farde L, Wiesel FA, Halldin C, et al. Central D2 dopamine receptor occupancy in schizophrenic patients treated with antipsychotic drugs. Arch Gen Psychiatry 1988;45:71–6.
15. Rifkind A, Doddi S, Karagigi B, et al. Dosage of haloperidol for schizophrenia. Arch Gen Psychiatry 1991;48:166–70.
16. Van Putten T, Marder SR, Mintz J. A controlled dose comparison of haloperidol in newly admitted schizophrenic patients. Arch Gen Psychiatry 1990;47:754–8.
17. Wolkowitz OM, Pickar DM. Benzodiazepines in the treatment of schizophrenia: a review of reappraisal. Am J Psychiatry 1991;148:714–26.
18. Fink M, Taylor MA. Catatonia. Cambridge: Cambridge University Press; 2003.
19. Foster P. Antipsychotic equivalence. Pharm J 1989;243:431–2.
20. May PR, Van Putten T, Yale C, et al. Predicting individual responses to drug treatment in schizophrenia. J Nerv Ment Dis 1976;162:177–83.
21. Tranter R, Healy D. Neuroleptic discontinuation syndromes. J Psychopharmacol 1998;12: 306–11.
22. Gilbert PL, Harris J, McAdams LA, et al. Antipsychotic withdrawal in schizophrenic patients: a review of the literature. Arch Gen Psychiatry 1995;52:173–88.
23. Day JC, Bentall RP, Roberts D, et al. Attitudes towards antipsychotic medication. The impact of clinical variables and relationships with health professionals. Arch Gen Psychiatry 2005;62:717–24.
24. Sharp HM, Healy D, Fear CF. Symptoms or side-effects? Methodological hazards and therapeutic principles. Hum Psychopharmacol 1998;13:467–75.

25. Joukamaa M, Heliovaara M, Knekt P, et al. Schizophrenia, neuroleptic medication and mortality. Br J Psychiatry 2006;188:122–7.
26. Saha S, Chant D, McGrath J. A systematic review of mortality in schizophrenia. Arch Gen Psychiatry 2007;64:1123–31.
27. Osborn DJ, Levy G, Nazareth Z, et al. Relative risk of cardiovascular and cancer mortality in people with serious mental illness from the United Kingdom's General Practice Research Database. Arch Gen Psychiatry 2007;64:1123–31.
28. Healy D, LeNoury J, Whitaker C, et al. Mortality for schizophrenia & related psychoses in two cohorts: 1875–1924 & 1994–2010. BMJ Open 2012;2:e001810. doi:10.1136/bmjopen-2012-001810.
29. Beddoe R. Dying for a cure. A memoir of antidepressants, misdiagnosis and madness. Sydney: Random House; 2007.
30. Watkins J. Healing schizophrenia. Using medication wisely. Melbourne: Michelle Anderson Publishing; 2006.
31. Christensen DC. Dear Luise. Portland, Oregon: Jorvik Press; 2012.
32. Vaughan I. Ivan. London: Papermac; 1986.
33. Cunningham-Owens DG. A guide to the extrapyramidal side-effects of antipsychotic drugs. Cambridge: Cambridge University Press; 1999.
34. Healy D, Farquhar G. The immediate effects of droperidol. Hum Psychopharm 1998;13:113–20.
35. Jones-Edwards G. An eye-opener. OpenMind 1998;September:12,13,19.
36. Healy D, Savage M. Reserpine exhumed. Br J Psychiatry 1998;172:376–8.
37. Healy D. Sitting on it. OpenMind 2000;March:18.
38. King DJ, Burke M, Lucas RA. Antipsychotic drug-induced dysphoria. Br J Psychiatry 1995;167:480–2.
39. Jones-Edwards G. On the receiving end. New Therapist 2000;7:40–3.
40. Belmaker RH, Wald D. Haloperidol in normals. Br J Psychiatry 1977;131: 222–3.
41. Kendler KS. A medical student's experience with akathisia. Am J Psychiatry 1976;133:454.
42. Drake RE, Ehrlich J. Suicide attempts associated with akathisia. Am J Psychiatry 1985;142:499–501.
43. Sullivan G, Lukoff D. Sexual side effects of antipsychotic medication: evaluation and interventions. Hosp Comm Psychiatry 1990;41:1238–41.
44. Healy D, Herxheimer A, Menkes D. Antidepressants and violence: problems at the interface of medicine and law. PLoS Med 2006;3:Sept. doi:10.1371/journal.pmed.0030372.
45. Healy D. Catatonia from Kahlbaum to DSM 5. Aust N Z J Psychiatry 2013;47(5):412–6. doi:10.1177/0004867413486584.
46. Healy D, Howe G, Mangin D. Sudden cardiac death and the reverse dodo verdict. Int J Risk Saf Med 2014;26:71–9.
47. Barnes TRE. Comment on the WHO consensus statement. Br J Psychiatry 1990;156:413–4.
48. Ayd FJ. Lexicon of psychiatry, neurology and the neurosciences. Baltimore, MD: Williams and Wilkins; 1995.
49. Bezchlinbnyk-Butler KZ, Jeffries JJ. Clinical handbook of psychotropic drugs. Toronto: Hogrefe and Huber; 1995.

SECTION 2
MANAGEMENT OF DEPRESSION

SECTION CONTENTS

The antidepressants

4

CHAPTER CONTENTS

INTRODUCTION

It is more difficult to specify what antidepressants do than it is to say what other psychotropic drugs do. Part of the problem lies in defining depression, and the terms mood and emotions. One way is to compare the relation of mood to emotions with the relation between climate and weather, or between the pedal and keys of the piano. The climate sets the frame within which weather varies, but it does not itself change much. The pedals colour the tone of a melody. In the same way, mood sets the frame within which emotions operate. Mood disorders are like a change in climate rather than an emotional outburst linked to a particular problem. When antidepressants work, our climate controls are reset, whereas tranquilisers act on bad weather – except that antidepressants do also have anxiolytic effects that are more like acting on bad weather.

Part of the problem lies in our changing views of depression brought about by the interaction between the development of antidepressants and the marketing strategies of drug companies. When first developed, these drugs were used to treat a condition called melancholia or endogenous depression, but the boundaries between this disorder and sadness have been obliterated, and many people now get antidepressants who shouldn't.[1]

Whilst it is difficult to specify what it is that antidepressants do, it is possible to describe their side effects fairly well and the risks associated both with taking and not taking them. These are laid out in detail. There are a great number of different antidepressants, most of which have slightly different side effects. For many people, it may make little difference which antidepressant they have, but for some it may make a considerable difference in terms of discomfort or adverse outcomes.

HISTORY

TRICYCLIC AND MAOI ANTIDEPRESSANTS

The tricyclic antidepressant (TCA), imipramine and the monoamine oxidase inhibitor (MAOI), iproniazid, were discovered in 1957 by Roland Kuhn and Nathan Kline respectively.[2] What was discovered, however, was not just a drug, but a disorder that the drug treated. There was no preconceived idea that these drugs should be antidepressant. Indeed, Kuhn thought he was testing out a new antipsychotic when he first gave imipramine to patients. Furthermore, there were a great number of stimulants available at the time, such as the amphetamines, but these did not appear helpful for severe hospitalised depression. What Kuhn and Kline did, as much as find the compounds themselves, was to make visible a condition that responded to these compounds – variously called biological or major depression.

In 1965, the Medical Research Council (MRC) attempted to compare the MAOI phenelzine with the TCA imipramine, electroconvulsive therapy (ECT) and placebo. Imipramine and ECT came out as superior to placebo and phenelzine. At the same time a serious hazard of the MAOIs, the cheese effect (see Chapter 5), had just been described. These joint findings put paid to the MAOIs, leaving the TCAs as the dominant antidepressants for more than two decades, and it is from the TCAs that the selective serotonin reuptake inhibitors (SSRIs) came.

Intriguingly, even this early family studies had shown that some people who respond to MAOIs do not respond to TCAs and vice versa. This holds true to this day with those not responding to SSRIs often doing better on MAOIs and these responses seem to run in families.

SELECTIVE SEROTONIN REUPTAKE INHIBITORS (SSRIS)

In the early 1960s it was discovered that TCAs blocked the reuptake of the neurotransmitters, noradrenaline and serotonin. Subsequently, it was demonstrated that the first two TCAs, amitriptyline and imipramine, broke down in the body to the tricyclic compounds nortriptyline and desipramine, which both turned out to be antidepressants. This suggested to some that these were, in fact, the real antidepressants, rather than imipramine and amitriptyline.

Nortriptyline and desipramine block noradrenaline rather than serotonin uptake, whereas imipramine and amitriptyline block both noradrenaline and serotonin reuptake. The logical conclusion was that depression involved a disturbance of noradrenaline rather than serotonin function. This observation led to the catecholamine hypothesis of depression, which states that depression involves a lowering of brain noradrenaline. This led to a belief that further antidepressants should act specifically on the noradrenergic system.

However, some clinicians had noted that drugs acting on the catecholamine system appeared to make people well by being energy enhancing, whereas imipramine and clomipramine, which also acted on the serotonin system, did something else.[3] This led Arvid Carlsson to make zimelidine in the 1970s, a drug that selectively blocked serotonin reuptake. This was succeeded by fluvoxamine, fluoxetine and a slew of others.

The term SSRI (selective serotonin reuptake inhibitor) was coined by the marketers of paroxetine. Selective means the drug does not act on the noradrenaline system – it does not mean 'clean' or 'specific'. Paroxetine and other SSRIs have as many indiscriminate effects on different brain systems as the older drugs, and none of the SSRIs are selective to the serotonin system. The term SSRI and the later SNRI (serotonin and noradrenaline reuptake inhibitors) are marketing rather than scientific or clinical terms.

What does it mean that SSRIs may be helpful for depression? First, the selective noradrenaline reuptake inhibitors, such as desipramine, make it clear that blocking serotonin reuptake is not necessary for an antidepressant action. Second, there is no correlation between how effective the SSRIs are at blocking serotonin reuptake and how effectively they help depression. Third, the SSRIs are ineffective in more severe or hospitalised depression. Finally, contrary to popular belief, there is no evidence that there is anything wrong in the serotonin systems of people who are depressed. Ideas of lowered serotonin or chemical imbalances are marketing creations.

What then do SSRIs do? Of the older drugs, clomipramine, which was the drug that had the greatest effects on the serotonin system, was also the drug that seemed to be in some way the most anxiolytic: it was found to be useful in phobic and obsessional states.[4,5] Since then the SSRIs have been licensed to treat social phobia, generalised anxiety disorder (GAD), panic disorder and obsessive–compulsive disorder (OCD), and more recently these drugs have been marketed very actively as anxiolytics. This suggests that blocking serotonin reuptake produces an essentially anxiolytic effect rather than anything else. If SSRIs are anxiolytics, this would explain why these drugs are relatively ineffective in cases of severe depression, which are much more likely to respond to older TCAs or ECT.

The anxiolytic effects of SSRIs are weather effects. The climate effect lies in breaking up a depressive syndrome, which takes anything from a few days to several weeks. The different kinds of antidepressant differ in their weather effects. Some can help break up a depressive syndrome by increasing energy levels (noradrenaline reuptake inhibitors) and others by producing an anxiolytic effect (SSRIs). Given that not all patients are equally suited to either of these effects, the art of treatment lies in matching patients to the most appropriate treatment for them.

It is also worth noting that most TCAs and SSRIs were derived from antihistamines and that many antihistamines have serotonin reuptake inhibiting properties. These antihistamines can be anxiolytic in just the same way as SSRIs and can also cause the irritability, aggression and even suicidality that SSRIs can cause.

OTHER ANTIDEPRESSANTS

The TCA trimipramine does not inhibit either noradrenaline or serotonin reuptake. It blocks noradrenergic and serotonergic receptors to produce tonic effects – increased sleep and appetite. It is similar in effect to mirtazapine, mianserin and cyproheptadine and has similarities to trazodone and agomelatine. This group offer an alternative to TCAs and SSRIs.

Table 4.1 lists the major classes of antidepressants.

A number of treatments for bipolar disorders are also used in depression (see Chapter 6 and Chapter 7). In addition, benzodiazepines such as diazepam and alprazolam, as well as antipsychotics such as flupentixol, are used. The serotonin S1a agonist, buspirone, is also marketed as antidepressant.

At the time of writing the greatest interest lies in increasing evidence that ketamine can be surprisingly effective for melancholic depressions that would otherwise only respond to ECT.[6]

Finally, ECT is also used. The use of ECT is not discussed in this book, but ECT has a clear role when antidepressants fail to work, and in addition it may be useful for mania, catatonia and some cases of schizophrenia.[7]

DEPRESSION

The discovery of the antipsychotics and the benzodiazepines were uncomplicated because these drugs bring about clear changes that are noticeable to the taker and to others within an hour. In the case of the antidepressants, the discovery happened only when these drugs were given to a particular group of patients, and even then it took several weeks of treatment before the effect became apparent in a specific illness. The antidepressants were not discovered because they obviously made sad people happy.

The illness has been called vital, biological or endogenous depression, or melancholia. There are a number of good descriptions of this syndrome.[8,9] This is a state characterised by the symptoms shown in Box 4.1.

Going through this checklist of symptoms should bring home the point that the condition that the antidepressants treated was not ordinary or even severe sadness, guilt or hopelessness. It was something different from what most people think of as depression. Indeed, the term depression really only came into being in the early years of the 20th century.

In cases of classical depression for which antidepressants are helpful, there will be some of the physical symptoms listed in Box 4.1. However, in most cases someone with melancholia will also show psychological symptoms,

Table 4.1 *The antidepressants*

Generic drug name	UK trade name	US trade name
Tricyclic antidepressants		
Amitriptyline	Tryptizol/Lentizol	Elavil/Endep
Imipramine	Tofranil	Tofranil
Nortriptyline	Allegron	Aventyl
Desipramine	Pertofran/Norpramin	Pertofrane/Norpramin
Clomipramine	Anafranil	Anafranil
Dosulepin	Prothiaden	–
Lofepramine	Gamanil/Lomont	–
Doxepin	Sinequan	Adapin/Sinequan
Trimipramine	Surmontil	Surmontil
Monoamine oxidase inhibitors (MAOIs)		
Phenelzine	Nardil	Nardil
Moclobemide	Manerix/Aurorix	–
Serotonin reuptake inhibitors		
Citalopram	Cipramil	Celexa
Escitalopram	Cipralex	Lexapro
Fluvoxamine	Faverin	Luvox
Fluoxetine	Prozac	Prozac
Paroxetine	Seroxat	Paxil
Sertraline	Lustral	Zoloft
Venlafaxine	Effexor	Effexor
Desvenlafaxine	Pristiq	Pristiq
Duloxetine	Cymbalta	Cymbalta
Vortioxetine	Brintellix	Brintellix
Vilazodone	Viibryd	Viibryd
Other antidepressants		
Bupropion	(Zyban – smoking cessation)	Welbutrin
Maprotiline	Ludiomil	Ludiomil
Mirtazapine	Zispin	Remeron
Reboxetine	Edronax	–
Trazodone	Molipaxin	Desyrel
Agomelatine	Valdoxan	Valdoxan

such as hopelessness, helplessness, guilt, ruminations, suicidal ideas or a wish to be dead and anxiety.

The antidepressants are commonly of little use for individuals who have these psychological symptoms in the absence of the physical symptoms listed in Box 4.1. They are not in other words 'anti-psychological problem pills'. This issue has become clouded somewhat by the increasing use of SSRIs in anxiety states, in lieu of benzodiazepines (see Section 5). As part of the marketing of the SSRIs, 'cases of Valium' have been transformed into 'cases of Prozac', and patients who until recently would have been seen as anxious, stressed or sad have been labelled as depressed instead. The fact that anxious people are also unhappy makes it easier to make this jump.

BOX 4.1 Core symptoms of vital depression

- Loss of energy
- Loss of interest
- Feeling physically run down or ill
- Poor concentration
- Altered appetite
- Altered sleep
- A slowing of physical and mental functions

These core symptoms are very physical in character, almost like having influenza. In addition to the core symptoms, other physical problems may come with a depression. These include:

- heartburn
- indigestion
- constipation
- ulcers of the gut
- dry skin, hair and mouth
- pins and needles
- aches and pains around the body
- headaches
- altered periods.

THE VARIETIES OF DEPRESSION

Until 1980 depression was divided into reactive and endogenous depressions. It was thought that 'reactive' depression, which comes on after a life event, was a milder, anxiety-based psychological problem that should not be treated with antidepressants. Endogenous depression was supposedly a more severe biological illness, not reactive to life events, that was accordingly more appropriately treated with pills.

These ideas were shaped by the development of ECT and the TCAs. It appeared that the more severe depressions, and in particular those with clear physical features, responded convincingly to these physical treatments whereas the response of states of anxious misery or morbid distress was much less convincing. The endogenous depressions came to be seen as conditions that were presumed to arise by virtue of some biochemical change in the brain. The reactive or neurotic depressions were presumed to arise in response to life crises.[2]

Probably to our detriment, these views have been superseded, in part because it was shown that the so-called endogenous depressions can be triggered by life events, and because antidepressants can appear to offer some benefits for many seemingly mild depressions. The terms endogenous and reactive depression have fallen out of use and have been replaced by major depressive disorder (MDD) and by dysthymia, which refers to a chronic low-grade misery.

In 1980 the Third Edition of the *Diagnostic and Statistical Manual* (DSM-3) introduced MDD and operational criteria as a means of getting over the divisions between those who saw depression as a psychological disorder and those who saw it as a physical problem. Whatever it was, we could supposedly agree that if you had five of nine symptoms from a mixture of the physical and psychological symptoms listed above, you had MDD. Some clinical judgement was also assumed so that someone who has poor sleep, listlessness and anxiety from being pregnant would not be diagnosed as depressed.

Now, however, when the criteria for different disorders are put on the Internet and most prescribing is in primary care, there is no clinical judgement and people find they have MDD, post-traumatic stress disorder (PTSD) and perhaps even a touch of Asperger's to boot. Also, some of those on antidepressants for MDD do not have anything that is major or depressive or a disorder.

NON-DRUG TREATMENTS

Another set of developments has been the demonstration that a number of brief focused psychotherapies, in particular interpersonal therapy (IPT) and cognitive behavioural therapy (CBT), can bring about a response in many depressions that might also be expected to respond to antidepressants.[10,11] The fact that the same depressions respond to a number of very different types of psychotherapeutic intervention suggests that there is not just one right way to treat a depression. It might be better, therefore, to regard the different treatments as offering antidepressant principles. Cognitive therapy, for instance, contains a number of different strategies, all of which may be helpful, such as problem solving, behavioural activation and cognitive restructuring. It seems that each of these components, rather than the whole package, may in fact work for some people. This is similar to the way in which tricyclic, MAOI and SSRI antidepressants offer a number of quite different therapeutic principles. The art of therapy with either drugs or psychotherapy involves finding the right principles for each particular person.

Finally, the patients given antidepressants first ended up in the hospital during the 1950s, 1960s and 1970s with severe depressions. However, these were in many respects atypical of the kinds of patients treated today who are being seen by general practitioners rather than psychiatrists. Studying this larger group of depressions has made it clear that depression often resolves spontaneously without physical treatments, with the average time to response being somewhere around 14 weeks.[12–14] In fact, even the majority of the most severe melancholias will resolve in 4–6 months without treatment.

DO ANTIDEPRESSANTS WORK?

It is now widely assumed that randomised controlled trials (RCTs) show whether a treatment works. But far from being a method to prove treatments worked, RCTs were initially designed to weed out treatments that did not work. For treatments that unquestionably do work, such as penicillin for bacterial endocarditis, RCTs are not needed. We are in much less certain waters than is generally realised when the outcome of trials makes it clear that it is neither possible to say that this agent does nothing on the one hand nor that it restores a significant number of people who take it to full health on the other.

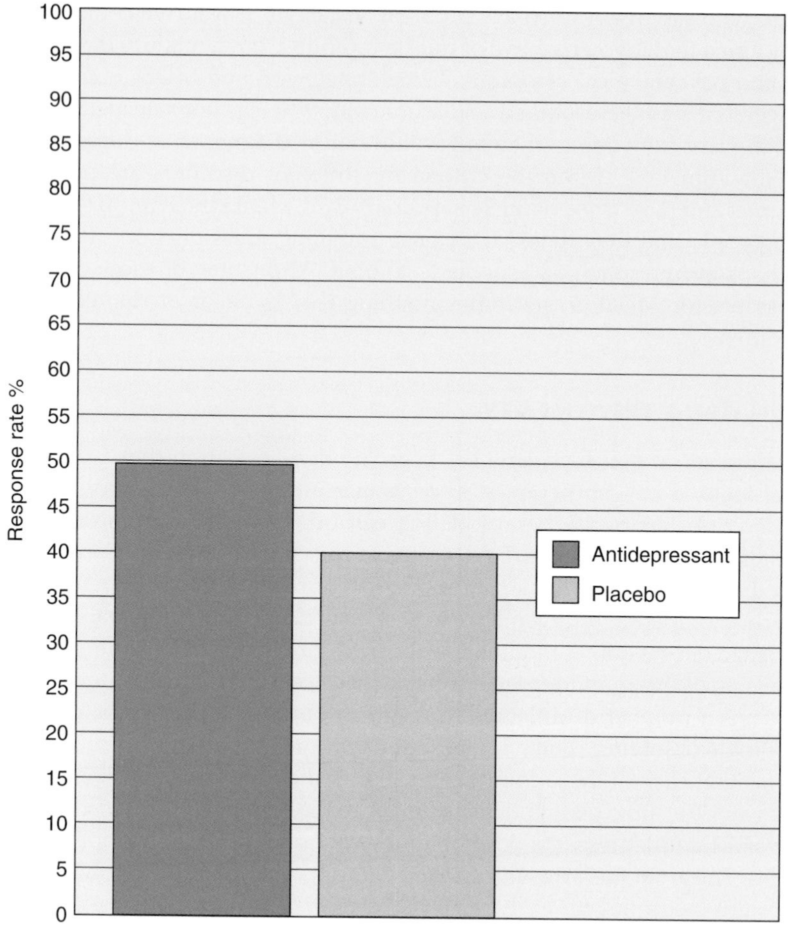

FIGURE 4.1 Antidepressants versus placebo. *Source: Stone M, Jones L. Clinical review: relationship between antidepressant drugs and adult suicidality. p. 31. http://www.fda.gov/ohrms/dockets/ac/06/briefing/2006-4272b1-index.htm, 2006.*

Data from a 2006 FDA analysis of all antidepressant trials (Figure 4.1) suggest that roughly 50% of patients entering published antidepressant trials have a response as measured on a rating scale like the Hamilton Rating Scale for Depression as compared with 40% of those who are given the placebo.[15]

A difference between active drug and placebo that is statistically significant is taken to indicate that the drug 'works'. However, if the trials are sufficiently large, even a minor difference of one or two rating scale points can be made statistically significant. As a result of this, a drug that is a little bit sedating or tranquilising will show up as 'working for depression' if the rating scale includes sleep or anxiety items. On this basis it would be possible to prove alcohol, nicotine vapes, benzodiazepines, stimulants, antipsychotics and many anticonvulsants are 'antidepressants'. The difference between this diverse group of drugs and more recent 'antidepressants' is that the SSRIs were patented for treating 'depression', whilst drugs like nicotine or the antihistamines were unpatentable for this purpose.

Such a claim sits uneasily with the supposed chemical imbalance that antidepressants fix. No-one claims nicotine, methylphenidate, diazepam or olanzapine fix this imbalance. There is little more than marketing myth to this chemical imbalance; a piece of biomythology just as notions of dopamine stabilisation on antipsychotics are (Chapter 2). In contrast with treatments from some other areas of medicine, antidepressant trials do not show evidence of lives saved or people back at work. The antidepressant data are best viewed as offering evidence that the drugs have an effect that might be consistent with them 'working' in some people.

An alternative way to read the data is that these trials allow us to quantify the contribution an antidepressant makes to treatment. Take the placebo response first. It is known that the natural history of depression means that many people will improve within a few weeks whether treated or not. It is also widely thought that sensible advice on matters of diet, lifestyle, alcohol intake and work and relationship problem solving may make a difference. It is suspected that patient perceptions that they are being seen and cared for by a medical expert may make a difference, and this effect may be enhanced by being given a substance they think will restore some chemical balance to normal – even if the imbalance is mythical. Simply presenting for treatment may make a difference. All of these factors are reflected in the placebo response.

These factors however also contribute to the therapeutic response for those on active drug. So four out of five (80%) of the patients who improve on antidepressants would have improved had they received the placebo. Only one out of five (20%) of responders have a specific response to the drug, and overall only one out 10 has a specific response to the drug. The number of patients needed to treat (NNT) to produce one specific drug response is 1/10% = 10. The rate of improvement amongst people on placebo is 40% (Figure 4.2). The NNT for the placebo group, therefore, is 1/40% = 2.5.

In practice, most clinicians and patients miss the fact that most responders are not responding to the drug. If we were really following the evidence, there would be a much greater use of placebos or judicious waiting, and in the case of responses, clinicians would generally caution patients that this may not be drug-induced. How do you tell if it's induced by the drug or placebo? Ask the person on treatment if they can detect anything the drug is doing they find useful – such as the right degree of emotional numbing on an SSRI.

The ambiguities here all stem from the word 'works'. A host of drugs from reserpine in 1955 through to the SSRIs have been shown in clinical trials to 'work', but at the same time a significant proportion of people taking them are not helped at all, and some may become suicidal. Even though superficially contradictory, there is no reason to disbelieve either the evidence from trials that some drugs work or from clinical experience that the same drugs may make many patients worse, if we realise that what, in fact, have been shown are average effects and that across a large number of patients it's just not possible to say this drug does nothing compared to placebo.

The problem we now have however is that journals and experts insist that the evidence from RCTs that antidepressants work trumps all other evidence such as the evidence clinicians and patients have from their own eyes that far from working a drug may be causing depression and suicidality.

FIGURE 4.2 Components of therapeutic response: specific drug versus non-specific placebo.
Source: Stone M, Jones L. Clinical review: relationship between antidepressant drugs and adult suicidality. http://www.fda.gov/ohrms/dockets/ac/06/briefing/2006-4272b1-index.htm, 2006.

In fact far from proving the drugs work, the data in Figures 4.1 and 4.2 are not inconsistent with the possibility that the drugs on balance do more harm than good. In the case of antidepressant and antipsychotic RCTs, there are in fact more dead bodies in the active drug than in the placebo group, which is not what would happen in a trial of penicillin for pneumonia. A further issue is that at present we have no way to know when patients walk through the door whether they are likely to respond to a serotonin or a catecholamine reuptake inhibitor. Up to 50% of people are being put on the wrong drug for them.

HOW LONG SHOULD TREATMENT CONTINUE?

In recent years an idea has gained ground that many people may need to stay on antidepressants for life. This might be true in occasional cases of severe recurrent depression but is quite wrong for most cases of depression. In the 1990s, the consensus view was that it is prudent for someone put on an antidepressant to stay on it for between 3 and 6 months after they have started feeling well. Given that depressions on average last for 3–4 months – even when left untreated – treatment approaches in the ordinary course of events should not endorse a much longer course of treatment than 3–6 months.

Indeed halting antidepressants immediately after recovery for some people can be done successfully. The risks of relapse from the illness seem to increase according to the number of previous episodes an individual has had and to the severity of those episodes. It is only if there have been a number of clear-cut previous episodes, severe enough to warrant hospitalisation, that the option of going on longer-term treatment should come up. Part of the current drift towards claiming that depression may need life-long treatment probably reflects a withdrawal problem. Antidepressant withdrawal effects may be

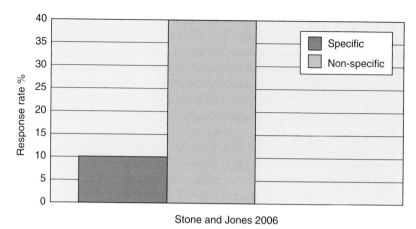

severe and may mimic the original illness and have almost certainly led both sufferers and physicians to believe mistakenly that treatment needs to be continued. Another part may stem from clinicians and patients mistakenly thinking that treatment rather than placebo factors have brought about a clinical response.

DRUGS OR PSYCHOTHERAPY?

The data from the antidepressant trials suggest that often neither drugs nor psychotherapy are needed. Watchful waiting may do the trick, and this, in fact, has the lowest relapse rates. Physical activity, structured routines and sensible lifestyle choices can all play a part in helping many depressive disorders. Compared with drugs, the therapies – CBT and IPT – offer a significant advantage in being less likely to produce withdrawal effects, but even if a depression has been cured with the latest psychotherapy without pills, it may relapse. The psychotherapies do not in this sense cure any more than the antidepressants. The more severe the depression, the more likely ECT or one of the older antidepressants, which combine a number of therapeutic principles, are able to make a clear difference. Even in the most psychotic depressions, however, it is worth noting that on average there will be a response within 6 months. The SSRIs do not work in severe or melancholic depressions.

Regarding the treatment of depression without pills, two points can be made. One is that it is not always the case that depressions can be treated without pills. Just as an SSRI may be the wrong pill for you, so also CBT may be the wrong therapy, and watchful waiting may not produce results. In the case of those depressions that fail to respond to waiting there is a case for combining both pills and therapy provided the pill is the right pill and the therapy approach is the right one. When they are the different mechanisms by which these work in principle should mean they are complementary.[2]

DO ANTIDEPRESSANTS CURE?

Many people think that antidepressants and ECT do not cure anything, that they only suppress problems or blunt reactions to some trauma until the individual has a chance to recover. However, the effect of antidepressants on depression, in this regard, is complex. In the case of classic endogenous or melancholic disorders, the treatment can come closer to being curative. With such kinds of depression, many people only ever have one serious episode. In other cases, depression seems to be a physical illness that clears up but may also come back, although each episode can be managed. Except for recurrent depression or dysthymia, depressions are not an illness like coronary artery disease or rheumatoid arthritis, which, once you have it, can never really be cured.

Whilst antidepressants often cure the illness they treat, relapse is possible even whilst the individual is on active treatment. This links into the vexed question of dependence.

Finally, antidepressants may also exert effects on people who are stressed rather than depressed. Taken chronically, SSRIs for example may produce a serenic effect in people under stress of different types – such as a stressful office situation. Should such people protest at office conditions instead of taking drugs? It is romantic to think that protest without resorting to pharmaceutical help is always the right answer.

WHAT DO ANTIDEPRESSANTS DO?

The principal theories about what the antidepressants do to biological systems in the brain have focused on their effects on noradrenaline and serotonin, leading to the amine theories, first put forward in 1965. These were based on the idea that drugs that lower noradrenaline or serotonin seemed to trigger depression, and the then known antidepressants appeared to increase the levels of these neurotransmitters. These theories have dominated discussion about depression in popular books or in articles from magazines such as *Cosmopolitan* or *Esquire*, giving rise to a language about chemical imbalances. The truth, however, is that despite more than five decades of work there is still no convincing evidence about what is wrong in depression. The drugs work on noradrenaline and serotonin systems, but there is no evidence for anything wrong in these systems in depression.

This lack of a convincing rationale for what is wrong in depression leads some people to have doubts about taking antidepressants. It should be borne in mind, however, that the questions of whether antidepressants work and how they work are quite separate. So, although there is little agreement about what is wrong in depression, there is good evidence that antidepressants can be helpful.

Clinically, for the first 2 weeks of treatment, the standard view is that antidepressants do very little except cause side effects. The change that then occurs seems to creep up on people rather than to sweep in on them. It seems to be rather like the kind of change that goes with influenza clearing up rather than the instant and dramatic changes brought about by anti-anginal tablets in cases of angina or bronchodilators in the case of asthma. What usually happens is that there is a slow increase in energy, a slow return of interest, a mild increase in appetite and an improvement in sleep. These occur gradually rather than clearly and they may be patchy, for example with one good night's sleep followed by a poor one the night after. Rather like a slow change of season – to return to the climate analogy.

For the most part, improvements in the sadness, hopelessness, guilt and suicidal thoughts that may go with depression seem to occur as a reaction to changes in things such as sleep, energy and interest. Sometimes sleep improves and energy and interest increase, but the individual may remain demoralised. The temptation in such cases is to increase the dose of the antidepressant; this rarely produces the hoped-for benefits.

Having made these points, we have given antidepressants to healthy volunteers – with surprising results. First, when the drug suited an individual, it was possible to make perfectly normal people 'better than well'. In the case of the SSRIs, this involved making a person more serene or mellow. For some people this can be unhelpful; for others it seemed to be something they appreciated. In the case of drugs active on the noradrenergic system, when these drugs were appreciated it was because they produced what the taker saw as a useful increase in energy and drive. All these effects were visible within 48 hours.[16]

This points to a number of things. One is that calling these drugs antidepressants is in a sense misleading. The drugs in the group differ and have effects on a wide variety of conditions and even on healthy people. Second, the first effects of 'antidepressants', good or bad, are likely to be visible within days rather than weeks. Against a background of a 50:50 chance that a person may have been put on the wrong drug for them, the first few days or weeks of treatment should be monitored carefully. The evidence that only 40% of people take antidepressants beyond a few weeks probably means many find the drug they have been put on unhelpful.

This runs contrary to traditional views of antidepressants, which is that unlike other drugs that act on the brain, whether tea or coffee, nicotine or alcohol, antipsychotics, minor tranquillisers or marijuana, antidepressants do not have an immediately obvious action. The only thing antidepressants obviously do in the short term is to produce side effects. The two views can be reconciled by suggesting that what people see happening at 2 weeks or longer is the depressive syndrome breaking up, but long before that it may be possible for someone to work out whether the pill they are on is suiting them or not.

This also runs contrary to the view that antidepressants only do anything to people who are depressed, unlike tea, coffee or antipsychotics, which have the same actions on everyone with or without mental disorders. In the case of the antidepressants, however, the puzzles about what happens may link to the effects these drugs have on personalities. Right from the first article on imipramine, through *Listening to Prozac* to the present, there are reports of patients getting better-than-well on these drugs, while on average the drugs seem barely better than placebo. This points to an unexplored interaction between these drugs and personality.

It does take several weeks to 'break up' a depression, but beneficial effects will often be apparent within 1–2 days if looked for. These may range from the tonic effects of some TCAs, which lead to an almost immediate improvement in sleep and appetite, to the anxiolytic or serenic effects with SSRIs, to drive-enhancing effects of noradrenergic drugs. This is very obvious when these drugs are given to healthy volunteers when the right effect for the right person may in fact even produce a better-than-well effect in a totally healthy person. On an SSRI, for instance, healthy individuals may become mellow, and this may suit them.

These effects are rather subtle compared with the effects of tea, alcohol, benzodiazepines or antipsychotics and, because of this, few people ask what is this drug doing to get a depressed person well, or what do we want a drug to do to get this person well. The assumption is that all antidepressants do much the same thing regardless of which brain system they work on. Nothing could be further from the truth.

Finally, antidepressants differ from the other drugs in psychiatric use in that in overdose many older antidepressants can be fatal in relatively small amounts, although this is much less the case with some of the more recently produced compounds.

ANTIDEPRESSANTS: FIRST CHOICE OR LAST RESORT?

Given that many depressions heal naturally, and given that psychotherapy can help, should people take antidepressants at all? Those who would argue that you should not take them commonly put forward three different objections. One is that antidepressants alter brain chemistry and this cannot be a good idea. Another is that antidepressants block messages in the brain and this cannot be a good idea. The third is that the use of antidepressants will interfere with the development of natural coping mechanisms.

ANTIDEPRESSANTS AND BRAIN CHEMISTRY

Antidepressants act on a multiplicity of receptors in the brain. They even bring about changes in brain receptors on which the drugs themselves do not act. Could this predispose individuals who take these pills to further episodes of depression by making them chemically unstable?

Unlike other drugs that act on the brain, the older antidepressants, but not the SSRIs, act relatively 'weakly' on the brain receptors they bind to. They neither vigorously act on nor comprehensively block anything. The changes they bring about tend to be within the range of circadian changes that are happening during the day anyway. Compared with the effects of coffee, tranquillisers or alcohol, for example, antidepressants are less likely to push the brain systems they act on beyond the normal range of circadian variation.

A further point is that severe depression – but not many primary care depressions – can also bring about changes in brain functioning. For example, severe depression causes an increase in levels of the stress hormone, cortisol. Prolonged increases in cortisol reset the central cortisol control mechanisms to a higher setting. This in turn is liable to lead to a raised cortisol level even when the person is not depressed. Increased cortisol synthesis may even, in time, lead to brain cell loss and premature ageing.

Whether through cortisol or another mechanism, severe depression predisposes to future depressive relapses and to increasingly severe episodes. Severe depressions can increase the risk for tumours and infections, and the presence of depressive symptoms after a heart attack is a significant factor in determining recovery and the likelihood of death in the following 12-month period.[17] Therefore, leaving depression untreated may not be as natural or as healthy as it might sound, but equally using antidepressants in conditions that will resolve spontaneously or involve normal misery rather than depression is likely to cause problems.

DO ANTIDEPRESSANTS BLOCK IMPORTANT MESSAGES?

Another reason given for not taking antidepressants is based loosely on the biochemical theories of how they work. The argument goes that they block impulses flowing from one brain cell to another. This never sounds like a good idea to anyone. However, chemical messages and psychological messages are not the same thing. As we age there are many fewer neurotransmitters whizzing around our brains, but psychologically we remain the same. Having said this, the mass use of antidepressants does raise intriguing questions about the nature of the self that have remained strangely unexplored.[18]

ANTIDEPRESSANTS AND COPING

A third argument goes: if antidepressants suppress or otherwise bring a halt to a depressive episode, surely the individual will not learn the coping skills that are necessary to handle depression and will therefore remain vulnerable to yet further depressive episodes. These latter depressive episodes will then increasingly have to be chemically controlled.

Regarding the question of whether antidepressants interfere with the development of coping mechanisms, this argument may hold for many of the conditions that are mistakenly labelled as depression and treated with antidepressants. However, severe depressions are demoralising disorders. They tend to be particularly demoralising the longer and more severe their course. Demoralisation is not something that antidepressants clear up. It typically resolves when the underlying depression resolves. At least, it does so when the underlying depression has not been particularly severe or long lasting.

We spring back naturally. Springing back does not come about because we have developed new coping skills. We simply do not need to be anxious and demoralised once normality has returned. We are less likely to spring back in this way if the underlying depression has lasted for a long time or has been severe. In this case, antidepressants may clear up the sleep and appetite disturbances and improve energy levels but leave the person miserable, unhappy and with an impairment of self-esteem that may be more or less permanent. This impaired self-esteem will also make further serious and lengthy depressions more likely as, should the person ever become mildly clinically depressed again, their impaired self-esteem will summate rapidly with the depression, leading to a very rapid evolution to severe depression.

Therefore, everything possible should be done to avoid demoralisation. The best method of doing this is to ensure that the depression a person has is as brief and as mild as possible and, in particular, that they are not exposed to a severe or long-lasting disorder. If it becomes clear the disorder is not going to be brief and self-resolving, some intervention is called for in order to prevent current coping skills from being lost in the face of demoralisation. This may be either a cognitive therapy or IPT or antidepressants or watchful waiting – but something rather than nothing. If demoralisation fails to respond to an antidepressant, consideration should be given to a psychological intervention rather than simply to more or longer courses of an antidepressant.

Another point also needs to be made is that people who improve on antidepressants should not conclude that the restoration of the self-confidence they have had is down to their antidepressant alone. Thinking this could lead on to a belief that one had to keep on taking the antidepressants to remain stable or to a belief that one is more vulnerable than the average person to further depression. Halting antidepressants, if this were the case, could be seen as the potential removal of a crutch and it could become quite threatening. Such an idea of what antidepressants do would rob a person of confidence in their own resources to handle further episodes of depression – and even to handle interpersonal difficulties generally.

One of the hardest things for people to do after they have been depressed, whether or not they have been treated with antidepressants, but particularly if they have been, is to let themselves get normally unhappy after they halt the drugs. We seem to assume that, because we have been cured, we should not get unhappy again. The first hint of a poor spell after stopping antidepressants may cause a serious panic.

However, returning to normal means returning to the normal ups and downs of life. What has to be relearnt is an ability to live with these ups and downs – as they cannot be stopped. Even on antidepressants, the normal ups and downs should continue. The greatest block to recovery may often be the person's own idea of what it means to be well: 'treatment should make me into someone who never has any ups or downs again'.

WHAT IF THERE IS NO RESPONSE?

Before concluding that there will be no response to an antidepressant, a subject should have been taking a full dose of the antidepressant they have been put on for up to 6 weeks – provided there are no indications that the drug is not suiting them. If there are indications the drug is not suiting, the switch should be made much earlier. If there is definitely no response, the options are:

- To change to another type of antidepressant, especially if there is any indication that the current antidepressant is not suiting.
- To go to a higher dose on the rare occasions that a biological factor makes a higher dose necessary (see doses in Starting Antidepressants).
- To add in a psychological therapy. Paradoxically, many resistant 'biological' depressions seem to need the addition of psychological interventions.
- To have a combination of antidepressants, for example, a TCA along with an MAOI or lithium or an SSRI with mirtazapine or lithium. This is termed an augmentation strategy. It should be rare outside of hospital settings.
- To discontinue antidepressants completely on the premise that, although the person is miserable and demoralised, they do not have the kind of problem that responds to antidepressants. In this case, psychotherapy may help, but concentrating on getting fit may do as much.
- To have ECT. This remains the most effective treatment for depression. Today it is usually used as a treatment of last resort, but, in fact, ECT has fewer side effects than many of the other treatments. It is used, for example, in the frail elderly or after heart attacks, where antidepressants may be contraindicated. As a treatment of last resort, however, ECT has often been given inappropriately to individuals who should never have been given antidepressants; giving ECT is particularly inappropriate in this case.

STARTING ANTIDEPRESSANTS

TCAs

The usual dose of most TCAs is 150 mg per day. In some cases, it is possible to start at 75 mg daily and increase to 150 mg per day within a few days. For others it is necessary to start at 25 mg per day and work up slowly. The more anxious the person, the slower the dose escalation. The entire 150 mg per day is also often given in one dose, usually last thing at night.

If there is no response to 150 mg a day, in some cases the dose may be increased to anything up to 300 mg daily, depending on side effects. For most non-responders such an increase will make no difference, but in some cases there is a failure to absorb the drug. Other factors that hinder recovery that may be overcome by a higher dose include high levels of cortisol, concurrent infections, concurrent treatment with contraceptives and obesity.

At present, the standard wisdom is that there is little point being on less than 75 mg per day of a TCA for full-blown depression. A little bit of an antidepressant is supposedly not even a little bit antidepressing. However, in clinical practice, TCAs such as dosulepin are often given in a 25 mg night-time dose and they work – at least in the sense of improving sleep in what may be cases of mild depression or anxiety.

MAOIs

In the case of the MAOI phenelzine the effective dose is between 60 and 120 mg per day. For moclobemide, the dose is 600–900 mg daily, in divided doses. These drugs are usually prescribed first thing in the morning rather than last thing at night, as they may be mildly stimulant and interfere with sleep.

SSRIs

Most SSRIs have been marketed in a convenient one dose fits all approach that may have accounted in part for their success. This has advantages but also disadvantages. It is clear that many people cannot initially tolerate the amount in even one pill; this is particularly true for people who are anxious. Company representatives warn physicians about the hazards of serotonin pick-up syndromes, even though officially the companies deny that this happens. This has led to a widespread practice of co-administering benzodiazepines for the first few weeks of treatment. There is lots of evidence that companies adopted a one size fits all strategy deliberately, ignoring evidence that doses a quarter of the standard dose would be adequate for many people. If treatment produces a bad reaction in the first few days, it may be worth dropping the dose down to a fraction of the usual dose.

STOPPING ANTIDEPRESSANTS

Even though the first report of withdrawal from antidepressants was published in 1961, for three decades the received wisdom was that antidepressants are non-addictive, and for many people there may be essentially little or no withdrawal reaction. It was conceded that rebound effects on halting TCAs or MAOIs, which may produce increased dreaming at night for one or two nights, could happen. However, it is now clearer that a number of individuals may become classically physically dependent on antidepressants and on halting may have difficulties lasting anything from days in mild cases to months in more severe cases. These dependence reactions have been associated predominantly with the SSRIs, but many TCAs also act on the serotonin system (see Chapter 23).

If starting an SSRI is more convenient than starting other antidepressants, stopping them poses greater problems. It is now clear that SSRIs may lead to significant physical dependence in more than 30% of takers. The commonest symptoms of this are anxiety and depression (which occur even in healthy volunteers stopping after only 2–3 weeks of treatment), dizziness, headache, sweating, fatigue and nausea, but a wide variety of problems can occur from electric sensations shooting up and down limbs to depersonalisation and muscle pain. The picture may resemble depression so that the problems that occur on stopping may be interpreted as illness relapse rather than withdrawal.[19–21]

No one knows at present the precise figure for the number of people affected by significant withdrawal problems. A majority of people now taking antidepressants are taking them chronically, often because they cannot stop. Many of those told by their physician that they may need to stay on treatment for the rest of their life are in fact physically dependent rather than suffering from a chronic illness. Women seem more likely to be affected than men – just as women seem more prone to tardive dyskinesia than men. Dependence and withdrawal can affect a person put on SSRIs for a relatively short period of time with a minor complaint that could have been handled without drugs or even someone treated with SSRIs for flushing for instance, who has no nervous problem.

For some experts addiction refers to a process whereby a drug transforms someone into a junkie. Antidepressants do not transform people into junkies. And so these experts say antidepressants are not drugs of addiction. However, for most people, addiction means being unable to stop a drug for one reason or another. In this sense antidepressants are addictive. This important point is developed further in Chapter 23.

Withdrawal is probably related to another phenomenon termed 'poop-out'. This was first described with SSRIs, shortly after their launch. It refers to the fact that in some cases, the drugs appear to stop working but can be made to work again by increasing the dose. This evidence of tolerance has now been demonstrated in clinical trials.[22]

MANAGING WITHDRAWAL

The recommendations for managing withdrawal are standard for all psychotropic drug groups. In all cases, antidepressants of whatever class should be tapered rather than discontinued abruptly. In cases of established or suspected withdrawal, the taper should be even slower. There are then options of switching the individual to a TCA with a lesser degree of serotonin reuptake inhibition, such as imipramine, and then tapering. Another option is to use a liquid form of the drug, allowing the dose to be lowered more gradually.

Side effects of antidepressants

5

CHAPTER CONTENTS

INTRODUCTION

For the first few weeks on an antidepressant, side effects rather than benefits often predominate. If the pill is ultimately going to be suitable for the person taking it, the side effects will generally be mild. Antidepressants should cause only tolerable side effects. If treatment makes someone clearly worse, it should be stopped until advice addresses the problem in hand.

It is sometimes said that the benefits do not appear for 4–6 weeks. This is wrong. The condition may not clear up for a few weeks, but the emotional numbing that can make a selective serotonin reuptake inhibitor (SSRI) helpful or the increased sleep and appetite and other effects that may make a tricyclic antidepressant (TCA) helpful may be there right from the first hour or two.

There may however be great difficulty in distinguishing the effects of treatment from some of the symptoms of the illness. Both drugs and illness may cause a dry mouth, headache, indigestion, anxiety, sleeplessness, feelings of unreality and even suicidality or aggression. The difficulties in discriminating what might be stemming from what are brought out beautifully in Rebekah Beddoe's *Dying for a Cure: A Memoir of Antidepressants, Misdiagnosis and Madness*.[23]

There is a number of other unusual aspects to the side effects of antidepressants. In severe depression, individuals are often much less sensitive to the effects of anything. They may not smell, taste or hear as acutely as before. Even three to four times the dose of a sleeping pill may not help the insomnia that goes with depression. The same people, a few weeks later when they have recovered, may be knocked out by a low dose of the same sleeping pill. This, however, is much less likely to apply to patients with a milder form of depression or anxiety, who are now most likely to be prescribed antidepressants. Those who are anxious may be more rather than less sensitive to the side effects of antidepressants. It is difficult, therefore, to predict the side effects that an antidepressant will have.

In addition, there can be huge variation according to personality type and ethnic background with certain personality types susceptible to certain side effects whilst others are not and some ethnic groups liable to difficulties that do not happen in others. Thus Japanese men seem prone to gynaecomastia on SSRIs whereas Caucasians are not.

The side effects listed here are the typical ones. Some of these occur in everyone to some extent, depending on the compound they are on, but they are usually mild and wear off after a few days. For the most part, these side effects are reversible on stopping the drugs.

As with the antipsychotics, there are two sorts of side effects to note: those that seem more like side effects, such as a dry mouth or sedation, and those that may feel like a worsening of the illness – like feeling more nervous or feeling strange and unreal, or even hearing voices. These latter side effects are the ones that need careful judgement and may pose the greatest risks.

User issues

The obvious side effects of antidepressants

Sedation

Many older antidepressants, especially amitriptyline, trimipramine, mirtazapine and trazodone, are very sedative when first taken, but almost all can be somewhat sedative. This sedation is similar to the effect from some antihistamines. Just as with antihistamines, about one-third of people who take these drugs are clearly sedated, whilst two-thirds are either slightly sedated or not sedated at all. Sedative effects may be quite unpleasant to begin with, but they usually wear off. In a minority of people, the sedation may persist, in which case the drug should be stopped, particularly if driving or work is compromised.

In the case of the SSRIs, there may be a paradoxical coexistence of feeling drowsy or fatigued, along with an inability to sleep. Even more clearly with the SSRIs, some people may be drowsy whilst others are unable to sleep so that for some the dose of an SSRI should be given in the morning and for others in the evening.

Arousal

In some people, rather than sedating, antidepressants may arouse and make sleep impossible. In this case it makes more sense to take the pill first thing in the morning rather than last thing at night. This is a problem more likely to happen with antidepressants acting on noradrenergic systems, such as desipramine, nortriptyline or reboxetine.

Monoamine oxidase inhibitors (MAOIs) are more likely than TCAs to cause arousal. For this reason they are usually given in the morning rather than at night. However, MAOIs may be heavily sedating in some cases and have to be given last thing at night.

In the case of the SSRIs, some are stimulated by them, but others are sedated. Even more unusually, the SSRIs sometimes cause a subjective drowsiness whilst at the same time bringing about what is normally seen as a more 'alert' performance on tests of cognitive function.

Dry mouth

Dry mouth is an almost universal side effect of antidepressants. This will usually be mild and after the initial effects wear off may be unnoticeable unless the taker has to talk at length. However, it may be severe to the point of feeling that the tongue is stuck to the roof of the mouth or that the inside of the mouth feels like sandpaper. The nose may also feel dry and congested.

Dry mouth is usually a minor inconvenience, but it can be more serious with long-term use as saliva protects against tooth decay and its lack may aggravate dental problems.

It has been traditional to put dry mouth down to the anticholinergic properties of antidepressants. However, the SSRIs, which have been supposed to have little or no anticholinergic effects, also produce a dry mouth.

Fainting

TCAs, MAOIs and mirtazapine all lower blood pressure. For most of us, abrupt changes in posture after getting out of bed or standing up from a chair can produce a feeling of faintness or a hint of seeing stars. On treatment, these postural changes may be exaggerated so that a minor change of posture may

Continued

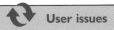

User issues—cont'd

cause a significant drop in blood pressure, leading a subject to topple over and potentially to serious injury. This is a greater hazard in older individuals for whom changes in posture are more likely to drop blood pressure with or without use.

Palpitations

Palpitations are one of the more unsettling effects of an antidepressant. Finding one's heart beating irregularly or thumping in one's chest is alarming. Despite being alarming, palpitations are usually harmless. They may simply stem from the heart trying to compensate for a drop in blood pressure by putting out more blood. All antidepressants can cause direct cardiac effects, which may be a real hazard for individuals with heart trouble and on treatments and for the rest of us if we have congenital QT interval prolongation, and for this reason, whilst ordinarily harmless, palpitations should be assessed rather than dismissed.

Urinary difficulties

Most antidepressants can cause trouble with urination. In the mildest cases, the subject will be aware of a slight delay before passing water. There may also be a feeling of distension around the bladder area, which causes a feeling of fullness just above the pubic bone. This may be uncomfortable and even painful. Textbooks usually list these symptoms as affecting only men, but they also affect young women. Occasionally the problem may be more marked to the point of having clear difficulty in passing water or even urinary retention. This latter is most common in older men with enlarged prostate glands. The concern for women is that they will get misdiagnosed as having a UTI.

Almost all drug information sources put this side effect down to the anticholinergic properties of TCAs. In fact, the problem stems from the action of these drugs on the noradrenergic system. Duloxetine, which inhibits both catecholamine and serotonin uptake, is also marketed as a bladder stabiliser, and atomoxetine (see Chapter 8), now used for attention deficit/hyperactivity disorder (ADHD), was also investigated as a bladder stabiliser. Neither have anticholinergic effects but both inhibit catecholamine reuptake.

Sweating

It is common for antidepressants to increase sweating. This is particularly common in hot weather. It may be most noticeable at night, leading to people waking up to find their sheets drenched. Increased perspiration may also be a feature of the serotonin syndrome (see Serotonin syndrome below).

Shake or tremor

Some people on an antidepressant may have a shake of their hand or arm. This is commonest at high doses. If it happens, it may mean that the dose is too high. In some individuals, because of differences in rates of absorption, the usual clinical dose may be too high and may need lowering. A shake is one hint that this may be the case.

Essentially, antidepressants – and in particular the SSRIs – can cause all the problems that the antipsychotics cause, from dyskinesias to dystonias, to akathisia and parkinsonian features (see Chapter 3). All these problems are likely to be more obvious when SSRIs are combined with antipsychotics, lithium, anticonvulsants, analgesics or oral contraceptives.

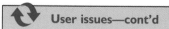

User issues—cont'd

Twitch or jerk

All antidepressants can cause twitches or jerky movements (myoclonus) of the head, arms or legs. These are commonest in the legs at night but may affect any part of the body at any time. This is a side effect of antidepressants rarely noted in any books, but it happens in up to 10% of takers. It may be commoner with drugs active on the serotonin system. It usually stops on switching to another treatment.

Tooth grinding (bruxism) and jaw locking (trismus)

Another rarely described side effect is tooth grinding. Many of us grind our teeth during sleep. Some antidepressants, in particular the SSRIs, may lead to tooth grinding during the day. This may get so intense as to cause marked gum pain. Those who can remove dentures do so, but at the cost of embarrassment. Occasionally the problem may be sufficiently severe to lead to a grinding down of the teeth and the need for them to be capped. Sometimes this problem can persist even after the drug is stopped.

There may be two distinct components to the problem: (1) abnormal movement of the jaw (a dyskinesia) and (2) an increase in tone of the jaw muscles (dystonia). In mild forms, this increased tone may be painful and, confusingly, may be experienced simply as a pain in the jaw area. In more severe forms, it can lead to lockjaw (trismus). The problems may also affect the throat and may be experienced as an acute sore throat (pharyngitis), leading the taker to believe they have a throat infection. In other cases there may be difficulty swallowing, as though the throat is constricted. Another variation on the phenomenon is forced yawning.

Although this problem is rarely described, up to 50% of the takers of an SSRI may experience these problems during the first week of treatment. Tooth grinding is the more likely to persist. This has the potential to lead on to tardive dyskinesia and perhaps should lead to treatment being halted.

Headaches are a common feature of depression and it may be difficult to be sure whether an antidepressant has caused them. An antidepressant headache is usually different to the one found in depression. Typically, antidepressants give a muzziness or feeling of painful fullness rather than the aching tension type of headache that most of us have had at some point or other. It may not be possible to distinguish these headaches, however, and if a new headache comes on after starting an antidepressant, or the old one seems to get worse, it is wise to seek advice. SSRIs can cause idiopathic intracranial hypertension, which if not checked can lead to blindness.

In rare instances, antidepressants may trigger migrainous headaches – headaches that have a throbbing, pulsating character that usually affects one side or other of the head and that may be accompanied by disturbances of vision and/or nausea and vomiting. The reason for this appears to be because most of these drugs act on the serotonin system, which regulates blood flow through the head and brain.

Headaches may be more serious in individuals who are on MAOIs and who have eaten food containing tyramine (see Cheese effect below), in individuals taking lithium, and in individuals taking combinations of antidepressants and antipsychotics, or either of these combined with lithium.

Continued

User issues—cont'd

Blurred vision

A further side effect of most antidepressants is blurred vision. This is commonest on TCAs, which have the most marked anticholinergic effects, but eyesight disturbances also happen with SSRIs. Whilst this is listed as one of the obvious side effects of antidepressants, it is surprising how often it leads people to make appointments to get their eyes checked. Any change of glasses should usually be deferred until after the drug has been discontinued.

Occasionally, individuals prone to glaucoma will have their condition exacerbated by treatment making it necessary to prescribe an antidepressant with minimal or no anticholinergic effects. Glaucoma presents with acutely painful eyes. This, however, is a rare occurrence, somewhat commoner when antidepressants are combined with anticonvulsants.

Weight gain

Depression often leads to a loss of appetite and weight. Successful treatment can therefore be expected to lead to some weight gain. For some, however, there is a more serious weight gain. They may put on up to 10 kg for reasons that are not fully understood but that are drug induced. Weight gain may be aggravated in individuals who are also taking lithium and antipsychotics.

In the short term, SSRIs can lead to weight loss through nausea and even vomiting. The nausea generally subsides within a few days, but a mild suppression of appetite may remain for a while. Taken over time, however, SSRIs often trigger marked weight gain.

While weight gain may seem like an obvious side effect of drug treatment, many individuals seem to be unaware that their drugs may be causing the weight gain, and accordingly, they may try to diet strenuously, encouraged by their doctor. Their inability to lose weight in the expected way may be quite demoralising.

Nausea

All antidepressants may cause nausea. They may also cause indigestion, constipation and a bloated feeling. The SSRIs, however, are far more likely to cause nausea and indigestion than other agents. Up to 25% of people who take these drugs may feel as though they are sea-sick. This usually wears off after a few days. In some cases, however, it may be quite severe, may lead to vomiting and may not wear off. In such cases the drugs have to be stopped. This seems to be a greater problem in Asian populations.

Rashes and infections

All drugs may cause idiosyncratic hypersensitivity reactions. The commonest sign of such a reaction is a skin rash. Skin rashes for the most part are not harmful and go quickly once the drug has been stopped. A more serious problem is recurrent fevers, with a sore throat and painful mouth. It may be necessary to take a blood test to check the white blood cell count to establish what is happening. Treatment may have led to a lowering of the white cell count predisposing to infection, especially in the elderly.

THE DISSOCIATIVE SIDE EFFECTS

The dissociative side effects of antidepressants include depersonalisation, derealisation and a number of other experiences that may be severe enough to produce frank confusion. The danger of these dissociative experiences lies in the fact that they may be interpreted by either the person taking the antidepressant or others as evidence that the illness is getting worse or that brain damage of some sort has been caused. If misinterpreted, such reactions can lead to suicide (see Antidepressants and suicide below). This risk, and the fact that a drug causing such reactions is most unlikely to cure depression, provide grounds for switching treatment.

DEPERSONALISATION

Depersonalisation refers to an experience of feeling strange and unusual, almost as though you are not really yourself anymore, or that you are operating in a kind of a dream or haze. It refers to the unreal feeling that many of us may have at interviews or other stressful situations where part of us seems to be functioning automatically and not under full control. Depersonalisation and derealisation are dissociative reactions that are relatively common on antidepressants.

DEREALISATION

Derealisation refers to a similar set of feelings and perceptions seen in depersonalisation, but in this case they apply to the world rather than to the self. This is a state in which the world seems strange or unreal; everything may seem far away or staged in some way – as though life is being watched rather than lived.

These feelings happen in anxiety states, but they also happen commonly in depression. If they start for the first time after taking an antidepressant or get clearly worse, treatment should be discontinued. The sensations will usually go within hours, or at the most days, after stopping treatment, but can sometimes be enduring. Like palpitations, these are very unsettling rather than directly dangerous experiences.

OTHER DISSOCIATIVE EXPERIENCES

- A feeling that time is standing still.
- Déjà vu experiences.
- Prominent nightmares or lucid dreaming – where the dreamer feels awake.
- Out-of-body experiences.
- Amnesia. In some cases an individual on antidepressants may find their memory clearly impaired. Subsequently, on discontinuing the drug, they may find it difficult to remember things that happened to them whilst they were on treatment.
- Auditory or visual hallucinations. These are more likely in the elderly but can happen to anyone. The biggest problem arises should the experience prompt someone to think that their illness must be getting worse because 'everyone knows voices are a sign of lunacy'.

CONFUSION OR DISORIENTATION

Also serious is the occurrence of confusion. This may be more obvious in older people but probably occurs in all age groups and is closely related to depersonalisation. In the case of depersonalisation, individuals ordinarily know that things are not quite right, yet are able to operate normally and appear to outsiders to be quite normal. One step further along this path lies confusion when it becomes obvious to others that something is not quite right. An affected subject may get to the stage of being disoriented and, as a consequence, quite agitated in a way that puts them at risk to themselves or to others.

Added to this is the fact that in rare instances, again especially in the elderly, TCAs and MAOIs can cause hallucinations. Combined with a confusional reaction, the occurrence of hallucinations may produce a picture of what looks like an almost full-blown insanity. The fact that it all clears up quickly once the drugs are stopped indicates that what is involved is a side effect of treatment rather than any change in the individual's mental balance.

SEXUAL SIDE EFFECTS

The sexual side effects of psychotropic medications are dealt with further in Section 8, but they are included here as impairments of sexual functioning are all too liable to be interpreted by depressed individuals as personal failings, providing further evidence of their inadequacy.

In men, antidepressants may cause difficulties in sustaining an erection, in ejaculating or with libido. In women, they may cause anorgasmia and loss of libido. Estimates have been creeping up recently, with suggestions that up to 50% of those on TCAs or MAOIs and closer to 90% of those on SSRIs have notable effects. The distress that this causes almost certainly leads some people to discontinue treatment, although delayed ejaculation can be helpful for men.

There is a further unusual effect on ejaculation, which is retrograde ejaculation. In this case, owing to altered sphincter tone, the seminal fluid passes backwards into the bladder on ejaculation rather than forwards in the usual manner. This effect may only be noticed later when the affected person notices that their urine is more cloudy than usual.

When SSRIs are taken to alleviate obsessional symptoms, many appear happy with the trade-off between an easing of their symptoms and changes in their sexual functioning, which can be managed by, for example, weekend breaks from treatment.

A delay in orgasm/ejaculation is the most immediately obvious effect. This may progress to difficulties with sustaining or having an erection with time or with increases in dose. These effects were described soon after the antidepressants were introduced. The effect of treatment on libido was for years less obvious as a reduction in libido is a common feature of severe depression. More recently, as these drugs have been used for longer periods, it has become clear that antidepressants can reduce libido.

It is now clear that treatment can have persistent effects on libido and sexual functioning. These persistent effects came into view in subjects who stopped treatment but were left with difficulties – persistent SSRI-induced sexual dysfunction (PSSD). Like tardive dyskinesia, this is a problem that can start on treatment when the taker may continue with treatment after misleading reassurances that the problem will resolve when treatment stops.[24,25] The frequency with which treatment leads to PSSD is unknown. It may happen to both men and women. The syndrome involves various combinations of lack of libido, anorgasmia and genital anaesthesia that may last for years after treatment stops. There are no good figures for how long PSSD is likely to last, nor for the proportion of those affected that make full recoveries. At present, there are no known cures. The issues are of particular concern in the case of prepubertal children or adolescents put on antidepressants as the effects of treatment in this case are simply unknown.

The reverse effects can also happen – persistent genital arousal disorder (PGAD) – and on withdrawal men and women can be left with premature ejaculation/orgasm.

Another side effect, primarily linked to trazodone, is priapism: sustained erection of the penis. If mild, this may be a welcome development, but in some cases the erection produced may be so full as to be painful or may be so sustained (12–24 hours) that it causes permanent damage to the tissues of the penis. Surgical relief is required if the condition is sustained beyond 12 hours. Trazodone may also enhance libido.

All antidepressants can cause a failure of orgasm in women in exactly the same way as they inhibit ejaculation in men. There is no reason to believe that it occurs any less frequently in women than in men. All can reduce libido in women, whilst trazodone is as likely to increase it in women as in men. PSSD in all likelihood occurs in women as often as in men.

Other possible changes involve disturbances to:

- the frequency and/or intensity of periods;
- changes in breast size and/or tenderness.

EMOTIONAL BLUNTING

There are good grounds for arguing that the SSRIs are primarily serenics or tranquilisers – drugs that produce an anxiolytic effect. They make individuals less reactive to triggers from the environment. When this effect kicks in, the individual feels more mellow, docile or sanguine. In many cases, however, either too much of this effect is produced or the effect is not appreciated by the taker, with complaints that the treatment is making them emotionally dead or emotionally blunted. This can be noticed in people who have failed to respond to treatment who report that they still cannot eat or sleep, but that they have at least stopped crying. In people who have recovered, it is common to hear complaints that everything would be great if they could only cry at sad movies or songs.

In some cases a lack of feeling may produce disinhibited behaviour. The disinhibition may even be extreme, being described as resembling the effects of a chemical lobotomy.[26,27] This disinhibition is probably what underpins many cases of apparent manic reactions on SSRIs, which clear up on discontinuation of treatment in a way that would not ordinarily happen with proper mania. Manic or psychotic reactions to antidepressants are now in fact one of the commonest causes of admission to a psychiatric unit.[28]

These effects seem to be dose dependent. In general a lower dose will reduce the level of emotional blunting to something more manageable and will make disinhibited or psychotic reactions less likely.

MANIC OR PSYCHOTIC REACTIONS

Intuitively it would seem that drugs that elevate mood could go too far and precipitate someone into a manic state. However, electroconvulsive therapy (ECT) and lithium are both antidepressants and at the same time are anti-manic. Maybe antidepressants could also stabilise moods? In some sense this is what underpins their use for prophylactic purposes.

Quite apart from mania proper, another possibility is that antidepressants will disinhibit or induce an emotional dysregulation or lability that may be mistaken for mania, as outlined above. It is also important to distinguish between a manic episode proper and the hyperactivity that may stem from mild confusion or a stimulant effect. If such reactions clear up quickly on discontinuing treatment, an adverse response to drug treatment should be considered.

Many antidepressants increase the availability of serotonin at post-synaptic S2 receptors and by stimulating this receptor can produce an LSD-like effect. In certain susceptible individuals, this mechanism may underpin a decompensation into psychosis. Whatever the mechanisms, manic and psychotic reactions have been noted in the trials of all SSRIs.

RESTLESSNESS, AGITATION AND TURMOIL: AKATHISIA

This side effect, common with antipsychotics, was once thought to be uncommon with antidepressants but is now widely recognised (see Antidepressants and Suicide below). It may occur within hours of starting treatment or take weeks to appear.

It is traditional to translate akathisia into the lay term 'restlessness', but this does not begin to convey all that may be involved. The first descriptions of this problem were in people taking reserpine for blood pressure problems. This led to quotes such as: 'increased tenseness, restlessness, insomnia and a feeling of being very uncomfortable', 'the first few doses frequently made them anxious and apprehensive ... they reported increased feelings of strangeness, verbalized by statements such as "I don't feel like myself" ... or "I'm afraid of some of the unusual impulses that I have"'. Or on 'the first day of treatment [he] reacted with marked anxiety and weeping and on the second day felt so terrible with such marked panic at night that the medication was cancelled'.[29] These quotes make it clear that a word such as turmoil is a better description of what is involved than restlessness.

This kind of turmoil seems most liable to happen in subjects who are anxious or agitated to begin with. It is particularly marked when antidepressants are given to patients who have panic disorder. Such patients may be made much worse if put immediately on a 75 mg dose of a TCA or a 20 mg dose of an SSRI. In the case of highly anxious patients, it seems better to start with a lower dose and to increase the dose slowly.

In addition to inner turmoil, this state may manifest itself on the outside as apparent tension rather than restlessness. The critical point is the person on the medication says is happening. Akathisia is an emotional state. Abnormal restless movements happening outside the subject's control are called dyskinesias rather than akathisia. The difference between akathisia and dyskinesia is that akathisia comes with a clear sense of turmoil or tension, whereas dyskinesia does not.[30,31]

ANTIDEPRESSANTS AND SUICIDE

Depression brings with it a risk of suicide. It has been widely noted that one of the times people are most likely to attempt to kill themselves has been around 10–14 days after starting antidepressant treatment. The rationale sometimes given for this is that depression causes both a slowing up (psychomotor retardation) of the affected individual and suicidal ideation. It has been claimed antidepressants clear up the retardation before they have reduced suicidal thoughts, leaving individuals with the drive and energy to effect their own demise in a way that was not possible when they were retarded. This paradoxical 'rollback' reaction was first described with ECT treatment, which was commonly given to severely retarded patients. Antidepressants are for the most part not given to such patients, and from the late 1950s clinicians described patients becoming unexpectedly agitated and suicidal on treatment in a manner they distinguished from the rollback phenomenon. It now seems likely that treatment-induced restlessness, tension, psychosis or dissociative reactions can trigger suicide attempts in that even healthy volunteers put on antidepressants can become suicidal.

In the case of depressed patients, it might be argued that subjects on antidepressants who find themselves feeling depersonalised or in turmoil sometimes reason that what is happening is that their nerves are getting worse. As this happens despite being on treatment, they conclude that they are incurable and that there is no option other than suicide. This is particularly likely to be the case in instances where the turmoil is intense. Impairments of sexual functioning of one sort or another are a further side effect that could conceivably produce a similar outcome.[32,33] However, the idea that people commit suicide just because they misinterpret changes caused by treatment does not readily account for healthy individuals becoming suicidal on SSRIs.[34]

The SSRIs and other newer agents are clearly safer in overdose than the older tricyclic compounds, and this initially led to hopes that their use might be associated with a lower incidence of successful suicide. However, clinical trials have now consistently shown that SSRIs produce a doubling of rate of suicides and suicidal acts in both depressed and anxious patients compared to placebo.[35,36] Older antidepressants cause suicidality also, but as they are more likely to be given in hospital under supervision, the risks may in fact be less than with SSRIs.[37,38]

SENSORY NEUROPATHY

It is becoming clearer that almost all psychotropic drugs can cause peripheral neuropathies. The classic symptom of this is burning feet (causalgia). Hands, mouths and other parts of the body can burn also or just be painful. Other features include a variety of bizarre sensations around the body or sensations of pain on temperature change or gentle touch. The paradox is that these drugs can also relieve pain. The worry is that they can end up treating conditions like the ones they were given for in the first instance.

Linked disturbances include tinnitus, visual disturbances like visual snow, altered taste perception and temperature dysregulation

SEROTONIN SYNDROME

Antidepressants, and in particular the SSRIs, may produce a picture that has similarities to the neuroleptic malignant syndrome (NMS) described in Chapter 3. This serotonin syndrome leads to a group of side effects, which all appear to stem from an excess of serotonin.[39–41] The occurrence of any one of these side effects on their own is not a cause for alarm; it is their conjunction that constitutes the serotonin syndrome.

The commonest feature of the syndrome is myoclonus (jerks and twitches), which occurs in up to 40% of cases. Tremors of the tongue or fingers occur in 25%, as do shivering and sweating. Up to 20% of subjects may become confused, agitated or restless. In 15% there may be evidence of hyperreflexia and in 10% diarrhoea. Little is known of the subjective nature of the state at present.

At least three of these symptoms should be present before making a diagnosis. Unlike NMS, this condition often simply responds to halting treatment and clears up without anything specific being done. However, the condition may also require hospitalisation, and fatalities have been suspected. It is not clear how often the condition actually occurs.

As the name implies, it is thought that the disorder stems from an excess of serotonin. It probably first began to occur when individuals were put on a combination of MAOIs and serotonin reuptake inhibiting TCA, such as clomipramine. It appears to have become more common with the availability of SSRIs. The SSRIs alone may cause the problem but are more likely to do so if combining with other drugs that act on the serotonin system.

EFFECTS SPECIAL TO THE MAOIs

CHEESE EFFECT

The cheese effect refers to a dangerous increase in blood pressure following an intake of cheese in people taking MAOIs. Cheese contains a substance called tyramine. This is normally broken down in the gut by monoamine oxidase (MAO) so that it does not get into the body. The MAOIs prevent this breakdown, and hence tyramine enters the body and leads to increases in blood pressure. The signs of the problem are headaches, neck stiffness, perspiration, flushing or vomiting. As increased blood pressure can cause a stroke, there is concern.

This means that anyone on an MAOI needs to avoid tyramine-containing foods, including all cheeses and dishes such as pizza, or pasta dishes with parmesan cheese on them.

These drugs come with lists of foods that contain tyramine and need to be avoided. Almost all wines and beers contain some tyramine. For the most part, except for some cheeses, pickled herrings, caviar and sausages, the amounts of tyramine in the foods typically listed are minimal. However, all tyramine-containing foods are usually held to be unsafe, and the effect of avoiding all such foods is a considerable interference with normal living.

There is no need for anyone to rush to hospital if they are on an MAOI and suddenly realise they have been having cheese and wine. Unless there is a clear onset of a headache or temperature or a stiffness of the neck, the odds are that there will be no harmful effect.

Moclobemide is a reversible inhibitor of MAO and is relatively free of the cheese effect. As a result, even cheese and wine in normal quantities can be taken safely – it would take extraordinary quantities to cause a problem.

User issues

Special conditions

Pregnancy

All serotonin reuptake inhibiting drugs (SSRIs, many TCAs and some antihistamines) risk causing birth defects and developmental delay in later life. They also increase rates of miscarriage. If pregnancy is contemplated, or if there is no clear need to continue with treatment, it may be wiser to stop, as there can be a real problem stopping if treatment is continued longer than necessary.

It is now clear that the SSRIs can cause heart defects in newborn infants and lung problems, such as pulmonary hypertension.[42–44] Premature birth and low birth weight are even more common effects – perhaps close to the norm on SSRIs.

There are claims that untreated depression can cause even bigger problems than treatment, and it is claimed that up to 20% of pregnant women are depressed. There is no evidence that depression causes problems or that 20% of women are depressed. The claim for 20% hinges on the fact that pregnant women may show sleep and appetite changes, as well as increased anxiety and irritability and lack of energy – they meet criteria for depression in other words. But meeting criteria and having depression are two different things and, in fact, few of the women labelled as depressed are likely to benefit from an antidepressant.

The claim for depression causing problems is that depression leads women to drink alcohol, take drugs and not look after themselves, but in fact there is better evidence that antidepressants increase alcohol and drug intake, cause diabetes and make the woman more likely to engage in risky behaviours.

A further problem with antidepressants in pregnancy is that after birth, infants may be precipitated into a withdrawal syndrome that could lead to convulsions amongst other things. The more general picture is one of restlessness, irritability and insomnia, lasting for a few days.

Both TCAs and MAOIs enter breast milk in small amounts but appear to be of little risk to babies being breastfed. Fluoxetine and citalopram are contraindicated in breastfeeding, and both paroxetine and sertraline come with warnings. SSRIs pose a risk of withdrawal if absorbed through breast milk.

Cardiac conditions

For all of us, TCA and SSRI antidepressants can be shown to have demonstrable effects on the electrical conduction of the heart, especially the QT interval. These effects can become a problem if the dose is increased, in those who have congenitally longer QT intervals, or when a person is put on a

Continued

User issues—cont'd

combination of drugs where each drug increases the QT interval to some extent leading to a dangerous increase. Pretty well all psychotropic drugs can cause some increase, so combinations of these drugs or their use with antibiotics is risky. There can be problems also in the elderly and in people with metabolic disorders such as young women with an eating disorder – where use of an SSRI to treat the problem could lead to a fatal arrhythmia.[45]

In anyone who has recently had a heart attack, has angina or another disturbances of cardiac rhythmicity, the effects of antidepressants are unpredictable, and extra care is needed.

Epilepsy

Owing to their effects on electrical conductivity, the tricyclic and MAOI antidepressants alter electrical thresholds. In the case of epilepsy this can actually be beneficial and make the occurrence of an epileptic fit less likely.

However, there can be a problem when the drugs are halted. The changing electrical thresholds that occur at this point in time may trigger a seizure. As halting can be accidental, as, for example, forgetting to take the drugs one night, this issue may be a problem for subjects with epilepsy. The SSRIs seem to be relatively free of this complicating factor.

Overdoses

Unlike benzodiazepines, antipsychotics and SSRIs, TCAs can be fatal in overdosage. Overdoses with a relatively modest amount of these pills can kill. Death is by interference with cardiac conduction, causing the heart to beat irregularly or to stop, or by causing convulsions.

Driving

With the development of the less-sedative SSRIs concern began to be noted about the possible behavioural toxicity of older antidepressants and, in particular, their possible role in causing road traffic accidents.[46] The risks associated with taking the older compounds have not yet been established. The risks posed by antidepressants in general are less than those posed by benzodiazepines and by antipsychotics, except in so far as SSRIs in particular can lead to increased cravings for alcohol and can increase blood alcohol levels.

Having made these points, individuals on a cocktail of drugs, those who are clearly sedated by their drugs or those who have just started a drug regimen should probably not drive without assessing responsibly whether their performance is affected. This applies particularly to the driver of heavy goods vehicles or coaches or other passenger-carrying vehicles. Whilst the legal responsibility to issue such warnings may strictly lie with the medical prescriber, in practice those who may be best placed to judge the extent of any risks, apart from the patient, may be friends, relatives or keyworkers.

Fractures

Whilst the SSRIs looked at one point as though they might be helpful in older subjects because they were less likely to cause postural hypotension and people were therefore less likely to fall over, it now seems as though the SSRIs can contribute to osteoporosis, and they are in fact associated with a higher incidence of fractures than older drugs.[47] Some of the older drugs, which also act in the same way on the serotonin system, may be as likely to produce this

User issues—cont'd

problem, but the TCAs were never used to the extent that a problem like this could be detected.

Haemorrhage
There is much more serotonin in the blood and gut than in the brain, and a further problem linked to SSRIs is that they increase the risk of bleeding. Bleeding on antidepressants has been reported regularly since the 1980s. It may be into the gut, into the womb or into the brain, in the form of a stroke. Aspirin and some other non-steroidal analgesics can also increase bleeding times, and the combination of these with an SSRI can increase the risk of a bleeding event six-fold.[48]

Alcohol
SSRIs can cause an intense craving for alcohol. This is not usually present from the first dose but develops over some weeks or months. The problem can escalate into full-blown alcoholism. Few people realise this can happen, and as a result doctors will usually try to keep the person on their antidepressant in the belief that treating an underlying depression can only be a good thing when in fact stopping the antidepressant can clear the problem up within days.[49]

SSRIs also appear in some people to raise blood alcohol levels in ways that are not at present understood so the person may be more drunk than they expect.

INTERACTIONS

Important interactions between antidepressants and other drugs are outlined in Box 5.1.

BOX 5.1 Antidepressants and drug interactions

- Barbiturates, benzodiazepines, alcohol and antipsychotics may all increase the sedative effects of antidepressants.
- Barbiturates, steroid hormones and oral contraceptives may all lower the plasma levels of antidepressants.
- Combinations of antidepressants and antipsychotics may increase the risk of antipsychotic-type side effects.
- MAOIs may react badly with a number of other drugs. These include cough medicines, pain relievers and cold cures, particularly those containing ephedrine, pethidine and anaesthetics. Anaesthetists should be informed before surgery – even dental surgery.
- MAOIs appear to enhance the effects of insulin and oral hypoglycaemic drugs. This may require either a change of antidepressant or a reduction in the dose of insulin or of the hypoglycaemic agent.
- SSRIs (and possibly a number of TCAs) interact with aspirin and other drugs that increase bleeding times to increase the risk substantially of bleeding into the gut, womb or brain.

REFERENCES

1. Horwitz AV, Wakefield JC. The loss of sadness. How psychiatry transformed normal sorrow into depressive disorder. Oxford University Press; 2007.
2. Healy D. The antidepressant era. Cambridge, MA: Harvard University Press; 1998.
3. Healy D. Let them eat Prozac. New York: New York University Press; 2004.
4. Beaumont G. The place of clomipramine in psychopharmacology. J Psychopharmacol 1993;7:383–93.
5. Healy D. The marketing of 5HT: depression or anxiety? Br J Psychiatry 1991;158:737–42.
6. Atigari O, Healy D. Ketamine and treatment resistant mood disorders. Aust N Z J Psychiatry 2013;47:998–1001.
7. Shorter E, Healy D. Shock Therapy. A history of electroconvulsive therapy in mental illness. New Brunswick: Rutgers University Press; 2007.
8. Styron W. Darkness visible. London: Jonathan Cape; 1991.
9. Wolpert L. Malignant sadness. London: Faber and Faber; 2000.
10. Beck AT. Cognitive therapy and the emotional disorders. New York: International Universities Press; 1976.
11. Klerman GL, Weissman MM, Rounsaville B, et al. Interpersonal therapy of depression. New York: Basic Books; 1984.
12. Blacker R, Clare A. Depressive disorder in primary care. Br J Psychiatry 1987;150:737–51.
13. Kessler RC, Berglund P, Demler O, et al. The epidemiology of major depressive disorder: results from the national comorbidity survey replication (NCS-R). JAMA 2003;289:3095–105.
14. Spijker J, de Graaf R, Bijl RV, et al. Duration of major depressive episodes in the general population: results from the Netherlands mental health survey and incidence study (NEMESIS). Br J Psychiatry 2002;181:208–12.
15. Stone M, Jones L. Clinical review: relationship between antidepressant drugs and adult suicidality. p 31, <http://www.fda.gov/ohrms/dockets/ac/06/briefing/2006-4272b1-index.htm>; 2006.
16. Tranter R, Healy H, Cattell D, et al. Functional variations in agents differentially selective to monoaminergic systems. Psychol Med 2002;32:517–24.
17. Frasure-Smith N, Lesperance F, Talajic M. Depression following myocardial infarction: impact on 6-month survival. JAMA 1993;270:1819–25.
18. Gold I, Ollin L. From Descartes to desipramine: psychopharmacology and the self. Transcult Psychiatry 2009;46:38–59.
19. Glenmullen J. Prozac backlash. New York: Simon and Schuster; 2000.
20. Glenmullen J. Coming off antidepressants. London: Constable and Robinson; 2006.
21. Rosenbaum JF, Fava M, Hoog SL, et al. Selective serotonin reuptake inhibitor discontinuation syndrome: a randomised clinical study. Biol Psychiatry 1998;44:77–87.
22. Baldessarini RJ, Ghaemi SN, Viguera AC. Tolerance in antidepressant treatment. Psychother Psychosom 2002;71:177–9.
23. Beddoe R. Dying for a cure. A memoir of antidepressants, misdiagnosis and madness. Sydney: Random House; 2007.
24. Csoka A, Shipko S. Persistent sexual side effects after SSRI discontinuation. Psychother Psychosom 2006;75:187–8.
25. Hogan C, Le Noury J, Healy D, et al. One hundred and twenty cases of enduring sexual dysfunction following treatment. Int J Risk Saf Med 2014;26:109–16.
26. Garland EJ, Baerg EA. A motivational syndrome associated with selective serotonin reuptake inhibitors in children and adolescents. J Child Adolesc Psychopharmacol 2001;11:181–6.
27. Hoehn-Saric R, Lipsey JR, McLeod DR. Apathy and indifference in patients on fluvoxamine and fluoxetine. J Clin Psychopharmacol 1990;10:343–5.
28. Preda A, MacLean RW, Mazure CM, et al. Antidepressant associated mania and psychosis resulting in psychiatric admission. J Clin Psychiatry 2001;62:30–3.
29. Healy D, Savage M. Reserpine exhumed. Br J Psychiatry 1998;172:376–8.

30. Cunningham-Owens DG. A guide to the extrapyramidal side-effects of antipsychotic drugs. Cambridge: Cambridge University Press; 1999.
31. Sachdev P. Akathisia. Cambridge: Cambridge University Press; 1996.
32. Creaney W, Murray I, Healy D. Antidepressant induced suicidal ideation. Hum Psychopharmacol 1991;6:329–32.
33. Healy D. The fluoxetine and suicide controversy. CNS Drugs 1994;1:223–31.
34. Healy D. Antidepressant induced suicidality. Prim Care Psychiatry 2000;6:23–8.
35. Healy D, Whitaker CJ. Antidepressants and suicide: risk–benefit conundrums. J Psychiatry Neurosci 2003;28:331–9.
36. Fergusson D, Doucette S, Cranley-Glass K, et al. The association between suicide attempts and SSRIs: a systematic review of 677 randomized controlled trials representing 85,470 participants. BMJ 2005;330:396–9.
37. Jick S, Dean AD, Jick H. Antidepressants and suicide. BMJ 1995;310:215–18.
38. Donovan S, Clayton A, Beeharry M, et al. Deliberate self-harm and antidepressant drugs. Investigation of a possible link. Br J Psychiatry 2000;177:551–6.
39. Dunkley EJ, Isbister GK, Sibbritt D, et al. The Hunter serotonin toxicity criteria. Q J Med 2003;96:635–42.
40. Lejoyeux M, Ades J, Rouillon F. Serotonin syndrome: incidence, symptoms and treatment. CNS Drugs 1994;2:132–46.
41. Sternbach H. The serotonin syndrome. Am J Psychiatry 1991;148:705–13.
42. Louik C, Lin AE, Werler MM, et al. First trimester use of selective serotonin reuptake inhibitors and risk of birth defects. New Engl J Med 2007;356:2675–83.
43. Healy D, Mangin D, Mintzes B. The ethics of randomized placebo controlled trials of antidepressants with pregnant women. Int J Risk Saf Med 2010;22:7–16.
44. Bérard A, Levin M, Sadler T, et al. SSRI use during pregnancy and major malformations: The importance of serotonin for embryonic development and the effect of serotonin inhibition on the occurrence of malformations. Reprod Toxicol 2015;in press.
45. Healy D, Howe G, Mangin D. Sudden cardiac death and the reverse dodo Verdict. Int J Risk Saf Med 2014;26:71–9.
46. O'Hanlon JF. Minimising the risk of traffic accidents due to psychoactive drugs. Prim Care Psychiatry 1995;1:77–85.
47. Richards JB, Papaiannou A, Adcock JD, et al. Effect of selective serotonin reuptake inhibitors on the risk of fracture. Arch Intern Med 2007;167:188–94.
48. Loke YK, Trivedi AN, Singh S. Meta-analysis of gastrointestinal bleeds due to interaction between selective serotonin uptake inhibitors and non-steroidal anti-inflammatory drugs. Aliment Pharmacol Ther 2008;27:31–40.
49. Brookwell L, Hogan C, Mangin D, et al. One hundred cases of alcoholism triggered by serotonin reuptake inhibitor intake. Int J Risk Saf Med 2014;26:99–107.

SECTION 3
MANAGEMENT OF BIPOLAR DISORDERS

SECTION CONTENTS

Management of acute bipolar disorder

6

CHAPTER CONTENTS

INTRODUCTION

In 1854, Jean-Pierre Falret and Jules Baillarger independently described a bipolar disorder in which affected individuals cycled between periods of elation or mania and depression. This was variously called *folie circulaire* or *folie de deux périodes*. It forms the basis for what later became manic-depressive disorder and is now often called bipolar disorder.[1,2] In 1896, Emil Kraepelin divided the major psychiatric illnesses into manic-depressive illness and schizophrenia. The former was primarily a disorder of mood, the latter a disturbance of cognitive functions. Manic-depressive illness usually followed an episodic course with individuals recovering to normal between episodes. Schizophrenia was more likely to become a chronic illness, with a majority of individuals never fully recovering. These distinctions held through to the mid-1990s when a number of pharmaceutical companies began to promote mood-stabilisers for bipolar disorder.[1]

Within the manic-depressive group, Kraepelin included all severe mood disorders, whether or not the person oscillated between manic and depressive poles. For this reason, until the *Diagnostic and Statistical Manual of Mental Disorders*, Third Edition (DSM III) in 1980 many individuals who only had recurrent severe depressions were diagnosed as having manic-depressive illness. But since 1980 there has been an increasing tendency to distinguish between bipolar and unipolar mood disorders. In bipolar mood disorders, individuals present with episodes of both mania and depression, in contrast to unipolar disorders in which there appears to be only depressive episodes. Unipolar mania is rare.

Until recently manic-depressive illness was a rare disorder – much less common than schizophrenia or depression. But now there are estimates that up to 5% of the population are bipolar. How did this happen?

Nothing distinguishes bipolar from unipolar disorders other than episodes of mania. When they are depressed, both groups look indistinguishable, both respond to the same treatments, and there are no biological markers that pick out one group from the other.

It's hard to know therefore whether a condition is a true unipolar disorder or a bipolar disorder that has hitherto presented only with depressive episodes. There are claims that between one-third and one-half of depressions are associated with an episode of mania at some point in a lifetime. The difficulties in being precise lie in depending on either the patient or their family or doctors for an accurate history of either manic or depressive episodes. The patient's partner, parents or children may have a more accurate view than the patient of serious or sustained periods of overactivity and disinhibition, and this can lead to a retrospective diagnosis of hypomania. But doctors who are committed to bipolar diagnoses will sometimes inappropriately diagnose mania on the basis of overactivity or bonhomie lasting no more than a few hours.

Distinctions are now also drawn between bipolar 1 disorders, where an individual has been hospitalised or severely incapacitated by a manic episode at some point, and bipolar 2 disorders, where there is a history suggestive of a period of elation, but the person may never have been admitted to hospital. There is also talk of bipolar 3, 4, 5 and 6 as well as bipolar spectrum disorders. These bipolar lite disorders make it possible to diagnose almost anyone as bipolar leading to claims that up to 5% of the population may have a bipolar disorder.

We are in the midst of a mania for bipolar disorder, driven by the fact that the antidepressants went off patent and to sell drugs companies have helped convert cases of depression into cases of bipolar disorder, cases of Prozac into cases of Depakote or Zyprexa.

Whether the patient has an old-style manic-depressive illness or one of the newer fashionable bipolar illnesses, treatment is increasingly likely to be with so-called mood-stabilisers rather than antidepressants. This chapter deals with drugs used to treat mania, now typically called mood-stabilisers. The issue of 'mood stabilisation' is picked up in Chapter 7.

Whilst the majority of people with mania present with an elated and euphoric mood or with disinhibited behaviour, not all do. Others may be irritable rather than elated and euphoric and paranoid rather than grandiose. Common to both groups is an increased level of activity so that hyperactivity is perhaps the most consistent diagnostic feature of mania. In addition, there is typically an increase in appetites and a decrease in time spent asleep.

In the case of a single manic episode, the US *Diagnostic and Statistical Manual* (DSM) requires a diagnosis of bipolar disorder. However, the

International Classification of Diseases (ICD) does not. Acute and transient manic episodes show a great deal of overlap with the acute and transient psychoses (Chapter 2). They do not recur. Some of us can have years between manic episodes without any indication they have a recurrent bipolar disorder. It is also far from clear that patients who are ordinarily depressive but have a 'manic' reaction to an antidepressant should be regarded as bipolar.

For these reasons the treatment of mania and the possibility of mood stabilisation should be separated, but they rarely are. In the case of an episode of possible mania, there is a default towards putting patients on mood stabilisers to ward off future episodes of what is presumed to be a bipolar disorder. These supposedly prophylactic treatments probably all bring about withdrawal syndromes, and this clouds the interpretation of what they actually do. Given these factors, whilst the treatment of mania very commonly slides into prophylaxis, the attempt to ward off future episodes may do more harm than good.

LITHIUM FOR MANIA

Lithium is used both as a specific treatment for mania and as a mood-stabiliser in the prophylaxis (prevention) of further episodes of either mania or depression. The issues of lithium's dosage and side effects are covered in Chapter 7 on prophylaxis.

In terms of managing acute episodes, many claim lithium is the most specific treatment for mania, bringing about a cleaner resolution of manic episodes than does treatment with antipsychotic drugs. According to this view, patients will sometimes need to be controlled with antipsychotics for the first days in hospital but, if they are prescribed lithium also, the mania will resolve much more specifically and cleanly than it would on antipsychotics alone – usually somewhere around day 10 after therapeutic blood levels have been reached.[3]

There have been great disputes about whether lithium is prophylactic or not, but what is not in dispute is that it can produce responses in mania. This is sometimes lost sight of, and patients are treated with antipsychotics instead. The reasons for this probably lie in the fact that using lithium involves a physical screen of the patient beforehand, which takes some days. In addition, the effects of lithium are slower in onset than those of antipsychotics, and the use of lithium is usually seen as involving a commitment to ongoing therapy that the patient may not be able to make in the acute stage of a manic illness.

Whether lithium is more specific to mania than other drugs remains uncertain. In addition, it is worth considering exactly what lithium does that is beneficial in mania. It is clear that the sedative and anti-impulsive effects of anticonvulsants and antipsychotics (see Antipsychotics for mania and Anticonvulsants for mania below) might be useful. Lithium is much less sedative than these other drugs, making the responses to it look at times as though they are in some way a more specific treatment for mania than the responses obtained from non-specific sedation. However, it has anti-impulsive or anti-irritability effects that have been relatively poorly characterised to date.

This returns us to the theme of this book – what we might find out if we asked people taking the different drugs what their drug was doing for them that they found useful. At present, the idea that drugs are mood-stabilisers acts as barrier to questions and to thought. Such drugs are supposedly correcting some physiological tendency to mania and to mood instability, and asking whether they also do something useful is seen by some as close to irrelevant. When a first mood-stabiliser fails to work, the response then is to add further mood-stabilisers so that the treatment of mania and the prophylaxis of bipolar disorder can end up with the patient on five or six drugs with all the risks that come with polypharmacy.

ANTIPSYCHOTICS FOR MANIA

In practice antipsychotics are often the first line of treatment for mania. In part this stems from the often pressing need to contain the behaviour of individuals with mania, and antipsychotics in moderate to large doses do this relatively quickly. Some of the largest clinical doses of antipsychotics are used for just this purpose.

However, whilst obviously useful to gain control of the clinical picture, antipsychotics are often the only treatment given for an episode of mania. The resolution of mania on treatment can suggest that antipsychotics are specific treatments for mania. Because antipsychotics are helpful in manic states, it is then argued that mania must involve a disturbance of dopamine neurotransmission. But this argument is clearly circular.

An alternative is that antipsychotics are therapeutically useful in mania without being specifically therapeutic. Just as attempts to engage depressed individuals in programmes of motivated activity will often assist a cure, so conversely the demotivating and immobilising effects of antipsychotics could be expected to assist the resolution of a manic episode by 'taking the wind out of the sails' of affected individuals. Indeed, it can be argued that antipsychotics may play a similar role to that which light plays in the treatment of depression. Arguably, when light therapy works for depression, it does so by activating the sufferer. The opposite treatment for mania might involve putting someone in a darkened room to deactivate them. In practice, large doses of antipsychotics may have a somewhat similar effect.[3]

A fall-back position would be that antipsychotics simply contain manic behaviour non-specifically, by virtue of their chemical strait-jacketing effect, until the episode burns itself out. This issue is not without importance for a number of reasons. One is that antipsychotics may have serious long-term consequences (see Chapter 3). Another is that the long-term treatment of a recurrent bipolar disorder requires engaging patients in the management of their own condition. This is something they are likely to be less willing to do if they have been chemically coshed.

Chlorpromazine was discovered in 1952 because of its effects on mania. Whilst antipsychotics have been used to treat mania ever since, they have also been used to 'stabilise' the person in between episodes with chlorpromazine being advertised as a stabiliser from the mid-1950s. The second-generation antipsychotics have introduced a new dimension to the issue. Clozapine, quetiapine and olanzapine are tricyclic agents from a class of drugs, many of which are antidepressant. When clozapine emerged in the late 1980s and seemed to raise some patients from the dead, some argued that many of the 'schizophrenic' patients who did best on it were schizoaffective or even had mood disorders misdiagnosed as schizophrenia.

The success of clozapine with this kind of patient and the obvious marketing opportunities that mania offered led the companies to undertake trials in mania for olanzapine, quetiapine and risperidone. In practice it is all but impossible for drugs of this type not to show some benefit in mania. Sedation will produce a rating scale benefit. But having received a licence for mania, the companies have moved on to claim their drugs are mood-stabilisers, a term that suggests these drugs will ward off future episodes of the disorder. There is no convincing evidence that this is the case. The reason older antipsychotics do not have clinical trial data to show some benefit in mania lies in the fact that until recently this condition was thought to be so rare that not enough people could be found for a trial. Furthermore, the patients were so ill that it would be unethical to recruit them to trials. The patients recruited to more recent antipsychotic trials have been much less severely ill.

The use of any antipsychotics, new or old, in the longer term for any patients who do not need them is problematic in that these agents have been linked to a high rate of suicidal acts, possibly because they cause akathisia, and there is increasing evidence of a general increased risk of premature mortality on antipsychotics (see Chapter 3).

ANTICONVULSANTS FOR MANIA

Whilst the antipsychotics have now become the front-line treatment for mania, anticonvulsants are also regularly used. Evidence that the anticonvulsants carbamazepine and valproate were useful in mania lead to the hypothesis that all anticonvulsants could help in mood disorders in just the same way that they help in epilepsy – by blocking kindling, that is the propensity of one fit to lead to the next. This idea implies that the anticonvulsants will be prophylactic for mood disorders but not that they will necessarily be any good for a manic episode.

CARBAMAZEPINE

Carbamazepine (Tegretol, Teril) came into widespread use for epileptic disorders, and in particular for temporal lobe epilepsy, in the 1960s. Compared with the barbiturates, which were then the first line of treatment, it was safer in overdose and not apparently addictive. In the late 1960s Japanese psychiatrists noticed that patients being treated with carbamazepine showed a lightening in their personalities that suggested some effect on mood. It was also noticed that patients with mood disorders given the sedative carbamazepine along with antipsychotics did well. This led to a series of trials confirming its usefulness in bipolar disorders.[4]

Carbamazepine is sedative, and as such just like the antipsychotics might be expected to be beneficial in mania. Combined with antipsychotics, its sedative effects may be particularly helpful. It is also used in lieu of lithium for mania and bipolar disorders characterised by dysphoria (irritability and paranoia) rather than elation, and it has some use in rapidly cycling affective disorders whereas lithium seems to trigger rapid cycling in some patients.

Carbamazepine is also used for a number of other purposes. It is used as a first line of treatment for trigeminal neuralgia, and for what is termed episodic dyscontrol syndrome. This term refers to outbursts of behaviour that appear to occur for no obvious reason. It has been argued that such outbursts in some cases may be epileptic without the normal convulsions rather than just temper tantrums. It seems more likely that carbamazepine is useful in such cases because of a more general anti-irritability action. Lithium also has an anti-irritability effect, but the similarities or differences between the two drugs in this respect have not been explored. In general those who do well with lithium seem to be a slightly different group to those who do well on carbamazepine, and we are no wiser as to why this might be the case.

SODIUM VALPROATE

Sodium valproate (Epilim) was also first used for epilepsy, and its use there led on to its use for mania. A recent re-formulation, semi-sodium valproate (Depakote), is marketed heavily for mood disorders. There no reason to think that sodium and semi-sodium valproate differ in any meaningful way. Both break down in the body to valproic acid, which is the therapeutic agent.[5] In the US, where valproate has been marketed particularly heavily as a mood-stabiliser, it has replaced both lithium and carbamazepine.[1]

Valproate is used for acute episodes of mania and can be expected to be useful if only because it's sedative. Its use in epilepsy however also suggested that it has some anti-impulsive effects and that it might be in some way 'personality strengthening'. Again these effects are unexplored, as if valproate is correcting some physiological abnormality such as kindling then such effects are irrelevant. There are suggestions that, as with carbamazepine, episodes of mania characterised by dysphoria and irritability rather than euphoria may respond better to valproate.

The use of valproate and other anticonvulsants is linked to what is a marketing concept – the notion of a mood-stabiliser. Valproate and carbamazepine gave rise to this concept, and their use and the use of other anticonvulsants now for mania is based on the loose idea that all anticonvulsants must in some way be mood-stabilisers, which as we will see is not right.

LAMOTRIGINE, GABAPENTIN AND OXCARBAZEPINE

Based on the effectiveness of valproate and carbamazepine, other anticonvulsants have been tried in both mania and for the prophylaxis of bipolar disorders.

Amongst these have been lamotrigine (Lamictal), which in contrast to the others is much less sedative and is of no use in mania. It may be somewhat more effective for depression, with a number of trials pointing this way but a large number of unpublished negative studies.[6] Its benefits in depression may stem from a sense of well-being it produces rather than the sedation the others produce. This is dealt with in greater detail in Chapter 7. Lamotrigine needs a slow titration upwards of its dose, which makes it unsuitable for front-line use for mania.

As with lamotrigine, the anticonvulsant gabapentin (Neurontin) came into use in bipolar disorders on the back of the mood-stabiliser concept. It has never appeared to be a stand-alone treatment for mania. Its role has become caught up in legal actions over the extent to which its makers Warner-Lambert promoted its use off-label in a series of ghost-written articles. What appeared to be vigorous off-label promotion came without good clinical trial evidence for benefits, and as a result gabapentin has fallen into disfavour. Gabapentin's benefits, if present, are likely to stem from a combination of anxiolytic and sedative effects.

Oxcarbazepine (Trileptal) is an anticonvulsant derivative of carbamazepine that has also been used as a mood-stabiliser. It is not used much in the front-line treatment of mania. There is little reason to think it differs from carbamazepine.

TOPIRAMATE AND VIGABATRIN

Topiramate (Topamax) and vigabatrin (Sabril) are two other anticonvulsants that in recent years have been tried in the management of mania and for the prophylaxis of recurrent mood disorders. At present, the data suggest a significant burden of side effects, including sleep disturbances, slurred speech, discoordination and impairment of concentration and memory, along with other problems in the case of topiramate, and disinhibition or emotional dysregulation and possible psychotic decompensation in the case of vigabatrin. These drugs have not found a place in the regular treatment of bipolar disorders and have little or no place in the management of either the manic or depressive poles of a bipolar disorder. The evidence from these two drugs suggests that a simple anticonvulsant action per se does not mean that a drug will be mood stabilising. If an anticonvulsant is helpful, it must therefore be doing something other than being anticonvulsant.[4]

ACETAZOLAMIDE

This anticonvulsant inhibits an enzyme called carbonic anhydrase. It is rarely used, and there have only been a few reports claiming that it may be useful. In particular, however, these reports have claimed that acetazolamide is of some use for the kind of dreamy confusional or cycloid psychoses that may occur postpartum or perimenstrually.

The possible benefit of acetazolamide was something of an oddity until the development of topiramate and zonisamide, which also inhibit carbonic anhydrase amongst other things (Chapter 7)

ELECTROCONVULSIVE THERAPY (ECT)

There has also been a tradition that ECT is both antimanic and antidepressant. In the case of mania, there are very few manic episodes that fail to respond to either lithium or antipsychotics and, accordingly, for a long time there was no satisfactory research evidence that ECT was specifically beneficial in mania. The rationale for using it, until recently, stemmed from the fact it was used widely in the era before lithium and antipsychotics were introduced and was noted to be useful. In recent years this situation has been remedied. It is now clear that ECT is as specific and as effective as lithium in the treatment of mania.[7,8]

There may be an independent effect of ECT on mania, but there is another aspect of the problem that should be noted. There is another bipolar disorder that exists in overactive and underactive forms: catatonia.[9] Up to 15% of patients with rapidly cycling or mixed affective states or dysphoric mania may, in addition to mania, have catatonic signs. ECT is the most effective treatment for catatonia. In cases that do not respond readily to lithium or antipsychotics, ECT may be an option for this reason.

BENZODIAZEPINES

In part, perhaps because the prevalence of catatonic features is so high in mood disorders, benzodiazepines such as clonazepam and lorazepam are used widely in the management of manic states in North America. As a first line of treatment for catatonia, benzodiazepines and barbiturates bring about a response in 60% of cases. The use of these drugs may therefore make sense in the early stages of the treatment of mania and may have arisen in North America because of perceptions of benefit stemming from this source.[9] Benzodiazepines are used much less explicitly for bipolar disorders outside of North America, other than as part of rapid tranquillisation protocols.

In fact, benzodiazepines are as anticonvulsant as any other anticonvulsant, and the first use of the term mood-stabiliser was for a benzodiazepine-like tranquilliser. Unlike other anticonvulsants, the benzodiazepines are the treatment of choice for an acutely convulsing patient. A good case can be made that there is little more to mood stabilisation than whatever it is benzodiazepines do.

DO ANTIDEPRESSANTS CAUSE MANIA?

There is a belief that antidepressants cause mania. It seems intuitively obvious that this should be the case. However, against this intuition is the fact that lithium, ECT, carbamazepine and many antipsychotics are in some sense both antidepressant and antimanic. Based on this, one might wonder whether all antidepressants might not also be antimanic. At present the only studies of tricyclic antidepressants given in mania suggest that they too may be antimanic.[10] Why, then, is there a belief that antidepressants cause mania?

The belief appears to arise partly because all mental-health professionals have seen people taking antidepressants become elated. However, there has always been a natural incidence of manic episodes following episodes of depression, even before the availability of the antidepressants or ECT. The opposite also appears to be true in that some people recovering from mania appear to become depressed. Many manic patients treated with antipsychotics appear to become depressed, but there is good clinical trial evidence that most antipsychotics can also be used to treat many cases of depression. Ordinarily such swings into mania and swings into depression tend to be relatively short lived and mild.

The effects of ECT and antidepressants in mood disorders appear to be to abort what might be lengthy depressive episodes much more rapidly than would otherwise have been the case. This may lead to the occurrence of a manic swing earlier than would have happened. Such swings occur even on ECT or lithium, which are effective antimanic treatments.[11]

However, when people become high, unlike with other problems our tendency is to see the treatment as causing the problem when it may not be.

Other factors can obscure the picture. Antidepressants can trigger dissociative reactions leading to confusion, agitation and hyperactivity (see Chapter 5), all of which may be diagnosed as mania. Such reactions resolve rapidly once the antidepressant is withdrawn, whereas a true manic episode lasts longer. There is however an increasing likelihood now that someone with such a reaction will find themselves on a mood-stabiliser without anyone waiting to see if the underlying state resolves naturally than would have happened some years ago.

In the case of the monoamine oxidase inhibitors (MAOIs), there can be an amphetamine-like stimulant effect, which again may resemble mania, but unlike mania it wears off once the MAOI is discontinued.

In the case of the selective serotonin reuptake inhibitors (SSRIs), it has been reported that up to 8% of hospital admissions for manic or psychotic presentations may be linked to a disinhibiting side effect of these drugs.[12] Again this is likely to resolve in many instances on discontinuation of treatment, unless a diagnosis of bipolar disorder is made.

BIPOLAR-MANIA

We are in the midst of an old style tulip-mania, except in this case the mania is for bipolar disorders. Lilly and other companies in their efforts to market antipsychotics have marketed bipolar disorder, suggesting that any poor responses to antidepressants stem from the fact that the person has a bipolar rather than a unipolar disorder and the answer might be a 'mood-stabiliser' rather than an antidepressant. One of the clear marketing goals has been to convert all primary care cases of depression and anxiety into cases of bipolar disorder.

This marketing of bipolar disorders has extended to childhood so that children diagnosed as hyperactive who fail to respond to stimulants are now likely to be portrayed as bipolar and put on drugs like olanzapine from ages as young as 2 or 3 years.[13] Books such as *The Bipolar Child*[14] have become best-sellers. Where there was once a concern that cannabis might be a gateway drug to harder drugs, in adults depression has become a gateway diagnosis to the harder diagnosis of bipolar disorder, and in the paediatric field attention deficit/hyperactivity disorder (ADHD) has become the gateway diagnosis that leads on to a supposed bipolar disorder.

The companies have helped support patient groups, educational material and disease awareness campaigns. As early as 2003, at an American Psychiatric Association meeting one-third of company symposia were on bipolar disorders – an unprecedented concentration of effort on one disorder. There are now journals and meetings devoted solely to bipolar disorders. This has all the characteristics of a stock-market bubble.

As a result, all sorts of conditions can lead on to a bipolar label now. The way into this market has been through the front-door of mania. Demonstrating a drug is useful in mania is spun into a message that it will be prophylactic against further episodes of related nervous problems – which for companies means treatment for life.

Given the evidence of harmful effects from SSRIs given to children and teenagers, which companies suppressed or reported in quite distorted terms, it would be wise to resist using any antipsychotics currently on patent for children with supposed bipolar disorders until there is a full disclosure of all results for the use of these agents in clinical trials in both adults and children. The consequences of a relatively indiscriminate use of agents such as olanzapine, risperidone and aripiprazole in this way, especially for children, are likely to be horrifying.

Mood-stabilisers

7

CHAPTER CONTENTS

HISTORY OF MOOD-STABILISATION

There are suggestions that the Greeks as early as the second century AD recognised that spring waters that were alkaline and as a result perhaps high in lithium salts were calming.[15–17] The Greeks did not recognise manic-depressive illness.[1]

Lithium itself was isolated by August Arfwedson in 1817. It was named lithium because it was found in stone – *lithos* being the Greek for stone. During the 1850s alkaline compounds such as lithium developed a reputation for treating rheumatic disorders and gout by interfering with the precipitation of uric acid in the blood and joints, and lithium was available in many countries through the 1970s for the treatment of rheumatism.

In the 1850s, mania and melancholia according to some were part of the same family of diseases as gout, and this led to the use of lithium for mania and melancholia also and the claim in 1880, by Carl Lange in Copenhagen, that it had a role in preventing episodes of periodic depression. At the same time, William Hammond in New York found the same thing.

Despite these discoveries, lithium slipped out of use for mood disorders and had to be rediscovered in 1949. In part this was because older world views that connected gout to manic-depressive illness vanished, and in part it was because of lithium's side effects – increased urine flow, tremor of the hands and difficulties with memory or concentration. Later, in the 1940s, when used as part of a salt restriction diet in the US, lithium was linked to cardiac problems, which led the Food and Drug Administration to ban its use.

In 1949, following observations that lithium had a tranquillising effect on laboratory animals, John Cade in Australia gave it to manic, depressive and schizophrenic patients. He noted that it was particularly beneficial in mania.

Cade's observations were followed up by Mogens Schou in Denmark, who confirmed in clinical trials that lithium was beneficial in patients with mania. This led to its subsequent spread for use in the treatment of mania.

The adoption of lithium, however, was slow and patchy for several reasons. One is that it can have serious side effects, so that blood lithium levels have to be checked regularly to ensure that its side effects do not outweigh its benefits. Second, lithium as an elemental compound is widely available and therefore no drug company stands to make much money out of it. It has certainly not been marketed as aggressively as other compounds. For 50 years, awareness of its usefulness depended largely on the efforts of Mogens Schou. Third, even for the treatment of mania, it took second place to the antipsychotics.

But in the 1960s, studies from the UK and Denmark appeared supporting Lange's 1880 claim that lithium may be useful in the prevention of recurrent episodes of mania or depression. These claims for a prophylactic effect caused a storm of controversy, which, in fact, may have helped market lithium.[1] One of the arguments of critics was that the results that showed people doing well on lithium and poorly off it might simply be the result of a withdrawal syndrome. This argument was dismissed by lithium's supporters at the time, but it now seems that there is indeed a dependence syndrome, although there appears to be benefits from lithium beyond those of avoiding withdrawal.

Lithium was not available in Japan during the 1960s. This led to an interest to try carbamazepine in mania and to the discovery that carbamazepine could produce useful inter-episode effects. The effects of valproate on mood were similarly discovered in France in the 1960s where lithium use never became widespread.[4,18,19]

In 1980, the example of valproate and carbamazepine led to the idea that anticonvulsants might help mood disorders in much the same way as they helped convulsive disorders – by reducing kindling. The notion was that each episode of a mood disorder kindled a further episode, in the same way that each epileptic fit increases the vulnerability to the next fit. This hypothesis led on to the systematic testing of every new anticonvulsant that has emerged on the market to see whether it might do something useful.

Even electroconvulsive therapy (ECT) it was argued increased seizure thresholds making further fits less likely. But little mention was made of the fact that lithium is pro-convulsant rather than anticonvulsant. Nor is any mention made of the fact that clozapine, which is widely thought to be in some way mood enhancing, is also pro-convulsant.

The kindling idea led to the concept of a mood-stabiliser. The term had first applied to oestrogen and progesterone and later clozapine and cannabis before it was picked up by the marketing department at Abbott to promote valproate. In 1995, even though only shown to be effective for mania, valproate was launched in the US as both Depakote and as a mood-stabiliser. There was no evidence that it stabilised moods. If Abbott had claimed Depakote was prophylactic, the FDA would likely have sued them, but they could claim it was a mood-stabiliser because the term has no definition. But it suggests prophylaxis – an ability to ward off future episodes. It suggested that Depakote, and all of the other drugs now called mood, are new forms of lithium.

There are two ways in which a drug might act as a mood-stabiliser. One would be to reduce kindling, in which case all anticonvulsants should help – but they don't. Lithium furthermore is not anticonvulsant. If mood-stabilisers worked by reducing kindling, the takers of these drugs should not notice anything useful about them other than that they reduced the frequency of episodes of mood disorder, in much the same way that patients on anticonvulsants for epilepsy do not talk about anything useful the drug does for them – they keep a record of whether they are having more or fewer fits.

The other way a mood-stabiliser might work would be if each does something useful. For instance, valproate is sedative, gabapentin is anxiolytic, carbamazepine has anti-irritability or anti-impulsive effects and lamotrigine produces a sense of well-being. If they all act in different ways, conceivably they each could suit different patients, and if the drug was helping, patients should be able to say this helps me because it does X or Y or Z. At present, however, there is no interest to pursue research like this that suits patients but not companies. Companies prefer the idea that if one mood-stabiliser doesn't work, you should be on several of them. But the more drugs a person takes, the harder it is to read the signals of what each might be doing.

Linked to the emergence of mood-stabilisation, there has been a trend to reinterpret personality disorders as mood disorders. Borderline, emotionally unstable and explosive personality disorders, some claim, involve an affective dysregulation at their core, and sustained treatment with a 'mood-stabiliser' helps. Many also argue that any patient with a recurrent mood disorder should be taken off antidepressants and put on mood-stabilisers instead.

These drugs are all called mood-stabilisers but it is by no means clear that drugs such as gabapentin are mood-stabilisers in the same sense as lithium is. Gabapentin is more anxiolytic than other compounds considered here. It is therefore not a surprise that patients with borderline personality problems may be helped by it. But the argument becomes circular if the response of borderline patients to gabapentin is taken to show that they have a mood disorder because gabapentin is classified as a mood-stabiliser. In this way the concept of bipolar disorder can expand to include almost everyone who has 'nerves' of any sort.

There is little evidence that anything except lithium is a mood-stabiliser. Indeed there is some evidence that despite the availability of so many more 'mood-stabilising' drugs now patients with bipolar disorder are doing worse than they were 100 years ago.[20] If the various different drugs do not correct an abnormality, then in fact they provide another physiological stressor (a pharmacological life event) to an already vulnerable system and are likely in the long run to destabilise and make things worse rather than better. There is therefore a need to make sure that people are on a drug that suits them and not just on a mood-stabiliser because that's what you do for people who have bipolar disorder. Calling something a stabiliser doesn't make it one.

LITHIUM AS A MOOD-STABILISER

Lithium affects such a large number of processes that 50 years after its introduction there is still no consensus on what its key physiological effects are. The surprise is that it acts so widely but yet has relatively specific clinical effects.

Since the early 1960s, there has been a clear body of evidence pointing to a role for lithium in the prevention of episodes of mania and depression in bipolar affective disorders. Many individuals who have been treated in hospital for mania are maintained on lithium for years or decades to prevent recurrences in what is known to be a recurrent disorder. The evidence that lithium prevents recurrences is better than the evidence for anything else.

Lithium has been linked to a lower rate of suicide than have other mood-stabilisers. This may stem from the fact that compliance with lithium may indicate someone who is generally more responsible and concerned about their condition and thus at lower risk of suicide. The same argument should apply to valproate and carbamazepine, but suicides in patients maintained on lithium seem lower than in these other two patient groups. Lithium probably doesn't prevent suicide, but it seems less likely to provoke suicidality.

There is some evidence indicating a role for lithium in recurrent depression. The current wisdom is that lithium is indicated if there are as many as two episodes per year or three episodes of depression over the course of 2 years. The efficacy of lithium, however, seems to fall off once there are more than four episodes of a depressive disorder a year.

The traditional wisdom had been that it was necessary to start prophylactic lithium after one manic episode, but now any patient with a manic episode is likely to be advised they need a mood-stabiliser. At the opposite end of the spectrum, lithium does not seem to help in what are called rapidly cycling mood disorders, where there are four or more episodes of a mood disorder per year. Overall, because of its withdrawal effects, there are estimates that patients have to stay on treatment for at least 2.5 years before they are likely to have had fewer episodes than they would have had had they not started lithium.

Table 7.1 gives the main lithium preparations.

DOSAGE

Unlike other psychotropic drugs, there is a clear window for lithium levels in the blood, below which level the drug appears not to work and above which its toxic effects outweigh its benefits.

In the acute treatment of mania or depression, a plasma level between 0.9 and 1.4 mmol/L is needed. Anything from 150 to 4200 mg of lithium per day may be needed to achieve these levels. For the prophylaxis (prevention) of affective episodes, blood levels between 0.4 and 0.8 mmol/L are adequate.[21] Because of the dynamics of lithium, blood needs to be taken 12 hours after

Table 7.1 *Lithium*

Generic drug name	UK trade name	US trade name
Lithium carbonate	Camcolit/Priadel	Eskalith/Lithobid
Lithium citrate	Priadel liquid/Litarex/Li-liquid	–

the last dose and 7 days after a change of dose to give plasma levels time to stabilise.

Because of its effects on the kidney, there was a tradition of giving lithium in divided doses. Concern about kidney toxicity also led to the production of slow-release preparations of lithium to give more even plasma levels. It became customary to give these slow-release preparations in a divided dose in the morning and the evening.

However, it now appears that a single pulse of lithium, giving a high plasma level at one point in the day and falling off to a lower steady-state level, may be less toxic than a moderate level the whole time. The implication is that lithium should perhaps be given as a single dose at one point in the day and that slow-release formulations are no better than conventional preparations.

There have been close to 50 different preparations of lithium on the market. In addition to conventional and slow-release forms, the main differences are between lithium citrate and lithium carbonate. Lithium carbonate is more common, but some prefer citrate to carbonate.

The list of lithium's hazards is fearsome. But lithium has the profile all drugs should have because there has been no company trying to hide the problems. Any symposia about lithium have typically been about its side effects and how to manage these, whilst symposia for the other drugs listed have been aimed at increasing sales rather than safety.

User issues

Lithium withdrawal and dependence

At present one of the most contentious issues in lithium treatment is whether there may, for some people, be a withdrawal syndrome on stopping treatment. In clinical practice, people who have just stopped their treatment seem to relapse with striking frequency but is this because they had begun to go high and therefore stopped treatment – after the new illness episode had started? This has led to a series of vigorous disputes.

Whilst it is difficult to control for all the factors that may be involved, the consensus of opinion on this issue at present would appear to be that some people, perhaps up to one-third or one-half, may have a withdrawal problem. This can be minimised by tapering the dose slowly.[22] Because of this lithium probably best suits those who will take it regularly and commit to it indefinitely. Early discontinuation may bring forwards the next illness episode so that it is necessary to commit to lithium for over 2 years to reduce the frequency of episodes.

User issues

Side effects of lithium

There is a considerable rate of non-compliance with lithium. The usual reasons given are that takers dislike the weight gain, poor memory, tremor, thirst and tiredness. Other reasons cited are that takers miss the highs that they normally get when not on lithium or that they feel well and therefore see no need to continue with treatment. Some discontinue because they are bothered by the idea of drug treatment itself.

Tremor

Individuals taking lithium may develop a fine rapid tremor. This is not ominous, although it may interfere with daily living by causing tea to spill from cups, for example. It will usually clear up when the lithium is discontinued. In occasional cases, it is persistent. It can sometimes be helped by the addition of a beta-blocker such as propranolol.

Thirst and urinary frequency

Lithium causes an inability to concentrate urine, which leads to the passing of greater volumes of urine than normal. This loss of water leads to thirst. Water is lost because lithium antagonises the action of vasopressin, antidiuretic hormone (ADH), which leads to an inability to concentrate urine, with a consequent loss of body water and thirst.

This leads to one of lithium's most troublesome complaints, which is having to pass water during the night. Up to 50% of those on lithium have this side effect. Some may even wet the bed. This is normally reversible once lithium is stopped. A small proportion of people may have a residual problem in concentrating urine when lithium is discontinued.

As lithium leads to fluid loss, it leads to thirst and a perception of a dry mouth. Paradoxically, however, it increases the production of saliva, so mouths are not actually drier than normal. It may also lead to an enlargement of the salivary glands.

Kidney problems

In a small proportion of people, lithium can produce chronic kidney problems involving the destruction of kidney cells and a permanent impairment of the ability to concentrate urine. These are more common in individuals who have been exposed to toxic doses of lithium at some point.

Kidney function should be tested before commencing lithium and 6-monthly thereafter, especially in people who develop urinary frequency, particularly at night. In such subjects a lower plasma level of lithium (0.4–0.6 mmol/L) is advisable.

Ordinarily, testing for urea and creatinine is a sufficient screening procedure for renal function. To avoid kidney toxicity, it is important to avoid inadvertent overdosing (see Lithium overdose and Drug interactions below).

Weight gain

Up to 50% of people put on lithium gain 5 kg in weight or more. The reasons for this weight gain are not clear. The thirst induced by lithium may lead people to drink more calories than they would otherwise do. If thirsty, people taking lithium should stick to water only.

Lithium may also increase appetite by reducing the effectiveness of insulin in the body, which stimulates appetite centres in the brain. Or it may lower basal metabolic rates so that less food is burnt off as energy during the day.

Diarrhoea

Diarrhoea is common early in a course of lithium treatment. Some people may continue to have loose stools for as long as they remain on the drug. In a minority of individuals taking lithium, there may be constipation.

Continued

User issues—cont'd

Diarrhoea is also a symptom of lithium toxicity. If an individual who has not been having diarrhoea develops diarrhoea, lithium toxicity should be considered. In the case of toxicity, the diarrhoea is likely to be accompanied by nausea, vomiting and tremor.

Nausea/abdominal discomfort

Up to one-third of people taking lithium have a certain amount of nausea or more vague abdominal discomfort for the first weeks of treatment. In occasional cases, this may be severe and lead to discontinuation of the drug. There may also be a sensation of bloating or painfulness in the lower abdominal area, one cause of which may be having a fuller than usual bladder owing to the effects of lithium on water concentration. Lithium, in occasional cases, may cause a loss of taste for food with a consequent loss of appetite.

Discoordination

A rarely mentioned but important side effect of lithium is that it may cause episodic discoordination or muscle weakness. Although rarely mentioned, it seems that this side effect is not infrequent. As one individual writing on psychiatric drugs has put it, the first thing she knew about lithium discoordination was when she fell down the stairs. What appears to happen is that there is a brief momentary loss of coordination and/or muscle strength. This leads to a feeling that a fall is imminent, a feeling that is often described as feeling dizzy or faint but in actual fact is neither dizziness nor faintness.[23]

Skin and hair changes

Lithium may cause a variety of skin rashes, eruptions or irritations. The commonest problems are a simple skin rash, pustules or acne. Occasionally there are more exfoliative irritations that, in the extreme, may amount to psoriasis. Changes in the texture of the nails, with pitting, may point to a predisposition to psoriasis and perhaps should lead to a discontinuation of treatment. These problems usually clear up once the drug is stopped but recur once it is restarted. They appear to happen because lithium accumulates in skin and sensitivity to that accumulation. Normally a tetracycline antibiotic would be given to treat acne, but tetracyclines are contraindicated with lithium because of kidney problems. Increased omega-3 fatty acids may be of some benefit.[6]

In about 5% of people there may be marked hair loss on lithium (alopecia). This usually clears even whilst remaining on the lithium, but occasionally it will resolve only once the drug has been discontinued.

White cells

Lithium increases the number of white cells in the blood. This will not be noticed by anyone taking lithium, but it may cause a doctor to wonder whether the person in question has an infection, as infections also lead to an increased white cell count. This effect of lithium is sometimes used in the management of leukaemias and other blood disorders.

Hypothyroidism

Lithium can lead to underactivity of the thyroid gland. The signs of this are dry skin, dry hair, hoarseness, weight gain, hair loss, sluggishness, constipation and sensitivity to the cold. On blood tests, there are low thyroid hormone

User issues—cont'd

(T_4 and T_3) levels and increased thyroid-stimulating hormone (TSH) levels, and the thyroid gland may enlarge to produce a goitre. The likelihood of either hypothyroidism or goitre is increased in women over the age of 45 years and in individuals who have thyroid antibodies (these are naturally present in up to 9% of the population). Before starting lithium, it is therefore routine practice to monitor both thyroid and kidney function, and both should be repeated at anything from 3-monthly to yearly intervals.

Hyperparathyroidism (overactivity of the parathyroid gland)
Lithium quite commonly leads to an increase in serum parathyroid hormone levels. This will in rare cases lead on to excessive calcium levels in the blood, the symptoms of which are similar to the side effects of lithium itself: thirst, increased urine, loss of appetite and nausea.

Tiredness
A relatively common complaint of patients on lithium is tiredness. In some instances, this may be quite marked. Trying to tease apart what is caused by depression and what is caused by lithium may be difficult.

Tension and restlessness
In a small proportion of cases, lithium may give rise to tense, restless feelings. It may be difficult to decide whether lithium is causing the problem or not if a taker is also on antidepressants or antipsychotics. A further reason, of course, is that tense restlessness may be part and parcel of a depressive disorder, or may occur naturally anyway.

Concentration and memory problems
There are a number of reports that lithium can interfere with memory and concentration. Again this is difficult to judge as disturbances of memory and concentration occur in depression anyway. On the other hand, in volunteers taking lithium, difficulties with memory and concentration have also been reported.

Confusion and distractibility
In toxic doses, lithium causes confusion and distractibility. Normally, toxic effects occur when lithium concentration goes over 1.5 mmol/L, but it is possible to have central nervous system toxicity in the presence of essentially normal plasma levels of lithium. In cases of toxicity, confusion and distractibility are likely to be accompanied by nausea and vomiting as well as a variety of involuntary movements such as tremor.

Toxicity is more likely if the subject has recently been put on some other drugs, particularly antipsychotics. It may also occur if they have developed an increased temperature or decreased their fluid intake because of an infection, and have become dehydrated. It can even happen if dehydration occurs because of an altered salt intake.

Headache
Recurrent headaches are a rare side effect of lithium. If they occur, they should be treated seriously. They may indicate raised intracranial pressure. This clears up once the lithium is discontinued but must be detected as early as possible.

User issues

Lithium overdose

Lithium becomes toxic at levels over 1.5 mmol/L with a risk of enduring damage when the levels are more than 2 mmol/L. The side effects most commonly found in toxic doses are nausea, vomiting, diarrhoea, tremor and confusion.

Toxicity may occur without the individual overdosing as such. Dehydration from excessive perspiration, a high temperature or restricted fluid intake may raise plasma levels. In addition, other drugs may increase plasma levels (see Drug interactions below). Inadvertent overdosage may come about simply by altering salt intake. In occasional cases, toxicity seems to occur even in the presence of an apparently normal lithium level.

The first treatment for toxicity is to give large volumes of isotonic saline (water with salt added to the level normally found in blood) intravenously. If lithium levels exceed 4 mmol/L, dialysis is usually indicated.

User issues

Contraindications to lithium therapy

Lithium is contraindicated or should be taken with caution in:

- Pregnancy. At present, studies in animals and surveys of babies who have been delivered by mothers who have been on lithium both at the time of conception and throughout gestation suggest that there is a small increased risk of birth defects and, in particular, a risk of heart defects in the child.

Later in the pregnancy, the risk to the foetus is less, but lithium has been linked to neonatal hypothyroidism. It also becomes difficult in pregnancy to know what plasma lithium levels mean, given that pregnancy brings about a large increase in body water.

There is a risk of lithium intoxication both to the mother and the baby after delivery, as the extra body water shrinks rapidly on delivery and may increase in plasma lithium levels. For these reasons, it may be prudent to discontinue lithium during pregnancy.

- Breastfeeding. Lithium gets into breast milk. Whilst it is not clear if lithium poses a risk to children reared on breast milk, this is clearly of concern. If breastfeeding whilst on lithium, it may make sense to take lithium once a day only and to ensure that feeds have taken place before the lithium dose to ensure the lowest possible level of lithium in the breast milk.
- Cardiac conditions. One-fifth or more of patients on lithium may have clear conductance changes (increased QT intervals) on electrocardiograph (ECG) recordings. This can be a significant problem if the person is also on another psychotropic drug as it too is likely to increase QT intervals.
- Neurological disorders, such as Parkinson's disease, Huntington's disease or any other organic neurological condition.
- Kidney disease.
- Thyroid disease.
- Ulcerative colitis or irritable bowel syndrome.
- Psoriasis, acne or hair loss.
- Systemic lupus erythematosus.
- Cataracts.

User issues

Drug interactions

Diuretics

Diuretics lead to water loss, which may lead to an increase in lithium plasma levels and accidental lithium toxicity. If it is necessary to use diuretics, the lithium dose may have to be reduced. Theoretically the best diuretic to use with lithium is amiloride.

Painkillers

Lithium should be combined cautiously with most common analgesics. Most of them increase lithium levels and risk lithium toxicity. For mild and occasional aches, pains and fever, the best painkiller or anti-inflammatory agent to use is probably paracetamol. For more severe painful or rheumatoid conditions, it appears that the best treatment is sulindac, which lowers lithium levels. All other drugs are usable with extra monitoring of plasma lithium levels.

Others

Lithium antagonises the effects of most social drugs. The effects of alcohol, cocaine, amphetamines and other stimulants are all reduced. Tea and coffee, however, and related drugs such as theophylline, which is used for asthma, may lead to a lowering of lithium levels.

Lithium may also interact with calcium channel blockers, used to treat angina, hypertension or cardiac arrhythmias, and with angiotensin-converting enzyme (ACE) inhibitors, used in the treatment of hypertension.

THE ANTICONVULSANT MOOD-STABILISERS

The role of anticonvulsants in mood-stabilisation begins with carbamazepine and valproate.

Carbamazepine was discovered by Teruo Okuma in Japan.[19] Both lithium and carbamazepine seem to have some anti-irritability action – carbamazepine is used in the management of aggression, in what are sometimes called episodic dyscontrol syndromes, and lithium has also been shown to be useful in aggression. Carbamazepine is also commonly used for, and can be remarkably beneficial for, chronic neuropathic pain syndromes, especially trigeminal neuralgia. Other anticonvulsants such as gabapentin seem to share this action.

It seems unlikely that common anti-irritability actions are what underpin the benefits of both carbamazepine and lithium in recurrent mood disorders, as the two drugs seem to be useful for different patients, with claims that lithium is more useful for the classical and purer forms of bipolar mood disorder and carbamazepine for more irritable, dysphoric forms of mania.[24] Carbamazepine, like lithium, seems to be more useful for manic than depressive states.

Valproate comes from valproic acid is an oil that was used as a butter substitute in Germany during the Second World War. Afterwards, it was used as a solvent for a variety of medicines. In this form its anticonvulsant properties were discovered in the early 1960s. Pierre Lambert discovered its mood-stabilising properties later in the 1960s.[18]

The use of valproate increased dramatically during the 1990s because of a vigorous promotion of semi-sodium valproate (Depakote – see Table 7.2) in the US. Sodium valproate (Epilim) and valproic acid (Convulex) were used elsewhere, and sodium valpromide is also available in France. All versions of this drug break down to valproic acid in the body. It is ethically difficult to run trials of either valproate or other anticonvulsants in patients with bipolar syndromes or other recurrent mood disorders because of the need to randomise patients at high risk of suicide to placebo for possibly several years to demonstrate a reduction in the rate of recurrences. Instead, agents such as valproate have been through trials in mania or depression, and their use as prophylactic agents has spread from there. Valproate has a clear antimanic action, possibly in large part because of its initial sedative effects.

Its popularity has meant that there are now large patient databases in which its use can be compared to that of lithium. Whilst these are not randomised trials, so patient selection factors may influence the results, at present lithium use is linked to a lower rate of suicides and suicidal acts than valproate. At the moment, as with other anticonvulsants, valproate is being used widely in borderline personality disorders, post-traumatic stress disorders, panic disorder, pain syndromes and dysphoric mood disorders with accompanying alcohol and drug misuse.[6]

MODE OF ACTION

The anticonvulsants can be divided by their mechanism of action into three groups – sodium channel blockers, gamma-aminobutyric acid (GABA)-acting drugs, carbonic anhydrase inhibitors and levetiracetam (see Table 7.2).

Even though they have different modes of action, the anticonvulsants have many effects in common. They induce suicidality, cause birth defects, lengthen QT intervals and have effects on skin. Teasing out the profile of effects of anticonvulsants is trickier than teasing out the profile of antipsychotics and antidepressants because these drugs are usually co-prescribed, and this may make it difficult to decide if anticonvulsants have extrapyramidal effects or effects on sexual function in their own right.

But the common problems are clear partly because these drugs are used for epilepsy and migraine as well as for mood disorders and these problems show up where there are no other confounding treatments and no psychiatric illnesses to confound the picture.

The common effects will be dealt with here and individual effects below.

SUICIDALITY

Just as the antidepressants and antipsychotics do, the anticonvulsants induce suicidal behaviour and ideation. In the case of the antidepressants, there is a better understanding of the mental states patients get into that leads on to suicide – the akathisia and disinhibition. This is less well understood for the anticonvulsants. They clearly cause a dysphoria but less obviously cause the kind of akathisia seen with selective serotonin reuptake inhibitors (SSRIs) and antipsychotics. Where the antipsychotics typically induce dysphoria and suicidality within hours or days, and the antidepressants typically do so in days

Table 7.2 *The anticonvulsant mood-stabilisers*

Generic drug name	UK trade name	US trade name	Mode of action
Carbamazepine	Tegretol/Teril CR	Tegretol	Sodium channels
Oxcarbazepine	Trileptal	Trileptal	Sodium channels
Lamotrigine	Lamictal	Lamictal	Sodium channels
Sodium valproate	Epilim	Depakene	GABA-ergic
Semi-sodium valproate	Depakote	Depakote	GABA-ergic
Gabapentin	Neurontin	Neurontin	GABA-ergic
Pregabalin	Lyrica	Lyrica	GABA-ergic
Topiramate	Topamax	Topamax	Sodium channels, GABA-ergic, carbonic anhydrase inhibitor
Zonisamide	Zonegran	Zonegran	Sodium channels, GABA-ergic, carbonic anhydrase inhibitor
Levetiracetam	Keppra	Keppra	Unknown

or weeks, the anticonvulsants are more likely to do so in weeks or months. Whilst doing so over weeks or months, others are more likely to describe personality change in the person taking the medication than with antidepressants.

These drugs are also likely to lead to aggressive behaviour and hostile or even homicidal behaviour with levetiracetam (Keppra) and topiramate appearing to be the worst. Keppra rage is well-known in internet chat groups.

BIRTH DEFECTS

The risk of birth defects with sodium valproate is well known, and its use is severely contraindicated in pregnancy. But in fact most if not all anticonvulsants appear to have a capability to cause a full range of birth defects, including severe neurological problems like spina bifida, but also mental impairment or developmental delay or what is increasingly termed autistic spectrum disorder. As with all drugs that cause birth defects, the anticonvulsants are linked to a high rate of miscarriages (spontaneous abortions).

The term foetal valproate syndrome (FVS) is now well known, but in fact foetal anticonvulsant syndrome (FACS) was described earlier than FVS.

SKIN PROBLEMS

The risk of Stevens-Johnson syndrome came to the fore with the use of lamotrigine for mood disorders. This lethal disorder in which the upper level of the skin peels away was new for mental health and grabbed the imagination. But all anticonvulsants can cause this problem or the closely related toxic epidermal necrosis. To complicate matters, all cause a range of skin rashes and eruptions and exanthema so both those on treatment and those looking after them, who typically know little about skin conditions, can become very alarmed and wonder if what they are seeing might lethal. It usually won't be lethal but has to be checked out.

CARDIAC EFFECTS

As with the antidepressants and antipsychotics, the anticonvulsants close to universally lengthen QT intervals. This effect is potentially more worrying in the case of mood-stabilisers as they are more likely to be combined with other drugs that also lengthen QT intervals. It may therefore be unclear which of several drugs is causing palpitations, tachycardia, an irregular pulse, heart failure or ECG abnormalities, but if any of these do happen, the treatment package will need close attention.

BURNING FEET

These drugs all cause peripheral sensory neuropathies. One of the classic signs of this is burning feet (causalgia). Hands, mouths and other parts of the body can burn also. Other features include a variety of bizarre sensations around the body or sensations of pain on temperature change. The paradox is that these drugs can also relieve pain. The worry is that they can end up treating conditions like the ones they were given for in the first instance.

Linked disturbances include tinnitus, visual disturbances like visual snow, altered taste perception and temperature dysregulation.

CARBAMAZEPINE AND OXCARBAZEPINE

There is a premium on finding who suits carbamazepine as the drug is not pleasant to take if it does not suit. On the other hand, carbamazepine is now off-patent, and there are no company efforts to defend its reputation. A derivative of carbamazepine, oxcarbazepine, is now more commonly used for prophylactic purposes than carbamazepine but with little reason to believe it offers significant advantages.

User issues

Side effects of carbamazepine and oxcarbazepine

The side effects of these two drugs include dizziness, unsteadiness, balance disturbances, drowsiness, nausea, abdominal discomfort and visual disturbances including double vision, nystagmus and eye pain. One strange effect is facial oedema so that a person's face can change shape.

They cause disorientation, confusion and cognitive decline up to pseudo-dementia levels. They can sedate heavily up to a semi-comatose level. Skin rashes occur in up to 15% of takers. For some, these can be very unpleasant drugs to take.

User issues—cont'd

Carbamazepine can cause almost any metabolic or blood parameter to change: low white cell counts, anaemia, hypothyroidism and low sodium levels, increased liver enzymes, increased bilirubin and frank jaundice.

At present, the evidence suggests that lithium is better in the more classical forms of manic-depressive illness. Carbamazepine has also taken something of a backseat to other more recent anticonvulsants. Its efficacy in some forms of aggression and especially for pain syndromes is, however, undoubted.

In general, a plasma level of between 4 and 12 mg/L is aimed for. The dose needed to produce such a level may vary considerably. It is customary to start on a dose of 200 mg per day and increase slowly – usually 200 mg per week – aiming at a dose of 800–1200 mg per day.

If there are signs of fever, sore throat or infection of any sort, a white cell count should be performed; if this is low, it may be necessary to discontinue treatment. In general blood counts and liver function tests should be carried out at something between monthly and 3-monthly intervals whilst carbamazepine is being taken, as carbamazepine is linked to agranulocytosis and aplastic anaemia.

User issues

Drug interactions
Carbamazepine induces liver enzymes. As a consequence, many other medications are metabolised more rapidly, notably the contraceptive pill. This may mean that a number of treatments do not work as well as before. Essentially almost all other agents will have their levels reduced by carbamazepine. Carbamazepine also blocks calcium channels and therefore it should be used cautiously with calcium entry blockers.

Contraindications to carbamazepine
In pregnancy, as with valproate, carbamazepine is linked to spina bifida and neural tube defects and to a higher than expected rate of congenital abnormalities. It gets into breast milk and can potentially lead to problems for the child ranging from sedation through to withdrawal.

SODIUM AND SEMI-SODIUM VALPROATE

User issues

Side effects of valproate
The common side effects are nausea, stomach cramps and diarrhoea, tremor, lethargy and weight gain. Up to one in six takers find that their hair thins or changes in texture, often becoming curly. This may be related to zinc deficiency, and it is common to co-prescribe zinc with valproate. Valproate also commonly leads to irregular menses in up to one-half of the women taking it, as well as gynaecomastia, polycystic ovaries (in over one-third of women) and an increase in testosterone levels in nearly one-fifth of women.[25]

Continued

User issues—cont'd

As with other anticonvulsants, there may be lethargy, tremor, discoordination and slurred speech. These side effects and others are more likely in combination with antidepressants or antipsychotics. In addition, facial flushing, skin rashes and a variety of blood abnormalities including anaemia are possible. Bruising of any sort should be investigated and possibly lead to discontinuation. Valproate has been reported to trigger systemic lupus erythematosus reactions and is contraindicated in anyone with liver disease – so it should be used with caution in individuals with alcohol or other substance dependency. It should be used with caution in both children and the elderly.

Dosages used in patients with mood disorders exceed those used for anticonvulsant therapy and range from 1200 to 2400 mg per day.

Drug interactions of valproate

Valproate inhibits liver enzymes, and this can lead to increases in co-administered drugs. For the most part, the co-administered drugs that have been looked at have been other anticonvulsants, but there also appear to be interactions with anticoagulants, salicylates, antibiotics, fluoxetine, sertraline, haloperidol, benzodiazepines and oral contraceptives.

Contraindications to valproate

Valproate is contraindicated in pregnancy because of FVS, which involves learning disabilities, dysmorphic facies, cardiac defects and limb malformations. Valproate also passes into breast milk, although at this point whether this is likely to be linked to problems for the child other than sedation is unclear.

LAMOTRIGINE

Just as with carbamazepine and valproate, lamotrigine began as an anticonvulsant. Like carbamazepine, it acts by blocking sodium channels on nerve cells and does so to an ever greater extent the more the cell is in use. Reports from clinical practice that lamotrigine seemed to induce a sense of well-being led to trials in depression, with some evidence that it can be beneficial, although only a proportion of trials undertaken were ever published.[6] Lamotrigine seems to be antidepressant rather than antimanic. It is now used widely, especially in North America, in the management of recurrent mood disorders but with little good evidence for a prophylactic effect.

The usual dose is 100–200 mg daily, with the dose built up by 25 mg increments every 2 weeks. Doses up to 500 mg per day are used in some centres.

User issues

Side effects of lamotrigine

The side effects of lamotrigine overlap heavily with those of carbamazepine – almost all those reported for carbamazepine occur with it also. The commonest initial problems are rashes and fevers. A real hazard is a skin condition called Stevens–Johnson syndrome. This occurs more often in children

User issues—cont'd

and adolescents than in adults and is more likely when the dosage is increased quickly. In order to avoid triggering this reaction, lamotrigine is usually increased slowly over a few weeks of treatment. This skin problem shows as a tingling or itch before it develops into a rash. If caught early, there is little problem. Left too late, the condition has been fatal. The occurrence of any rash early in treatment should lead to an evaluation and possibly discontinuation of treatment.

These skin reactions are hypersensitivity reactions. However, hypersensitivity can occur without an obvious skin reaction. The signs in this case are fever, swollen lymph glands, puffiness of the face and abnormalities of liver function. Other side effects include headaches, dizziness, lack of coordination, nausea, blurred vision and either drowsiness or insomnia.

Combinations with valproate are likely to lead to an increase in lamotrigine levels and consequent toxicity. Carbamazepine, in contrast, lowers lamotrigine levels. When added to another anticonvulsant, in addition to changes in the dosage levels, there may also be a multiplication of neuropsychiatric side effects, with blurred vision, discoordination and other similar side effects becoming more common.

Lamotrigine is a risky drug to take even if there is a benefit. It should not be taken just because it is supposed to be a mood-stabiliser.

GABAPENTIN AND PREGABALIN

Gabapentin and pregabalin are essentially the same drug. Gabapentin breaks down to pregabalin in the body. Unlike lamotrigine or valproate, neither gabapentin nor pregabalin have been shown to be effective in clinical trials for mania or depression. Despite this, their use for recurrent mood disorders has increased dramatically. This may stem from an anxiolytic profile, which is appreciated by many patients. These drugs are quite benzodiazepine-like. Both can also produce significant dependence.

Many people with substance-abuse and chronic personality-based problems now receive one of these drugs, with claims of benefits – leading to a circular argument that these patients must lie on a bipolar spectrum. The marketing of pregabalin has targeted women with fibromyalgia – low-grade chronic pain conditions are one of the biggest markets in medicine.

User issues

Side effects of gabapentin and pregabalin

The common side effects are drowsiness, dizziness, discoordination, visual disturbances, headaches, tremor, nausea and vomiting, slurred speech and throat pains of various sorts. Pancreatitis, liver problems and Stevens–Johnson syndrome have also been reported. Many people taking them, however, find them almost free of side effects and quite agreeable – which may be risky in terms of dependence.

Continued

User issues—cont'd

The usual dose of gabapentin and pregabalin for convulsive disorders is up to 900 mg per day, but up to 3600 mg has been used in mood disorders. Withdrawal reactions have been reported and therefore tapering should be gradual. 'Poop-out' – an apparent loss of effect – has also been reported.

TOPIRAMATE AND LEVETIRACETAM

Even more than other anticonvulsants, these two drugs lead to a wide range of behavioural changes that are in fact neurological or semi-neurological problems. The taker can become discoordinated, clumsy, slurred and disoriented. Almost anything can happen as the Alice in Wonderland syndrome linked to topiramate indicates – where the person sees objects changing size or shape in front of their eyes. Whilst all anticonvulsants can lead to agitation and aggression, levetiracetam is linked to a well-known Keppra rage.

The clinical picture may look like hysteria in part because the events reported can seem bizarre or like catatonia because it actually does contain catatonic features like echolalia or echopraxia. There is a risk that what happens may be viewed as part of an underlying illness and lead to inappropriate treatment rather than a removal of the triggering treatment. With these two drugs, families or carers are more likely to report the person has had a change of personality.

User issues

Side effects of topiramate and levetiracetam
In addition to the above, topiramate is linked to visual problems from glaucoma to retinal changes including macular degeneration. It is particularly likely to be linked to facial pain and eye pain and, on the other hand, a range of odd sensations around the body including numbness.

Where other anticonvulsants all cause skin problems, levetiracetam in addition is linked to acne and other facial problems such as burning mouth and painfully cracked lips.

ANTIPSYCHOTICS AS MOOD-STABILISERS

Almost all the second-generation antipsychotics have sought to position themselves as mood-stabilisers – especially olanzapine, risperidone, quetiapine and aripiprazole. The only drug with a licence for this purpose is olanzapine, gained on the basis of trials that may be better interpreted as showing olanzapine causes dependence and continuing treatment minimises withdrawal.[26]

In practice, for the past 50 years antipsychotics have been used in bipolar disorders during both remission and acute phases but in lower doses during remission. A judicious use of an antipsychotic with lithium on a pragmatic basis seemed useful in some cases, but nobody called these antipsychotics mood-stabilisers. The recent marketing of second-generation antipsychotics misleadingly suggests that the use of recent antipsychotics in bipolar disorder is curative in a way that older antipsychotics were not.

There is clearly a place for antipsychotics – for real manic-depressive illness. It may well be that some of the most dramatic responses to clozapine happen in patients who are bipolar. This being said, the risks of using drugs like olanzapine, which cause dramatic weight gain, induce diabetes, cause akathisia and precipitate suicide, must be questioned in anything but the most severely ill patients.

The marketing of these antipsychotics has aimed at trying to persuade prescribers that almost any nervous problem in primary care might be bipolar disorder, especially in those who fail to respond to antidepressants or have substance misuse and personality problems. Once a person becomes bipolar the implication is that they need to stay on a mood-stabiliser for life. There is no evidence that this is a good idea.

The data behind aripiprazole offers a cautionary tale.[27] This was licensed for mood-stabilisation on the back of a multicentre study involving US and Mexican hospitals. It turns out that there were no differences between it and placebo in the over 20 US hospitals recruiting patients, but in the two Mexican hospitals it was wonderfully effective and placebo without effect. It was only after adding the Mexican 'data' in that anything could be shown.

User issues

Side effects of antipsychotics

When used as mood-stabilisers, the antipsychotics have all the side effects outlined in Chapter 3, including dyskinesias, dystonias, parkinsonism, demotivation, akathisia, tardive dyskinesia, weight gain, metabolic syndrome and diabetes. The hazards outlined here focus on certain key areas where the antipsychotics compare with other mood-stabilisers.

One of the major issues with mood-stabilisers outlined above is the risks posed by treatment in pregnancy and breastfeeding. In contrast to valproate, carbamazepine and lithium, the risks to the foetus at one point seemed less with older antipsychotics. But this lack of evidence may hinge on the fact that until recently anyone given these drugs had schizophrenia and were much less likely to get pregnant. Wider use of these drugs may bring the risks more clearly to light. It typically takes a decade or two for the risks of a treatment in pregnancy to emerge.

All antipsychotics except clozapine increase lactation, but in general they are incompatible with breastfeeding because of the risks of dependence and withdrawal posed to the baby.

This is a particular issue in women with bipolar disorders, who are at a much higher risk of postpartum psychosis than any other group. The very first manifestation of bipolar disorder may in fact be in the form of a postpartum psychosis. The best possible management of such episodes may be of considerable importance therefore to the future well-being of both mother and child.

COCKTAIL TREATMENT

In the 1980s, the big issue in schizophrenia treatment was megadoses of antipsychotics. The issue in bipolar disorder is cocktail treatment. Patients who are 'resistant' to one mood-stabiliser often end up on cocktails of six or seven 'mood-stabilisers'. This practice rests on a misinterpretation of what clinical trials show. Trials are portrayed as showing that anticonvulsants or antipsychotics 'work' for bipolar disorders, when in fact the trials have only shown usefulness in mania and even in mania the correct interpretation is that these trials have shown that it is not correct to say this drug does nothing more than placebo. Exactly what the benefit is, is less certain, and may be little more than a sedative effect.

Putting people on five or six drugs that have all been shown to work if they aren't responding sounds reasonable to many people and might overcome their scruples about drugs or concerns as to whether they were really ill enough to be on this many drugs. Putting people on five or six drugs, regarding the effects of each of which we are deeply uncertain, is a very different matter. But none of these drugs, except perhaps lithium, has been clearly shown to reduce the frequency of episodes. Because they are called mood-stabilisers, however, the assumption is that this must be what they do. If the drugs can't be shown to reduce episodes, the sensible basis for taking them would lie in the taker being able to identify something useful a particular drug does for them. Few people, however, are likely to be able to pick out a useful something like this from a particular drug if they are five or six different drugs.

In the case of rapidly cycling mood disorders or other resistant mood disorders, treatment may often be part of the problem. Many of the mood-stabilisers interfere with a variety of vitamins such as folate, or essential minerals such as zinc, making a clinical response much less likely. Rather than add to cocktails, an earlier consideration of adding diet and hygienic manoeuvres to a drug would seem a better bet.

All of these 'stabilisers' cause significant withdrawal problems in at least a proportion of cases. Dose reduction therefore must be gradual. Convulsions and a range of other problems have been produced by over-rapid cessation.

CODA

There are two further issues to consider here. There is a good reason to doubt that many 'mood-stabilisers' do much good, but there is no reason to doubt they have a psychotropic effect. The problems may stem from efforts to shoehorn these effects into a categorical model of disease that assumes mental disorders are like bacterial infections and that the role of drugs is to eliminate them. This is the way companies are forced to bring their drugs on the market at present. The alternative is that the drugs interact with dimensions of our personalities, so that some agents will suit one person and others will suit another, in which case the task becomes one of identifying what the drugs do for the patient and maximising effects that are useful.

A second issue is that although there has been an explosion of interest in bipolar disorders in recent years, and apparently a lot more drugs and a lot more information, in fact the quality of that information is extraordinarily poor with few studies being done for purposes other than marketing and few of the data publicly available.

REFERENCES

1. Healy D, Mania A. Short history of bipolar disorder. Baltimore: Johns Hopkins University Press; 2008.
2. Pichot P. The birth of the bipolar disorder. Eur Psychiatry 1996;10:1–10.
3. Healy D, Williams JMG. Moods, misattributions and mania. Psychiatr Dev 1989;7:49–70.
4. Harris M, Chandran S, Chakraborty N. Mood-stabilizers: the archeology of the concept. Bipolar Disord 2003;5:446–52.
5. Balfour JA, Bryson HM. Valproic acid. A review of its pharmacology and therapeutic potential in indications other than epilepsy. CNS Drugs 1994;2:144–73.
6. Aubry J-M, Ferrero F, Schaad N, et al. Pharmacotherapy of bipolar disorders. Chichester: Wiley; 2007.
7. Fink M. Electroshock: restoring the mind. Oxford: Oxford University Press; 1999.
8. Small JG, Klapper HH, Kellams JG. Electroconvulsive treatment compared to lithium in the management of manic states. Arch Gen Psychiatry 1988;45:727–32.
9. Fink M, Taylor MA. Catatonia. Cambridge: Cambridge University Press; 2003.
10. Healy D. The antidepressant era. Cambridge, MA: Harvard University Press; 1998.
11. Angst J. Switch from depression to mania – a record study over decades between 1920 and 1982. Psychopathology 1985;18:140–54.
12. Preda A, MacLean RW, Mazure CM, et al. Antidepressant associated mania and psychosis resulting in psychiatric admission. J Clin Psychiatry 2001;62:30–3.
13. Healy D, Le Noury J. Paediatric bipolar disorder. Int J Risk Saf Med 2007;19:209–21.
14. Papolos D, Papolos J. The bipolar child. New York: Broadway Books; 2000.
15. Johnson FN. The history of lithium. Basingstoke: Macmillan; 1984.
16. Johnson FN. Depression and mania: modern lithium treatment. Oxford: IRL Press; 1987.
17. Schou M. Phases in the development of lithium treatment in psychiatry. In: Samson F, Adelman G, editors. The neurosciences: paths of discovery, vol. II. Boston, MA: Birkhauser; 1992. pp. 149–66.
18. Comité Lyonnais pour la Research et Therapie en Psychiatrie. The birth of psychopharmacotherapy: explorations in a new world, 1952–1968. In: Healy D, editor. The psychopharmacologists, vol. 3. London: Arnold; 2000. pp. 1–54.
19. Okuma T. The discovery of the psychotropic effects of carbamazepine. In: Healy D, editor. The psychopharmacologists, vol. 3. London: Arnold; 2000. pp. 259–80.
20. Harris M, Chandran S, Chakroborty N, et al. Service utilization in bipolar disorder, 1890 and 1990 compared. Hist Psychiat 2005;16:423–34.
21. Abou-Saleh MT. The dosage regimen. In: Johnson FN, editor. Depression and mania: modern lithium treatment. Oxford: IRL Press; 1987. pp. 99–104.
22. Goodwin G. Recurrence of manic-depression after lithium withdrawal. Br J Psychiatry 1994;164:149–52.
23. Blaska B. The myriad medication mistakes in psychiatry: a consumer's view. Hosp Community Psychiatry 1990;41:993–8.
24. Greil W, Ludwig-Mayerhofer W, Erazo N, et al. Lithium versus carbamazepine in the maintenance treatment of bipolar disorders – a randomised study. J Affect Disord 1997;43:151–61.
25. Ernst CL, Goldberg JF. The reproductive safety profile of mood-stabilizers, atypical antipsychotics and broad-spectrum psychotropics. J Clin Psychiatry 2002;63(Suppl. 4):42–55.
26. Tohen M, Calabrese JR, Sachs G, et al. Randomized, placebo-controlled trial of olanzapine as maintenance therapy in patients with bipolar I disorder responding to acute treatment with olanzapine. Am J Psychiatry 2006;163:247–56.
27. Rosenlicht N, Tsai AC, Parry PI, et al. Aripiprazole in the maintenance treatment of bipolar disorder: a critical review of the evidence and its dissemination into the scientific literature. PLoS Med 2011;8:e10000434.

SECTION 4
STIMULANTS AND DRUGS FOR CHILDREN

SECTION CONTENTS

Stimulants and drugs for children

8

CHAPTER CONTENTS

One of the most striking changes since the first edition of this book has been the growth in use of psychotropic drugs for children. This began with the stimulants, moved on to the antidepressants, and now embraces the antipsychotics. This chapter begins with the use of stimulants and then takes in the principles underlying psychotropic drug use in children.

THE HISTORY OF THE STIMULANTS

Up to a century ago, there was a general understanding that treatments for 'nerves' could aim at strengthening weak nerves or depleting or settling overactive or irritable nerves. The way to strengthen nerves was with 'tonics'. Settling typically involved damping down behaviour – or sedation. Strengthening might lead to convulsions; settling was more likely to be anticonvulsant.

The tonics included arsenic, strychnine, camphor and coca (later cocaine). Strychnine and camphor cause convulsions, as do lithium, clozapine, ketamine and of course electroconvulsive therapy (ECT). These are pro-convulsant drugs. The tonic group also includes stimulants.[1]

In a famous natural experiment, a flood in Pavlov's laboratory in Leningrad in 1924, which nearly drowned his experimental dogs, left many of them nervous. The shock in each case was the same, and dogs had what Pavlov called a traumatic neurosis. But what intrigued him was that there was a difference in their response to treatments: some were helped by sedatives and others by tonics. This raises the possibility that quite different drugs could be effective for the same condition, depending on the constitutional type (the personality) of the individual.[2]

These ideas were later elaborated into a sophisticated theory of personality by Hans Eysenck, who, taking a concept first outlined by Carl Gustav Jung, distinguished between introverts and extraverts. According to both Jung and Eysenck, introverts handle their fears internally and in so doing predispose themselves to phobic and obsessional disorders, as well as neurotic anxiety. Extraverts handle their difficulties in the interpersonal space so that their difficulties become problems for both themselves and others. They are predisposed to hysteria and psychopathy.

These dimensions of introversion and extraversion were, for Eysenck, biological realities, shaped by our genes rather than our upbringing. In support of this, he pointed to a differential sensitivity between introverts and extraverts to the effects of stimulants and sedatives. Answers on the Eysenck Personality Questionnaire can, in fact, predict how much anaesthetic will be needed to put someone to sleep for surgery: introverts need much more than extraverts. Similarly, extraverts are much more sensitive to the effects of stimulants, which can have apparently paradoxical effects on them.[3]

Almost at exactly the same time as these ideas took shape, the amphetamine series of molecules were first made and elaborated.[4] It took some years for chemists to appreciate their stimulant properties. Exploring these further led to the discovery of dexamphetamine in 1935, an amphetamine with much more marked stimulant properties than other amphetamines. This quickly swept away the use of other stimulants. Dexamphetamine was tried out in a range of conditions and found to be helpful, including narcolepsy, anxiety disorders and a condition that has since come to be called attention deficit/hyperactivity disorder (ADHD).

In 1937, Charles Bradley reported on the beneficial effects of benzedrine on a series of disturbed children in care in the following terms: 'to see a single dose of benzedrine produce a greater improvement in school performance than the combined efforts of a capable staff working in a most favourable setting, would have been all but demoralising to the teachers had not the improvement been so gratifying from a practical viewpoint'.[5]

In succeeding decades as the use of these drugs for children grew, stimulant use was increasingly linked to violence, aggression, dependence and drug abuse. The amphetamines were viewed as crystal meth (another stimulant) is viewed now. In the early 1970s the stimulants were made controlled drugs, and their use plummeted. No one could have imagined their comeback.

THE EMERGENCE OF ADHD

Amongst the range of difficult and disturbed children in institutional care in the 1930s, it was only a small group whom Bradley reported as responding to stimulants – others were given and responded to sedatives. But the response to stimulants led to a slow increase in the usage of the drugs. In 1954, another stimulant appeared: methylphenidate (Ritalin), which appeared effective for the same group of children Bradley had looked at. This helped trigger the emergence in the late 1950s of the concept of minimal brain dysfunction (MBD) to explain what appeared to many to be a paradoxical response – overactive children becoming calmer on a drug that agitated many adults. There was considerable speculation about the origins of MBD, with proposals ranging from minor birth injury through to allergic responses to food additives. Children with MBD were often said to have hyperactivity.

MBD in turn became ADHD in the *Diagnostic and Statistical Manual of Mental Disorders*, Third Edition (DSM III) in 1980.[6,7] But this name, rather than indicating a well-understood disorder, simply describes a state in which some children may be overactive and others may be inattentive. Given the fluid nature of both inattentiveness and overactivity, there is an inevitable risk that diagnoses will lead on to treatment with a problem group of drugs when it should not. With the creation of ADHD and suggestions of MBD, Ritalin, which had been available for 25 years before that, exploded into popular consciousness.[8–10]

Initially, these results from the US were discounted in Europe. In Europe, until recently the story was that there are a small number of children, mostly boys, who are intensely hyperactive, on whom stimulants can have an almost miraculous effect. These children typically grow out of the problem in adolescence.

In the US, the first explanations were in terms of something wrong with the brains of hyperactive children so that drugs that in normal children abolished appetite, interfered with sleep and stimulated produced the opposite effects in these 'hyperactive' children. Then, Judy Rapoport demonstrated that similar effects could be shown in non-hyperactive children. This introduced the notion that there was a paediatric response to these drugs that differed from the responses of adults. This idea has also since been discarded, leaving us with two options. The stimulants work because they correct ADHD, a brain disorder, or they have useful effects in extraversion, a constitutional predisposition that many people have that makes them more sensitive to the calming effects of stimulants. (There is a third option, which is that the effects of stimulants depend in part on the baseline activity rates of the person or animal taking them, leading to slowing down effects against a background of high activity rates and a stimulant effect against a background of low activity rates.)

There are a number of extraordinary features of this history. One is that the stimulants breached the taboo of giving psychotropic drugs to children. As a result, children, especially in North America, are now being given cocktails of psychotropic drugs on a vast scale. When up to 15% of children in some areas are diagnosed with ADHD, it becomes very difficult to believe they all have a clear-cut disease.[11,12]

Second is that there is a lack of pharmacological distinction between the drugs being used – Ritalin and dexedrine – and banned agents such as cocaine and speed (amphetamine sulphate). It seems we can look at a group of drugs and both see them as harmless and as a major threat to society.[9,10]

Whilst the response of overactive children to stimulants was once seen as paradoxical, and this for some pointed strongly to the pathological basis of the condition, it is now clear that many adults, unsurprisingly, report benefits from stimulants. This has led companies to promote the idea of adult ADHD – we were supposedly mistaken in thinking everybody grew out of their ADHD. There is a trend to recognising milder forms of difficulties in adults that might respond to stimulants. It is increasingly common to hear of college students for instance seeking scripts for stimulants around times of examinations and attributing their ability to master the concentration problems that come with large paper loads to treatment of their illness, where in fact this is simply a quite normal response to stimulants – that comes with a very predictable set of attendant problems (see Chapter 18).

Beyond this, a number of clinicians in recent years in books like *Shadow Syndromes* have very actively promoted the idea of adult ADHD and the use of stimulants for such people. Some people will unquestionably find a benefit from this, but benefits do not make a diagnosis, and there are other ways to interpret what is happening as is outlined above and further below.

STIMULANT TREATMENT FOR ADHD

There is little doubt, based on the clinical trial evidence, that stimulants can produce dramatic behavioural changes in some children. Treatment may transform children's lives so that they are enabled to get on with socialising and other developmental tasks. In other cases, whilst the superficial effects may be clear, there is much less evidence that these benefits actually translate into improved school performance or better socialisation.

Any prescription of stimulants to children, adolescents or even adults with 'ADHD' should still be viewed with caution. The effects should be monitored to ensure that there are clear superficial benefits and, ideally, indicators of deeper improvements.

Having made this point, an equal but opposite one also needs to be made, namely that refusing to prescribe on the basis that non-drug approaches are in some way ethically preferable is difficult to defend given the significant improvements for the individual and their families that can be produced by the judicious prescription of stimulants. If the interests of the child are to be paramount, then all therapeutic options need to be on the table.

A more recent addition to the stimulant armoury is modafinil. This was patented in 1990 for the management of narcolepsy. It was given orphan drug status by regulators on the basis that narcolepsy was so rare no company stood to make much money from its treatment. Its makers claim it has the alerting properties of dexamphetamine without the euphoriant properties or the activity-increasing effects and that it has much less potential for addiction. But such statements are typical of all new drugs, and with time the profile of modafinil has become ever harder to distinguish from classic stimulants. It leaked into use for children with ADHD and was also promoted for 'excessive daytime sleepiness'.

NON-STIMULANT DRUG TREATMENTS OF ADHD

Whilst the very wide use of stimulants in recent years has led to a certain familiarity, these drugs were nevertheless made controlled drugs in the 1960s owing to their abuse potential. As a result, clinicians treating 'ADHD' have experimented with a variety of other agents, in particular antidepressants. From amongst the antidepressant group, it had become clear in the 1970s that noradrenaline reuptake inhibitors such as desipramine were more useful than serotonin reuptake inhibitors.

Eli Lilly ran with this notion in developing atomoxetine as a non-controlled drug treatment for ADHD. Atomoxetine in fact began life as an antidepressant but performed poorly in trials and was rerouted first as a possible treatment for urinary incontinence, before finally finding a niche for ADHD. It has nothing to recommend it over other noradrenaline reuptake inhibitors or stimulants, but its use does perhaps help focus some of the complexities in this area. When disturbed children previously responded to noradrenaline reuptake inhibitors, were they responding because they were depressed? Or did some children we saw as depressed because they responded to an 'antidepressant' really have ADHD? Our abilities to establish what might be going on in these cases is heavily compromised by company efforts to market diseases such as ADHD or depression. If some children respond to drugs active on the noradrenaline system whilst others respond to drugs active on the serotonin system, is this evidence of two different diseases or as evidence of differences in their physiology that have links to the development of temperament and personality?

When stimulants or antidepressants failed in children, some clinicians were always liable to turn to anticonvulsants or antipsychotics. In recent years this has been justified by claims that childhood hyperactivity may stem from the fact that they are bipolar (Chapter 6 and Chapter 7). Another option found in Europe but not at the moment in the US is that the child has DAMP (deficits in attention, motor control and perception), a notion created by Gillberg in Sweden.[13] This condition supposedly lies somewhere in between ADHD and Asperger's and is typically treated with an antipsychotic, most commonly risperidone. There is a great deal of biomythology or figleafing here. The key issue to monitor is whether the treatment helps or not, and even when helpful, a careful eye needs to be kept out for the appearance of side effects.

NON-DRUG TREATMENTS OF ADHD

In addition to non-stimulant drugs, there is a variety of behavioural techniques that can be helpful in the management of children who have conditions that may be diagnosed as ADHD. The majority of these focus on family management programmes, not in the belief that families have caused the problem but that the condition, even when treated with drugs, can be improved by secure boundaries and consistency. Over the longer run, the evidence from the biggest study comparing drug and non-drug treatments suggest that these programmes do as well as drug treatment.[14]

There is in fact a huge overlap in behaviours between children who might be diagnosed as having ADHD and children who might otherwise or who might formerly have been diagnosed as having conduct disorder or oppositional defiant disorder. ADHD has often seemed to descend to the level of a blanket diagnosis for children causing trouble. There is good evidence that elements of conduct disorder and other intra-familial problems can be helped by appropriate strategies that do not involve drug treatments and that can lead to significantly reduced levels of what could be termed hyperactivity.[15]

OTHER USES OF STIMULANTS

ADULT ADHD

At present we are witnessing a very aggressive marketing of the notion of adult ADHD. This condition, once thought to occur in children only, we are now told may persist into adulthood and be responsible for marital breakdown, career failure and drug abuse. Until recently there was a clear consensus that children grew out of ADHD, and the results of studies like the MTA study (Multimodal Treatment Study of Children With ADHD) still point this way.[14] One of the striking features of the current situation is that where four out of every five children with supposed ADHD are male, more than half of adult ADHD cases are female. This may be the only disorder in medicine that changes gender ratio like this with age.

A further aspect to the growing use of stimulants is that stimulant and psychotropic drug use in the US, especially for children, has often been a middle-class phenomenon, suggesting the drugs are being used in the belief that they will confer some sort of competitive advantage. In contrast, in Europe the use of psychotropic drugs has been much more often to sedate social problems. Even in Europe, adult ADHD appears very American in that it seems to be a much more middle-class thing. It has links to questions of cognitive enhancement (Chapter 18).

STIMULANTS IN ANXIETY AND DEPRESSION

The stimulants were traditionally distinguished from the antidepressants on the basis that they supposedly had little effect on depression. However, the depression on which they had little effect in the 1940s and 1950s was melancholia or the severe endogenous or psychotic depressions that led to hospitalisation. These depressions somewhat paradoxically responded to sedative drugs – the tricyclic antidepressants.

In contrast, through the 1950s, 1960s and 1970s stimulants were used regularly for tired-all-the-time states, depressive neuroses and anxiety disorders. The first placebo-controlled clinical trial in medicine involved the use of dexamphetamine in depression and schizophrenia; this demonstrated that dexamphetamine helped patients with depression but not those with schizophrenia.[16] There is, indeed, considerable evidence that stimulants are just as good as selective serotonin reuptake inhibitors (SSRIs) for primary care nerves.[17] Given that the SSRIs have never been shown to be effective for melancholic depressions of the kind that responded to the first antidepressants, if this group of drugs had been introduced in the 1950s or 1960s, there is every reason to think that they would not now be called antidepressants either.

The basis for using stimulants for these nervous states is the same as that outlined above for their use in children, namely that at least part of the contribution to the nervous problems that many adults end up with stems from temperamental inputs, which can be expected in the case of extraverts to respond to stimulants. In the past, this response to stimulants in adults would never have led to a diagnosis of adult ADHD, but times have changed, and these 'depressions' or nervous states are now being diagnosed as ADHD on the basis of a response to stimulants.

In addition to use as 'antidepressants', stimulants have also been used as adjunctive therapies with other antidepressants, in some cases possibly by clinicians nervous about using them on their own.

The doses and side effects, when used in this way, are the same as those for ADHD.

STIMULANTS IN SCHIZOPHRENIA

In any consideration of the dopamine hypothesis of schizophrenia, one of the arguments put forward is that amphetamines lead to mental disorders characterised by prominent paranoia and a stereotyped thought disorder. This state has similarities with some schizophrenic states. As the stimulants increase dopamine and the antipsychotics block dopamine neurotransmission, this suggested that schizophrenia must involve increased dopamine functioning and, accordingly, giving a stimulant to someone with schizophrenia would not be a good idea.

However, the picture in real life is more ambiguous. In the first place, there is a substantial amount of evidence that up to one-third of individuals with 'schizophrenia' actually do well on stimulants.[18]

Second, there are good grounds for suggesting that not all individuals who are labelled as having schizophrenia, or who get antipsychotics, actually have schizophrenia. There is some evidence that a proportion of individuals who have suffered from hyperactivity in childhood may present with a psychotic disorder later in life,[19] at which point they are likely to be given antipsychotics, which do the opposite to stimulants, and may in fact make the psychosis worse.

Third, the collapse of the dopamine hypothesis of schizophrenia removes some of the worry that hindered the use of stimulants in psychoses. This hypothesis made it impossible to prescribe stimulants to people with psychosis, even when clinically there were clear benefits.

Aside from the beneficial effects that stimulants might have for some psychoses, they ameliorate a number of antipsychotic side effects.[20,21] In practice, whilst amphetamines may lead to psychotic breakdowns and admissions, this is usually linked to high dosage and chronic use. Most mental-health staff, however, will know of people taking amphetamines, whilst also taking antipsychotics, who do well. The books will claim that the antipsychotics prevent amphetamine use from leading to a psychosis, but the alternative view that amphetamine use may be reversing side effects of antipsychotic therapy seems reasonable in many cases.

For example, antipsychotic-induced demotivation can be helped by a combination of lowering the dose of the antipsychotic and adding a stimulant. Weight gain on antipsychotics may also be counteracted by stimulants. Antipsychotic-induced increases in levels of the hormone prolactin, which lead to menstrual irregularities, increased breast size and the production of milk even in men, may respond to a stimulant or a dopamine agonist such as bromocriptine. Motor side effects, which are unresponsive to the usual antidotes, may also respond well.

In general, stimulants are more likely to benefit the subgroup of us who appear to be sensitive to the dopamine-blocking effects of antipsychotics (probably 5–10% of us), for whom antipsychotics, even in relatively low doses, produce marked motor side effects and/or demotivation, so much so that the taking of these drugs may be quite distressing and in the long run possibly harmful to mental health.

STIMULANTS AND COGNITIVE ENHANCEMENT

Following on from the increasing use of stimulants during the 1990s, from 2000 onwards this use migrated into efforts to enhance academic performance with students using these drugs to help them focus, maintain wakefulness and work for exams. This has led to widespread concern with the British Medical Association issuing an ethics paper on this use of stimulants (see Section 7).[22]

OTHER STATES OF OVERACTIVITY

There is a place for the stimulants in a range of brain disorders from Alzheimer's disease and other dementias, especially subcortical dementias, to head injuries and Parkinson's disease. In subcortical dementias and following head injury, the benefits may stem from a simple speeding up of cognitive functions. In the case of Alzheimer's disease and other cortical dementias, their use can lead to a 'paradoxical' inhibition of excess activity.

This paradoxical inhibition of excess activity even extends to mania. A number of clinicians have given dexamphetamine or other stimulants to manic patients and have found that it calms them down – temporarily. This links into a neglected line of work on the stimulants, which emphasises the fact that the results obtained with stimulants may depend in part on the baseline level of activity of the person to whom they are given.[23]

Finally, stimulants are also used to treat narcolepsy, a disorder that involves falling asleep abruptly (see Section 6).

DOPAMINE AGONISTS

Stimulants work on the dopamine system. This makes them relatives of the dopamine agonists used for Parkinson's disease. Cabergoline, pramipexole and ropinirole are the best known of these. The key points that the dopamine agonists bring out are that drugs that stimulate dopamine can cause stereotyped or compulsive behaviours (see below). These include compulsive gambling and sexual activity, so this is not harmless. It is also clear that the dopamine agonists for some people come with a serious dopamine agonist withdrawal syndrome (DAWS). This has brought into greater relief the question of whether people become dependent on stimulants and suggests that yes they do.

User issues

Side effects and interactions

The stimulants (Table 8.1) are given in slowly increasing doses, with dexamphetamine and methylphenidate being given in doses from 5 to 60 mg and other stimulants in the equivalent dose range. These medications have a short half-life and therefore have to be given in twice or thrice daily doses. This has led to an increasing use of slow-release preparations.

The side effects include an increasing hyperactivity, leaving an individual with too much motor energy and drive. The energy is relatively unfocused, so that, rather than getting lots of useful things done, the person is left pacing up and down. They may be unable to sleep properly and may become increasingly anxious, even paranoid. Side effects such as this should lead to a discontinuation of treatment. Related to these effects may be an increase in nervousness, palpitations, increased irritability and aggression and an increased number of tics. If any of these effects appear, they are likely to get worse with continued treatment.

Amongst the most famous side effect of stimulants are stereotypies. This has a range of lay descriptions such as punding. It can lead to the compulsive behaviours that are very obvious in the case of the dopamine agonists, such as compulsive gambling and sexual activity. In general the risk is a loss of judgement as the person goes on something of an auto-pilot.

The dopamine hypothesis of schizophrenia was born from the idea that amphetamines could trigger a schizophrenia-like psychosis. They can unquestionably cause hallucinations and delusions, but the clinical picture is more of a paranoid psychosis rather than schizophrenia proper.

Stimulants classically suppress appetite in the short term. This may lead to a reduced rate of growth in children. This delay in growth may be overcome by a drug holiday, for instance during the school holiday, but it is not something to take lightly. Over the longer run, stimulants have been linked to weight gain in some.

When the amphetamines were banned, the question of whether they cause dependence and a withdrawal syndrome was unresolved. Some said they didn't. The dopamine agonists have brought the nature of stimulant withdrawal more clearly to light. These drugs do cause dependence, and the problems that remain afterwards can endure for a considerable time. There is, at present, no known treatment. Many people will be diagnosed as being depressed rather than in withdrawal and given an antidepressant, which is unlikely to help.

Yet another group of problems are the development of tics or motor disturbances. Children on stimulants have a high rate of verbal or motor tics, which may show themselves as minor facial twitching or grunting. When tics develop, unless there is a very clear benefit to treatment, ongoing use of the stimulant should stop. However, it is not uncommon instead to find children put on drugs such as clonidine or antipsychotics such as risperidone or olanzapine to manage these problems.

One of the problems in the field of childhood psychotropic drug prescription is the enthusiasm of many prescribers. Born in part from a desire to help, prescribers who sometimes see themselves as having to battle against forces hostile to the drug treatment of children do neither their patients nor their

Continued

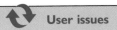

User issues—cont'd

cause any good by refusing to give up in the face of non-response or a frank deterioration in the child's state. In some cases this means that children who become overactive on a stimulant will be co-prescribed a sedative or an antipsychotic where treatment might be better discontinued.

Perhaps the most serious problem on both stimulant and related medication in children is the occurrence of fatal cardiac problems. There is a significant number of children prescribed stimulants, antidepressants, or antipsychotics who simply drop dead on them. This may be linked in some instance to pre-existing cardiac problems, but in a significant proportion of cases it is likely to stem from dopaminergic input to the regulation of the cardio-respiratory system and to the effects as well of the drugs on QT intervals. If anything, perhaps because they are more active or prone to infections, children seem more at risk from QT lengthening problems than other age groups.

Stimulants potentially interact with monoamine oxidase inhibitors (MAOIs) and some antihypertensives. But in the main their use is relatively uncomplicated by interactions.

Table 8.1 ***Commonly used stimulants***

Generic drug name	UK trade name	US trade name
Dexamphetamine	Dexedrine	Dexedrine
Dexamphetamine and d,l amphetamine		Adderall
Methylphenidate	Ritalin	Ritalin
Dexmethylphenidate		Focalin
Slow-release formulations		
Dexamphetamine		Adderall XR
Methylphenidate	Concerta Equasym Medikinet	Concerta Equasym Medikinet
Non-controlled 'stimulants'		
Modafinil	Provigil	Provigil
Atomoxetine	Strattera	Strattera

PSYCHOTROPIC DRUGS AND CHILDREN: GENERAL PRINCIPLES

In the main, the first clinical trials undertaken to get a drug on the market are not done on children. This means that when new drugs become available they have not been tested on children. This throws up two issues. One centres on the issue of whether a drug which works for adults will also work for children. The other centres on the issue of safety of usage in children.

In general across medicine, clinicians who have a treatment that works for a condition in adults, when faced with a comparable condition in children will use that treatment. For instance, clinicians faced with a convulsing child will not hesitate to use an anticonvulsant even if the drug they choose has not been shown to work in children. This use depends on an understanding that the condition being treated is the same in children and adults.

The same principle can apply in the case of nervous problems in children. Obsessive–compulsive disorder (OCD), for instance, is a condition known to begin as early as 3 or 4 years of age and to last through to adulthood, and there is no reason to believe that the condition in adults differs from that in children so that in severe cases of OCD, a drug treatment that works in adults can be considered for children also. In just the same way, it might be reasonable to consider using drugs like lithium for a severe bipolar disorder in adolescents or even a treatment like ECT for a severe depressive disorder or catatonia.[24]

That being said, the use of drug treatments in children is fraught with uncertainties. A number of conditions that may have similar names in adults and children do not appear to be the same conditions. For example, what are often termed psychotic or schizophrenic disorders in children may, in fact, be pervasive developmental disorders rather than prodromes of an adult psychosis. Whilst full-blown and severe bipolar disorder can occur in adolescence, this in fact is rare, and the use of treatments for bipolar disorders in adolescents should be correspondingly rare and should not happen in children. Children get depressed, but until recently it was thought these depressions were better regarded as distress rather than early onset depressions of the type that happen to adults, and the resort to antidepressants should be much more cautious as a consequence.

THE CHANGING PICTURE

Vigorous company marketing in recent years has added to the complexities in this area. When a drug company gets a licence to market a drug for ADHD, depression or bipolar disorder, this does not mark the point at which clinicians become able to use these drugs for children, but rather the point at which the companies are enabled to start converting aspects of childhood into disorders and to build pressure to have these disorders treated with drugs. This marketing underpins the current mania for diagnosing bipolar disorders. In the case of many children with difficulties, what this means is that if a diagnosis of ADHD and a prescription for stimulants fails, the child is likely to be rediagnosed as bipolar and put on a prescription for sedatives such as olanzapine or valproate.

Where once we were concerned drugs such as cannabis might be gateway drugs leading onto harder drugs, now we have gateway diagnoses like ADHD or depression in children, where failure of treatment does not lead on to rethinking the problem but rather a move to a harder diagnosis like bipolar disorder and a corresponding treatment. Clinical problems such as suicidality on SSRIs have become marketing opportunities for companies pushing compounds that are even more problematic in paediatric settings.

In addition to ever wider use of drugs for children, there is a new safety issue. Until recently, clinicians treating children with psychotropic drugs had standard rules of thumb for working out the best doses of treatments. Whilst clinical trials will not have been used to set these doses, there is every reason to believe that older ways of approaching these issues in children were safer in that they inevitably led to a gradual dose escalation based on close monitoring for side effects. Pharmaceutical companies in contrast at this stage have a clear track record in making doses available through clinical trials that suit their marketing interests rather than the best interests of the child.[25]

In recent years, this mix of competing interests has been disturbed by the regulators who since 1990 have been requesting companies to undertake trials in children to establish drug safety profiles. This has led to an extensive series of clinical trials, most of which have either not been reported or when reported have been couched in grossly misleading terms so that whilst on the one hand we seem to be moving into an era where there is apparently more data that might inform clinical judgement, in fact there is a greater need than ever to be concerned about the quality of that data.

It has been difficult for companies to show their drugs work for childhood disorders. But rather than informing clinicians of this or seeking a licence that would make their data public, they have taken to producing grossly misleading articles and having academic staff make presentations at medical meetings on the reality of childhood illness and the benefits of the company's medication. The lecture fees for professors come to a lot less than paying the salary and pension costs of a sales staff.

The changing picture does not stem solely from company marketing. Other factors have helped transform the picture. First, getting a diagnosis for a child, whether of autism, ADHD or another condition, has become a means in some cases to get the child other social supports and in some cases disability payments.[26] Second, there is a general perception from the adult field that clinical trials have proven the treatments work, and if they work and as a result reduce the risks for children that stem from an untreated condition, many parents will feel compelled to accept treatment. Third, there is a perception that the drugs do not have side effects and clinicians do little to deter this perception. Fourth, in some instances parents do want to sedate their child and this need has meant there has always been some use of psychotropic drugs for children. Fifth, there is a profoundly disturbing use of antipsychotics in particular amongst children in foster care and with learning disabilities that has been happening for a long time but has escalated in recent years.

A further important factor is the use of operational criteria. In 1980, the DSM III introduced the notion of operational criteria to overcome the profound divides between biological psychiatry and psychodynamic approaches. We might not agree on the cause of a problem or even its correct treatment, but we could surely agree if five clinical features were present or not, and in the case of depression the presence of five out of nine agreed features meant you 'met criteria' for the disorder.[2] Meeting criteria for a disorder is not the same thing as having it though. For instance, pregnant women or any of us who have influenza would often meet criteria for depression – if we lose sleep, have altered appetite, feel more anxious than usual, are more fatigued than usual and lose interest in things. In 1980, it was assumed that clinical judgement would mean that if there was another explanation for why a person had particular symptoms, they would not be diagnosed as depressed. But once criteria began to be put up on the internet, often by drug companies, many people doing their own research have found them and find they meet criteria and come to the conclusion that they or their children have some condition that they do not in fact have. I have had people with successful careers in public life, who have accessed the Internet in this way, tell me they have Asperger's syndrome and ADHD or possibly bipolar disorder. This is just simply wrong.

THE USE OF ANTIDEPRESSANTS FOR CHILDREN

For a long time the conventional wisdom was that antidepressants did not work in children.[27] Despite the failure to show benefits in repeated clinical trials, however, the use of antidepressants, especially SSRIs, continued to grow through the 1990s. At the prompting of the Food and Drug Administration (FDA), companies undertook trials in OCD, social phobia, panic disorder and depression.[28] Most of these trials on fluoxetine, sertraline, paroxetine and venlafaxine remained either unreported or reported in misleading or fraudulent terms.[29] Suicidal acts were coded as emotional lability whilst aggression, including homicidal ideation, was coded as hostility. At the end of the day, the SSRIs could be shown to produce some benefits in OCD and in social phobia but not in depression or generalised anxiety.

These trials also brought hazards to light. Across all these conditions, SSRI use was associated with children becoming suicidal. The fact that children became suicidal was missed by many of those reading the academic literature, who did not realise that articles describing emotional lability as a side effect of SSRI use were in fact referring in code to children who had become suicidal. There was also clear-cut evidence of children becoming aggressive on SSRIs, but again what was happening was not clear from articles in the academic literature that simply described children as becoming hostile.

Based on these findings, in 2003, the regulators in Britain and elsewhere advised strongly against the use of antidepressants in children on the basis that the hazards were not balanced by clear-cut benefits, in contrast to the situation in adults where there was some benefit. The evidence pointed to a doubling of suicidal acts on these drugs compared to placebo.

There remains grounds to consider the use of SSRIs for children – in OCD for instance. Whilst behaviour therapy is the best treatment to try first for conditions like this, in some instances drug treatment may make good sense.

In terms of treating children, the use of these drugs needs to be monitored to ensure the child gets the benefit of treatment without undue risk. All of the side effects outlined in Chapter 5 are likely to be found in children, with an extra concern linked to our lack of knowledge as to what effect treatment will have on the developing brain and sexuality.

There are further issues. Children on SSRIs show a slowing in their rate of growth. Also a number of adults show reduced levels of sexual hormones and, in some cases, a persistent loss of sexual function on SSRIs in particular. We have no idea what effect this might have on the processes of puberty (see Chapter 5 and Chapter 20).

THE USE OF ANTIPSYCHOTICS FOR CHILDREN

Until recently antipsychotics were used sparingly in children. This has changed for a number of reasons. First, these drugs have been used to manage the side effects of stimulants given to children. Second, they have been used in the current mania for bipolar disorders in some cases even for preschool children. Third, they have a growing use in research and in clinical practice by clinicians who believe that this use might prevent a psychosis from developing in those thought to be at risk of developing schizophrenia. Fourth, the drugs are being used for newly minted conditions like DAMP or disorders like autistic spectrum disorder. In almost all instances, these various usages involve the use of newer rather than older antipsychotics.

A large number of the trials of these drugs have been undertaken in children across diagnoses. The results have been dismal, with the trials often ending early and being left unreported. So there are no good data on the frequency with which the side effects appear in children, but there is every reason to believe that children will display an increased sensitivity to weight gain, diabetes and the full range of problems found in adults with additional effects consequent on the impact of these drugs on the developing brain.

Unless a child's problem is very severe and/or the child's response to treatment shows clear and substantial benefits, it is difficult to justify the use of antipsychotics in children, other than on a short-term basis. A number of other points can be made. First, there is something of a global consensus at present that bipolar disorder does not exist in children. It rarely starts before adolescence. Second, although these drugs are called antipsychotic, there is little reason to believe they are likely to forestall the emergence of a psychosis. Third, their use to manage the side effects of other treatments, such as tics or hyperactivity, is injudicious. It would be preferable to stop the provoking agent. Fourth, these drugs are used to manage difficult behaviour in children, sometimes under a diagnosis of hyperactivity. Whilst some efforts to sedate difficult children have always happened, the process is open to abuse and the use of antipsychotics is particularly abusive. Fifth, children may be even more sensitive than adults to the weight promoting and diabetes inducing effects of these drugs and at least as sensitive to the effects of these drugs on the heart.

REFERENCES

1. Atigari O, Healy D. Ketamine and treatment resistant mood disorders. Aust N Z J Psychiatry 2013;47:998–1001.
2. Healy D. The creation of psychopharmacology. Cambridge, MA: Harvard University Press; 2002.
3. Claridge GC. Drugs and human behaviour. London: Allen Lane; 1970.
4. Rasmussen N. On speed. New York: New York University Press; 2008.
5. Bradley C. The behavior of children receiving benzedrine. Am J Psychiatry 1937;94:577–85.
6. Klein R. Children and psychopharmacology. In: Healy D, editor. The psychopharmacologists, vol. 3. London: Arnold; 2000. p. 309–32.
7. Rapoport J. Phenomenology, psychopharmacotherapy and child psychiatry. In: Healy D, editor.

The psychopharmacologists, vol. 3. London: Arnold; 2000. p. 333–56.
8. Diller L. Running on Ritalin. New York: Bantam; 1998.
9. DeGrandpre R. Ritalin nation. New York: Oxford University; 1998.
10. DeGrandpre R. The cult of pharmacology. Durham, NC: Duke University Press; 2007.
11. LeFever GB, Dawson KV, Morrow AL. The extent of drug therapy for attention deficit-hyperactivity disorder among children in public schools. Am J Public Health 1999;89:1359–64.
12. Lefever-Watson D, Arcona A, Antonuccio D, et al. Shooting the messenger: the case of ADHD. J Contemp Psychother 2014;44:43–52.
13. Gillberg C. Deficits in attention, motor control and perception: a brief review. Arch Dis Child 2003;88:904–10.
14. Jensen PS, Arnold EL, Swanson JM, et al. Three-year follow-up of the NIMH MTA study. J Am Acad Child Adolesc Psychiatry 2007;46:989–1002.
15. Hutchings J, Gardner F, Bywater T, et al. Parenting intervention in Sure Start services for children at risk of developing conduct disorder: pragmatic randomised controlled trial. BMJ 2007;334:678–81.
16. Dub LM, Lurie L. Use of benzedrine in the depressed phase of the psychotic state. Ohio State Med J 1939;35:39–45.
17. Chiarello RJ, Cole JO. The use of stimulants in general psychiatry. Arch Gen Psychiatry 1987;44:286–95.
18. Lieberman JA, Kane JM, Alvir J. Provocative tests with psychostimulant drugs. Psychopharmacology (Berl) 1987;91:415–33.
19. Bellak L, Kay SR, Opler LA. Attention deficit disorder psychosis as a diagnostic category. Psychiatr Dev 1987;5:239–63.
20. Bowers MB, Swigar ME. Psychotic patients who become worse on neuroleptics. J Clin Psychopharmacol 1988;8:417–21.
21. Huckle PL, Thomas R. Pemoline and neuroleptic induced side effects. Ir J Psychol Med 1991;8:174.
22. British Medical Association Ethics. Boost your brain power: ethical aspects of cognitive enhancement, <www.bma.org.uk/ap.nsf/cognitiveenhancement>; 2007.
23. Robbins TW, Sahakian BJ. 'Paradoxical' effects of psychomotor stimulant drugs in hyperactive children form the standpoint of behavioural pharmacology. Neuropharmacology 1979;18:931–50.
24. Healy D, Nutt D. British Association for Psychopharmacology consensus on childhood and learning disabilities – psychopharmacology. J Psychopharmacol 1997;11:291–4.
25. Healy D, Mania A. Short history of bipolar disorder. Baltimore: Johns Hopkins University Press; 2008.
26. Diller L. The last normal child. Westport Connecticut: Praeger Press; 2006.
27. Healy D. Let them eat Prozac. New York: New York University Press; 2004.
28. Sharav VH. The impact of FDA Modernization Act on the recruitment of children for research. Ethical Hum Sci Serv 2003;5:83–108.
29. Healy D. Manufacturing consensus. Cult Med Psychiatry 2006;30:135–56.

SECTION 5 **MANAGEMENT OF ANXIETY**

SECTION CONTENTS

The anxiety disorders

9

CHAPTER CONTENTS

DRUGS USED IN ANXIETY

Six groups of drugs are used to manage anxiety, as shown in Box 9.1.

TYPES OF ANXIETY

To understand how these drugs may be useful, it is necessary to understand the types of anxiety. The term anxiety covers four sets of experiences, expressed in a variety of symptoms.

First is mental anxiety, which roughly translates as worry or a preoccupation with things that might go wrong. This may also include intrusive ideas, thoughts or impulses of a distressing nature. This form of anxiety may be present without many physical symptoms such as increased muscular tension, heart rate, sweating or shaking. Antipsychotics, opiates and selective serotonin reuptake inhibitors (SSRIs) tend to work on this component of anxiety.

Second is physical tension, which consists of a knotting of the various muscles around the body. This probably results from an inhibition of action. When we get emotional or worried, we review possible things to do to sort

BOX 9.1 Groups of drugs used to treat anxiety

- The antipsychotics. These are considered in Section 1.
- The antidepressants. These are dealt with in Section 2 and Chapter 11.
- Minor tranquillisers of the benzodiazepine type. These are covered in Chapter 10.
- Drugs active on the serotonin system, which are discussed in Chapter 11.
- Beta-blockers such as propranolol, which are considered in Chapter 12.
- Stimulants. These are dealt with in Section 4, Chapter 8.

our problems out and in the process prepare our muscles for action – tensing them up. If all we do is think about things and do nothing, that tension is not discharged and may become chronic. Physical relaxation or activity, alcohol and benzodiazepines work on this component of the anxiety spectrum.

Third is a set of physical symptoms, such as increased heart rate and increased intensity of the heart beat – palpitations – a shake in the hand, sweating, feeling faint, butterflies in the stomach and sometimes nausea, loosening of the bowels that may lead to diarrhoea, and a tendency to breathe more shallowly and quickly. This hyperventilation can produce symptoms such as tingling in the hands and legs, pins and needles, light-headedness and visual disturbances. Beta-blockers have been thought to help some of these features of anxiety.

Related to the symptoms produced by hyperventilation, there is a fourth form of anxiety called dissociative anxiety. The cardinal features of this are:

- Depersonalisation – a feeling of being detached or removed from oneself or as though one's body is not operating normally (see Chapter 5).
- Derealisation – an impression that the world seems unreal, flat or as though everything is happening on a stage (see Chapter 5).
- Out-of-body experiences that relate closely to depersonalisation and derealisation.
- Hallucinations – either auditory or visual.
- Recurrent waves of emotion or recurrent short-lived black moods.
- Episodic feelings of being numb, either mentally or physically, to the point where one can cut oneself and not feel any pain.
- Amnesia for past events – whether the happenings of the day or episodes in one's past life.

FORMS OF ANXIETY

In addition to the types of anxiety mentioned above, there are a number of situations in which anxiety arises and according to which it is categorised and treatment given.

STAGE FRIGHT

This is the kind of anxiety that everyone gets when faced with an interview or having to perform for others. Typically stage fright leads to increased muscular tension, sweating, butterflies, a tremor in the hand and palpitations, as well as a feeling perhaps of being unreal or out of touch. In other words, some aspects of all of the forms of anxiety mentioned above may be experienced.

Stage fright can often be helped by either minor tranquillisers or beta-blockers. The basis for a response to these drugs appears to lie in an interruption of the feedback from increased heart rate or muscular tension to the mental state. When we worry about something and our heart rate increases, our hands shake and we begin to perspire; these symptoms can in turn lead us to be more anxious. If these signs of anxiety are blocked, we appear to assume that we are less anxious and as a result we become less anxious. This tricking of ourselves is a legitimate manoeuvre and is undoubtedly what human beings have been doing for millennia, mostly by using alcohol to abolish the manifestations of anxiety – giving us Dutch courage.

There are two problems with this approach. One is that it is normal to feel anxious before a performance of any kind and some anxiety probably helps us to perform at a higher level than otherwise. People who are too relaxed may lose a certain amount of 'edge', and in this manner over-zealous tranquillisation may impair performance.

The second pitfall lies in starting treatment too early. In the case of a concert, a speech or an interview, treatments should be used only on the day of the performance or the night before. Danger arises when performances come close together and an individual is self-medicating for too long before each performance so that they slide into a routine of constant medication. This may produce dependence in the case of drugs such as alcohol or benzodiazepines.

Another problem is that whilst it is legitimate to use drugs of this sort if they are found to be effective, there is an inevitable tendency to rely on the drugs rather than to develop the skills to help manage activities such as interviews, or performing in front of others. A judicious use of anxiolytics to combat stage fright, on the other hand, may enable the taker to go on stage and perform and in the process to become accustomed to performing in front of others. In other words, anxiolytic drugs can lead, if used properly, to their own discontinuation.

NEUROTIC ANXIETY

We all become acutely anxious on occasions. If the anxiety is intense or long lasting, or if it catches us at a vulnerable time, there is a tendency for it to organise itself into a neurosis. A neurosis is a relatively long-lasting and self-perpetuating maladaptation to anxiety.

For example, someone who has a shock whilst out shopping may perhaps be left nervous. They may then, when they come to go shopping next, find that they are apprehensive about going out. If they do not go out to the shops, perhaps by getting someone else to go instead, the nervousness about going shopping may become established. Not going shopping to avoid becoming anxious about shopping leads to an inability to go shopping and damage to your self-image. Such problems can be self-perpetuating.

Sometimes the difficulty may clear up spontaneously. Many neuroses also respond very well to behaviour therapies, which act on much the same principle as telling someone who has just fallen off a horse to get up and ride again as quickly as possible. Blocking avoidance responses and exposing oneself to the thing that one is afraid of are the basic behavioural methods for handling neurosis. They work extremely well and are, broadly speaking, the optimal therapy for phobic and obsessive–compulsive neuroses.[1]

However, there are other treatments and anxiolytics that are commonly used for various neuroses. To understand their place, we will first lay out the different kinds of neuroses and then indicate where and why drug treatments may also be employed.

PHOBIC NEUROSIS

There are both general and specific phobias. A general phobia of going out is termed agoraphobia. The specific phobias involve phobias of a particular thing such as a fear of spiders, snakes or thunder and lightning.

Exposure therapy is the treatment of choice for specific phobias and for phobic disorders uncomplicated by depressive illness. Antidepressants are also often used for agoraphobia but rarely for specific phobias. One rationale for using antidepressants in these conditions is that many people who are agoraphobic will also have a depressive disorder, and if this is tackled, the neurosis may clear up. However, in addition to the clearing up of a depressive disorder, the SSRIs and monoamine oxidase inhibitors (MAOIs) appear to be independently anxiolytic, and treatment with these drugs can produce benefits for those who are phobically anxious but not depressed.

PANIC DISORDER

Panic attacks are episodes of intense anxiety that can come on in company, out of doors or indoors at home alone. The primary experience is usually intensely physical – acute awareness of a thumping heart and shaking hands, with feelings of nausea, weakness and shortness of breath, but there are usually also thoughts of impending doom. Panic disorders typically seem to come out of the blue. These attacks may lead secondarily to a phobia of going shopping if, for example, the first attack happened in the supermarket.[2]

There have been vigorous attempts to market anxiolytics, particularly the benzodiazepine alprazolam, for panic disorder. Most of the antidepressants have also been tested in panic disorder and shown to have a certain amount of usefulness.

Exposure therapy is used widely to manage panic disorder, as is cognitive therapy.[3] Briefly, the behavioural and cognitive approaches propose that people who panic interpret symptoms such as palpitations, breathlessness or weakness as indicators of an imminent stroke, loss of control, heart attack or outburst of some sort. They then take evasive action to avoid such an outcome. A person worried about a heart attack will, for example, sit down – just as any reasonable person who actually thought they were having a heart attack would do. This sitting down and taking things easier, however, perpetuates the problem. Treatment aims to get the person to do the opposite to what they have been doing and to try to get hold of the thoughts that come to their mind during episodes of panic, so they can recognise what is happening. Over and above this, the cognitive approaches further emphasise the thinking style of affected individuals.

SOCIAL PHOBIA

Three forms of social phobia are described. The first is a specific form that involves fear of performing in front of others, sufficient to lead to avoidance. Second, a generalised form of social phobia involves avoidance of most occasions of interaction with others. This may range from avoidance of shopping because of difficulties in asking for things to crossing the street when aware of the approach of anyone who might want to engage in conversation. This phobia involves extreme self-consciousness: affected individuals evaluate themselves as boring. Finally, there is a condition termed 'avoidant personality disorder', which, as the name implies, is a state where an individual's freedom to act is heavily constrained by their interpersonal difficulties. In its extreme form, individuals with this condition may become housebound. There is a high incidence of alcohol abuse and other phobic disorders, panic disorder or depression, with social phobia, so these problems are far from trivial.

Until the 1970s, social phobia was unrecognised in the West, although it is commonly diagnosed in the East. It is still likely to be viewed by many as a form of shyness, in other words not as something that should lead someone to seek medical help so that it neither presents in primary care nor is detected by primary-care physicians.[4] Some estimates claim 3% of the population are affected, but such estimates and efforts to ensure the condition is detected and treated have been seen by many as a classic instance of disease mongering.[5]

MAOIs and SSRIs may bring about some improvement in the condition and may do so for individuals with severer forms of the disorder, even in the absence of any obvious depressive disorder. Beta-blockers or benzodiazepines appear to be of limited usefulness. There are a number of specific behavioural and cognitive strategies for social phobia also.

Whilst the condition is real and may be severe, in recent years it has become a symbol of how pharmaceutical companies market diseases. Creating awareness of the condition will lead many people who are shy to seek help; the problem is that treatments often do more harm than good.

OBSESSIVE–COMPULSIVE DISORDER (OCD)

OCD may present three fairly dissimilar ways. First is a general indecisiveness and inability to take action. Second is an obsessional and ritualised checking on things, such as whether one's hands are clean or whether one has locked the back door, turned off the gas – things we all do, but which in OCD are done to an extraordinary and disabling extent.[6] Third is having images of oneself shouting out obscenities in public or impulses to pick up a knife and skewer one's children. The fear that such imagery or impulses may generate can be extreme.

The drug for which most research has been done is clomipramine (Anafranil).[7] Based on its success, studies were undertaken of the SSRIs for OCD, and broadly speaking all these drugs seem to take the edge off intrusive mental worries or imagery – see Chapter 11.

In addition to being anxiolytic, there may be an underlying depressive disorder, the stress of which has precipitated the full-blown OCD. Resolution of the underlying depression may bring about an improvement of the neurosis or make the person more accessible to a behavioural programme.

Is the usefulness of the SSRIs in OCD down to some anxiolytic effect of serotonin reuptake inhibition, or are these drugs in some way specifically anti-obsessional?[8] In favour of the idea that the SSRIs help because they are non-specifically anxiolytic is the fact that these drugs also seem to be useful in panic disorder, social phobia and other anxiety states. This raises the question of whether any other anxiolytics may be useful for OCDs. The simple answer to this is that we do not know. No proper clinical trials have been done on any other agents. It seems unlikely that beta-blockers or benzodiazepines would be particularly useful as there are no prominent physical symptoms of anxiety in OCD.

However, there is often a marked degree of agitation and, on this basis, one might imagine that antipsychotics would be useful. Before the recent vogue for using SSRIs, antipsychotics were used quite widely and successfully in OCD.

The main form of treatment for OCD is behavioural management, for both OCD involving rituals or intrusive imagery and impulses. Behaviour therapy is much less successful for OCD characterised solely by indecisiveness or slowness. The principle behind a behavioural approach in these disorders is to expose the sufferer to the thing that is frightening them the most and to block, at least temporarily, their avoidance of what they have been avoiding. This forces the individual to encounter the stimulus to their fears and to habituate to it. Such an approach may produce a brief spell of intense anxiety, but it appears to be an effective way of breaking obsessive cycles of behaviour.

HYSTERICAL OR DISSOCIATIVE DISORDERS

At one time, hysteria was the commonest diagnosis in medical circles for patients with nervous problems. It has fallen out of favour for a variety of reasons. It remains the case, however, that there are a number of patients who have classical hysterical disorders leading them to, for instance, seemingly become paralysed in a leg or an arm or to go blind in an eye without there being any apparent physical basis for the problem. Ordinarily these problems are triggered by some sort of psychological shock or ongoing stress. Less dramatically there are innumerable patients in medical settings who have medical symptoms without a clear physical cause, such as repetitive stress injuries.[9] These presentations are commonly termed somatisation.

Whilst gross hysteria or somatisation can unquestionably happen without the affected individual also being depressed, a depression may underpin cases of hysteria. Effective treatment of any underlying depression may therefore help clear up a hysterical neurosis.

Hysteria is also commonly called dissociative disorder or conversion disorder or somatisation today rather than hysteria.[10] Simply put, dissociation means that psychological functioning is in some way split by pressure or stress. For example, the idea of how to use your arm is cut off from the actual arm itself so that whilst there may be nothing wrong with your arm, you may not be able to use it – it may effectively be paralysed. Under strain or stress, people may often be cut off from memories of things that happened in the past, even so profoundly cut off as to be unable to remember their own name or how they got to where they are. This is not uncommon in people before interviews or exams.

At the turn of the 19th century, Sigmund Freud, Pierre Janet and others argued that hysteria arose in response to trauma. Many of the features of hysteria as they described it then correspond well with what is now termed post-traumatic stress disorder (PTSD). PTSD officially came into being in 1980. It is a condition linked to trauma, whether rape, physical violence, sustained mental torture or disasters. These traumas lead to a split within the individual so that they are in part cut off from what happened to them, which returns in experiences of recurrent intrusive images of what has happened or awarenesses of something that they may be afraid happened to them, but which they cannot clearly remember, or uncertainties regarding things they feel they ought to have done during the traumatic episode, such as struggle more in the course of a rape. These experiences alternate with episodes of numbness, blankness and amnesia.

Long-standing wisdom suggests that if caught soon after the initial trauma, tranquillisation with benzodiazepines or barbiturates may help. Quite commonly, people who have a PTSD also develop a depressive disorder at points during the course of their post-traumatic state. Antidepressants in this case may be helpful for the depressive component of the picture. SSRIs in principle should be helpful, even in the absence of depression, because of their anxiolytic effects. At present the evidence is mixed – a large number of failed trials remain unpublished, and there are few data on the drugs being useful for men.

PTSD was recognised in the early 1980s, and a number of attempts have been made to produce techniques such as debriefing to manage the intrusive images and episodes of emotion that happen in this disorder. At present these techniques seem unhelpful, and the condition seems more likely to resolve (at least temporarily) if the subject can actively engage in doing new things and getting on with life.

When the condition has become chronic, it is common to find that sufferers resort to alcohol or minor tranquillisers to numb the distress they feel. Whilst these may work very effectively in the short term, and may even in the short term assist in the resolution of the disorder, neither works well in the long term.

Finally, whilst stressors such as war have always been recognised to bring problems in their wake, the term PTSD is used much more widely now than just for trauma of the kind found in war or after rape, for instance. It is almost certainly the case that many cases now designated as PTSD would be better seen as instances either of anxiety or depression rather than PTSD.

A further condition called borderline disorder or borderline personality organisation would once also have been labelled hysteria. Present research links this condition to trauma or neglect in childhood, which leads to recurrent dissociative experiences and later unstable interpersonal relationships and self-injurious episodes. Individuals with this disorder have been diagnosed under a range of headings from schizophrenia to brief recurrent depressive disorders.

Antidepressants may sometimes be of use in these states, but in many instances they may aggravate the depersonalisation and derealisation to which such individuals are prone, and in clinical trials for these conditions, the SSRIs in particular seem unhelpful or indeed more likely to aggravate rather than help. Antipsychotics may help to reduce impulsive behaviour, such as self-mutilation. Benzodiazepines appear to be the most reliable means of bringing to an end the acute episodes of dissociation or extreme agitation that accompany this disorder but are not suitable for chronic use.

HEALTH ANXIETY OR HYPOCHONDRIASIS

Another condition, whose former name now has pejorative associations, hypochondriasis, has been renamed as health anxiety. Both depression and anxiety may produce a range of physical sensations, some of which may be extremely uncomfortable and may give the impression that there is something physically wrong. Googling sensations of weakness and the odd sensations that may come about as a result of anxiety, in particular after hyperventilation, would be quite likely to lead many of us to diagnose ourselves with something like multiple sclerosis.

It may be very difficult to shift an individual from such a diagnosis. Besides which, the medical profession has a reputation for not telling patients when they have got something seriously wrong with them such as cancer, schizophrenia or multiple sclerosis. Accordingly, the fact that a doctor does not confirm the diagnosis for many people may not be very reassuring.

A number of other factors may play a part in the generation of a health neurosis. One is that attention to a physical complaint is likely to aggravate that complaint by giving it greater salience. Such attention may have a defensive quality to it. When any of us are under stress, one mechanism for coping with the problem is termed a displacement reaction. This is what happens when, for example, we have to study for an exam or write an awkward letter, and somehow a range of other things seem easier to do – tidying the pens in the holder, clearing out the drawer in the desk, etc. In the same way, attention to a physical problem may be a means of not facing something more stressful. Prolonged displacement on to the supposed physical problem may lead to an ongoing focus on health functioning long after the original stressor has been resolved.

An unhelpful focus on aspects of health is more likely in someone who has particular ideas about their health. Thus, someone who believes that their bowels must move at least once per day, and that there are serious consequences for their health if they do not, may get very preoccupied by the constipation that often goes with depression or antidepressants. Chronic insomnia can be viewed as a form of health anxiety, often made worse by fixed ideas about the need for a regular 8 hours' sleep. Fixed ideas like this tend to run in families.

Far from being a mild disorder, health anxiety will often lead to repeated visits to doctors or alternative therapists. And visits to the doctor will result in the person being put on antihypertensives, lipid-lowering or other drugs that will produce symptoms in their own right, many of which the doctor may deny could be linked to treatment. The disorder can become extreme, with an individual becoming paralysed by their concerns and their incessant complaints leading to alienation from family members, doctors and others.

There are a number of cognitive strategies for health anxiety[11] that resemble those in use for panic disorder (both conditions involve a misinterpretation of physical symptoms). Behaviour therapies have not been as effective as in obsessive or phobic disorders. A general anxiety management strategy may help, particularly if there is any evidence that some of the symptoms come on after episodes of hyperventilation.

GENERALISED ANXIETY DISORDER (GAD)

This is what used to be called anxiety.[12] It involves unrealistic or excessive anxiety and apprehensive expectation about two or more problems, such as worry about possible misfortune to one's child (who is in no danger) and worry about finances (for no good reason). For a diagnosis of GAD, a person must be bothered by these concerns for more days than not.

This is a form of anxiety that combines worry with signs of motor tension, autonomic hyperactivity and of increased vigilance and arousal. The symptoms of motor tension include trembling, shakiness, muscle aches or soreness, restlessness and easy fatigability. Those of autonomic hyperactivity include shortness of breath or smothering sensations, palpitations, sweating, cold clammy hands, dry mouth, dizziness or light-headedness, nausea, diarrhoea or other abdominal distress, hot flushes or chills, frequent urination and trouble swallowing or a 'lump in the throat'. The symptoms of increased vigilance and arousal include feeling keyed up or on edge, exaggerated startle responses, difficulty concentrating or finding one's mind going blank because of anxiety, trouble falling asleep and irritability.

In practice there is considerable overlap between GAD and panic disorder, PTSD, social phobia and depression, with regard to both symptoms and the fact that many individuals may present with a phobic neurosis one year, GAD the next, and perhaps OCD the following year. If one of the worries is about health, then distinguishing GAD from health anxiety may be very difficult. A book by Patricia Pearson gives a vivid account of what it can be like to suffer from states like this and how drug treatment can make things worse.[13]

However, broadly speaking, GAD refers to the large number of anxious states in which individuals appear globally or diffusely anxious, in which there has been no crystallising of the anxiety into a clear phobic or obsessive state or preoccupation with health as the sole focus of concerns. For these reasons, it may be difficult to see a point of entry for cognitive or behavioural strategies. GAD, therefore, is the anxiety state for which general practitioners and others have tended to resort to the use of minor tranquillisers and for which they have been blamed for an inappropriate tranquillisation of distress. They are now likely to use SSRIs on the basis that these drugs supposedly do not produce dependence, are anxiolytic and that behind a GAD there may often be a depressive disorder and anxiety that, according to pharmaceutical companies, stems from a serotonergic imbalance.

The problem with GAD lies in the maladaptive or habitual nature of the anxiety or in its severity. Very often the sufferer may have very real problems that are relatively intractable, and 'out of sympathy' a doctor will prescribe something to try to calm the person down or to take the edge off their distress.

This may lead, when the pills fail to work, to an increased level of prescription or to the addition of yet other drugs into the cocktail. The person in question has their distress dulled – but often at a cost.

When not disablingly severe, GAD is the form of anxiety that lends itself most readily to interpretive approaches. These may include an identification of the real stresses that the individual may be under, such as an unsatisfying marriage, isolation from family or friends or pressures at work. The identification of such stresses and the institution of appropriate anxiety management strategies may be all that is needed to bring about considerable change.

CATATONIC ANXIETY

Catatonia is covered at various points in the chapters on antipsychotics, antidepressants and mood-stabilisers, where it has not been portrayed as an anxiety state. But in fact this state is one that features high levels of internal anxiety in the sufferer, and it is highly likely that there are briefer forms of the condition going undetected at present where the person affected is precipitated acutely in to a state of very high anxiety lasting hours or days, either out of the blue or linked to stress – a kind of extended panic attack. Anna Karenina had all the features of catatonic anxiety as she walked to her death.[14]

These states are often misdiagnosed as panic attacks or severe mood disorders and given antidepressants or antipsychotics when they are much more likely to respond to high doses of benzodiazepines given for a few days.

THE NOTION OF AN ANXIOLYTIC

The first treatments for nerves were generally sedating and were termed sedatives. There was no notion that there was anything else to do with nervous problems other than sedate the affected person. The first breach in this way of thinking came when it was found that stimulants could be used for nervous problems. Whilst they made many people more anxious or unsettled, they settled others. This fits with theories of nervousness stretching back centuries that suggested these problems arose because of lack of tone in the nervous system.

In 1955, Frank Berger launched meprobamate, the first non-barbiturate sedative. In the course of developing this drug, which had pronounced muscle relaxant properties, Berger argued that it should be possible to produce a drug for nervous problems that was not sedative – a drug that might work by producing muscle relaxation without sedation.

To distinguish meprobamate from the older sedatives, Berger used the term tranquilliser. Meprobamate and the benzodiazepines ended up termed minor tranquillisers, to distinguish them from the major tranquillisers such as chlorpromazine.

The benzodiazepine dependence crisis of the 1980s turned the term tranquilliser into a problem. As a consequence, pharmaceutical companies have been careful to call the SSRIs anxiolytics rather than tranquillisers, a term that, for the moment, does not have the connotations of a tranquilliser. However, there is no reason why the benzodiazepines could not also be called anxiolytics.

Benzodiazepine anxiolytics

10

CHAPTER CONTENTS

INTRODUCTION

The dust is beginning to settle on the benzodiazepine controversies (Table 10.1).[15] There are a number of excellent histories of these drugs.[16,17] When they were first introduced, these drugs were seen as being of major benefit. They were regarded as extremely safe and effective. They were popular with physicians, consumers and the pharmaceutical industry. However, during the 1980s the benzodiazepines came to be described as one

Table 10.1 *Commonly used benzodiazepine anxiolytics*

Generic drug name	UK trade names	US trade names
Diazepam	Formerly Valium	Formerly Valium
Chlordiazepoxide	Librium	Librium
Lorazepam	Ativan	Ativan
Bromazepam	Lexotan	Lexotan
Oxazepam	Serenid	Serax
Alprazolam	Xanax	Xanax
Clobazam	Frisium	Frisium
Medazepam	Nobrium	Nobrium
Clorazepate	Tranxene	Tranxene
Clonazepam	Rivotril	Klonopin

of the greatest menaces to society in peacetime. They were seen as the epitome of the psychotropic drug juggernaut. A group of drugs that was more difficult to stop than heroin.

As these things played out in the media in the late 1980s and early 1990s, benzodiazepine dependence was portrayed as the only case of drug dependence in which the dependent person was viewed with sympathy. He or she was portrayed as a victim of forces beyond their control rather than as the author of their own destiny.[18] The benzodiazepine crisis marked a point where consumers first took up arms against the medicopharmaceutical complex, rather than simply against the dangers of a particular group of drugs.

On the other side, doctors and industry claimed these drugs remained remarkably safe, that reports of dependence and withdrawal reactions were exaggerated, and that problems were probably more linked to the personality of the sufferer than to the pharmacology of the drugs.

These opposing views became polarised making it difficult to write an account of the benzodiazepines. The position taken here will be that the benzodiazepines are safer for most people than they were perceived to be some years ago, and they have crept back into secondary care use for this reason. But there remains a large group of individuals who, through no fault of their own, will encounter enduring difficulties after exposure. The enduring withdrawal issues are real. There is great overlap with selective serotonin reuptake inhibitors (SSRI) protracted withdrawal syndrome (see Chaper 23). Whilst these problems remain to be explained there will continue to be hostilities between patients and medicine/pharma. In so far as clinicians continue to deny these problems, they will be tarred with an industry brush.

Another way to frame this issue is that to the public and primary care doctors benzodiazepines seem like a darker drug than SSRIs, so much so that the brand name Valium has been withdrawn, but in fact the SSRI group of drugs almost certainly pose greater hazards to takers than Valium ever did. Most lay people if forced to take Valium or Prozac for a year would take Prozac, but most secondary care staff, if forced to choose, would likely choose Valium.

When the benzodiazepines arrived in 1960, the alternatives were the barbiturates or the antipsychotics. The barbiturates caused excessive sedation, marked dependence and fatalities in overdose. The antipsychotics, whilst not afflicted with these problems, had their own drawbacks, as outlined in Section 1, and their prescription was seen as inappropriate for milder disorders. The irony now is these same drugs are being blithely prescribed to children from infancy onwards.

The benzodiazepines had none of the side effects of the antipsychotics. Compared with the barbiturates, they produce a relatively mild sedation, seem to cause less physical dependence and, most of all, are safe in overdose. They became increasingly popular and widely prescribed. A wide-scale chemical tranquillisation of anxiety ensued.

We now recoil from what happened during the 1960s and 1970s. There is evidence that many patients do as well with brief counselling from general practitioners as they do on benzodiazepines and that they are as happy with such counselling. General practitioners today often squirm in the face of such findings, but before the large-scale prescription of benzodiazepines, there was a great deal of chemical management of anxiety disorders with barbiturates and painkillers, and there is now a wholly comparable use of SSRIs for just the same problems. The question of finding a balance in this area seems to be an issue that is with us always. Hence, it may be somewhat naive to ascribe the dark side of the benzodiazepine story solely to the pharmaceutical industry following the siren call of the profit motive.

MECHANISM OF ACTION OF THE BENZODIAZEPINES

We know more about how benzodiazepines work than we do about almost any other psychotropic drug. The first development in our understanding of the benzodiazepines came with the discovery that a compound called γ-aminobutyric acid (GABA) is one of the most plentiful neurotransmitters – more common than serotonin or noradrenaline. It is the brain's principal inhibitory neurotransmitter. Benzodiazepines modulate normal functioning of the GABA system by binding to one of three types of benzodiazepine receptor, BZ1, BZ2 and BZ3, which mediate sedative, myorelaxant and anxiolytic effects, respectively.

It has emerged that there are a number of natural compounds within the brain, the β-carbolines, which bind to the same sites on the GABA receptor as the benzodiazepines. One surprising finding has been that β-carbolines may both alleviate anxiety and produce relaxation just as benzodiazepines do, but also that other β-carbolines may cause anxiety, tension and convulsions. This finding changed our understanding of how neurotransmitters and receptors work naturally. It had previously been thought that neurotransmitters act on receptors and that drugs may either mimic this action or antagonise it. It now seems clear that some compounds may produce opposite actions at the same receptor site. Where actions on benzodiazepine receptors are concerned, we can now produce compounds that relieve anxiety, compounds that increase anxiety and compounds that block both of these effects. These three types of compounds differ, but all act at the same receptor.

Another interesting feature of the benzodiazepines is that in contrast to other neurotransmitters such as noradrenaline, dopamine and serotonin, which are found in single-celled or quite simple organisms, benzodiazepine receptors are confined mostly to cortical areas of the brain and have emerged only in higher animals.

CLASSES OF BENZODIAZEPINES

By convention the benzodiazepines are divided up according to their half-life – the length of time it takes for the amount of the drug in the blood to decrease to half its initial level after a standard dose. There was a great deal of interest in this concept during the 1970s, as it was thought that producing a benzodiazepine with a short half-life might overcome hangover sedation apparent with some of the longer-acting compounds. The half-life of some of the earlier compounds was so long that taking the pills regularly meant that a first pill had not washed out of the system by the time a second was taken, and so on. This led to an accumulation of the drug, which in the elderly was a problem. However, even in the case of the supposedly shorter-acting compounds, it should be kept in mind that whilst the duration of action depends on the chemical make-up of the compound, it also depends on how much of the drug is given: a large amount of a short-acting compound will act for a long time (see Box 10.1)

CLINICAL USES FOR BENZODIAZEPINES

Benzodiazepines give a relaxing warm glow, like alcohol. There is a sense of muscular release and a soothing feeling that many (but not all) people describe as pleasant. In one sense the benzodiazepines are one of the 20th century's greatest inventions. After 2000 years of trying to improve on alcohol, they represent success in some respects. Like alcohol, they can be used for general relaxation purposes, as anti-anxiety agents for acute crises such as interviews or whatever, and they are just generally pleasant without causing liver, heart, joint or gut problems.

ANXIOLYSIS

Benzodiazepines are anxiolytic but by no means universally anxiolytic. They are of benefit in anxiety states that have a significant muscular tension or

BOX 10.1 Benzodiazepines classified by duration of action

Long	Intermediate	Short	Ultra-short
Chlordiazepoxide	Flunitrazepam	Alprazolam	Midazolam
Clorazepate	Nitrazepam	Lorazepam	Triazolam
Diazepam	Lormetazepam		
	Oxazepam		

dissociative component to them. The anxiolytic effect of benzodiazepines appears to resemble most the effects of alcohol. This effect differs from the 'anxiolytic' effect of the antipsychotics, which work best in distraught and agitated rather than in anxious states. Benzodiazepine anxiolysis also differs from the anxiolysis brought about by beta-blockers, which work best in states characterised by increased heart rate, palpitations, butterflies in the stomach and shakes of the hand. It also differs from the serenic effect produced by SSRIs and other compounds acting on the serotonin system.

The above description of the anxiolytic effects of benzodiazepines is only approximate. Greater precision is not possible at present, which seems remarkable given that so many benzodiazepines have been prescribed and taken in the past 50 years. One might expect that there would be a better appreciation of just what kind of anxiolysis they bring about. This is a major indictment of the way we develop drugs at present.

ANTICONVULSANT

In addition to being anxiolytic, the benzodiazepines are anticonvulsant. They are not used widely for epilepsy because carbamazepine, valproate, lamotrigine and others are preferred for chronic use. In states of intractable epilepsy, however, the benzodiazepines may often be used in conjunction with these other compounds, and in status epilepticus diazepam is the drug of choice. Clobazam is also used more widely in epilepsy as it provides an anticonvulsant effect without producing the sedation associated with most benzodiazepines. Another benzodiazepine, clonazepam, is also used for the management of epilepsy, restless leg syndrome, myoclonic jerks and a range of other neuropsychiatric indications.

SEDATION

Benzodiazepines are sedative but less so than barbiturates that work on the same receptor. The sedation, however, varies from individual to individual and from benzodiazepine to benzodiazepine. With regular ingestion of benzodiazepines, tolerance to these sedative effects develops quite quickly. The sedative effects of benzodiazepines provide the basis for their use as hypnotics (see Section 6). Whilst the use of benzodiazepines as anxiolytics has fallen dramatically in the past 10 years, their use as hypnotics has not. They are prescribed for sleeping purposes as regularly now as they were 10 years ago.

MUSCLE RELAXANTS

The muscle relaxant properties of benzodiazepines that makes them anxiolytic can also be used for patients with spasticity, dystonia and multiple sclerosis.

AMNESIA

The benzodiazepines can produce an amnesia that resembles the effect of alcohol on memory. Essentially, they impair the registration and subsequent recall of events. This seems to be most marked for short-acting agents such as lorazepam, midazolam and triazolam. It is also more marked when the drugs are given intravenously. For this reason, short-acting benzodiazepines are given before operations to produce amnesia regarding the events of surgery. Something like this effect may also be partly responsible for complaints from people hooked to benzodiazepines for years who claim that periods of their lives seem indistinct or blotted out.

The effects of benzodiazepines on memory are at present the subject of much investigation. In general, it has been believed that stimulants improve memory, whilst sedatives impair it. This appeared to apply to the benzodiazepines, until it has more recently become clear that many amnestic effects of these drugs occur in periods after the sedative effects have worn off. The amnestic effects also seem to be better linked to the rate of binding to benzodiazepine receptors rather than simply to receptor binding.

ABREACTION

Paradoxically, the benzodiazepines may also be used for abreaction, a technique used to recover memories. Abreaction involves getting individuals to remember scenes from their past life in great detail. In the course of such remembering, it is hoped that hints about or glimpses of a significant event will be recovered. Abreaction can be conducted without pharmacological intervention of any sort, but commonly the relaxation produced by a tranquilliser helps, and mystique is introduced by hints that remembering is being assisted by a truth drug.

A partial reconciliation of the amnestic effects of benzodiazepines and their role in bringing back buried memories lies in the fact that the amnesia induced by these compounds is for events that happen after they have been taken, rather than for events that may have happened in the past. It is, for example, reasonable to work for an oral examination for weeks and then take a benzodiazepine the night before or morning of the oral without the homework done being wiped out. What is more likely to happen is that memory of the exam itself may be hazy.

ALCOHOL WITHDRAWAL

The benzodiazepines are the standard first-line treatment for alcohol withdrawal. The early institution of a comprehensive benzodiazepine regimen for such individuals has all but abolished the rigours of alcohol withdrawal and prevents individuals going into delirium tremens on withdrawal. Before the benzodiazepines, delirium tremens had a high level of fatalities. The benzodiazepines can then be tailed off over the course of a week or two.

CATATONIA AND NEUROLEPTIC MALIGNANT SYNDROME

In recent years the benzodiazepines have become the first-line treatment for catatonic syndromes and for neuroleptic malignant syndrome (see Chapter 3). Lorazepam is used most often, in doses of up to 16 mg per day, but diazepam or other benzodiazepines in high doses are equally likely to be effective.[18]

It seems highly likely that there are many milder forms of catatonic anxiety presenting to clinicians and being misdiagnosed as panic attacks for severe mood disorders that would be much more likely to respond to high doses of benzodiazepines given for a few days than to antidepressants or antipsychotics.[14]

MANIA

Benzodiazepines are regularly prescribed in mania, particularly in North America. There seems to be no clear theoretical rationale, but it may be that the high incidence of catatonic features in bipolar disorders leads to a noticeable benefit and that this perceptible benefit underpins the practice (see Chapter 6).

RAPID TRANQUILLISATION

Concern has developed in recent years about deaths that have occurred during the course of the rapid tranquillisation of those showing disturbed or violent behaviour with antipsychotics. The intramuscular use of antipsychotics has been implicated. These concerns have prompted a fresh look at regimens for rapid tranquillisation and a consensus has emerged that benzodiazepines have a place. The agent most commonly used at present is lorazepam (0.5–2.0 mg) because its short duration of action makes it less likely to accumulate. This will often be given alone or in combination with an antipsychotic.[20]

The primary hazard in the use of benzodiazepines for rapid tranquillisation is respiratory depression. If this occurs, it can be reversed by flumazenil (Anexate), which can be given continuously (200 μg intravenously, up to 600 μg) or administered in a glucose or saline solution.

User issues

Side effects of benzodiazepines

Sedation

Sedation is a feature of all benzodiazepines except clobazam. It can impair normal daily functioning. It was to avoid such effects that the intermediate- and short-acting benzodiazepines were synthesised. The impairment of daily functioning that can occur with tranquillisers such as diazepam or with sleeping pills such as nitrazepam are comparable to the effects produced by alcohol. These compounds also impair reflex reactions and car-handling ability. Surprisingly, however, given current concerns with alcohol and driving, there is no ban against driving under the influence of benzodiazepines.

The sedative effects of benzodiazepines depend on the state of arousal of the individual. For a subject who has never had benzodiazepines before, 5–10 mg of diazepam may be heavily sedating. For an individual used to benzodiazepines, 5–10 mg of diazepam may produce a noticeable but not undue sedative effect. The same individual having a tooth extraction or going to an interview may be

Continued

User issues—cont'd

able to take 30–40 mg without significant sedation. Up to 100 mg of diazepam may be necessary in some agitated states to produce noticeable sedation.

Rebound anxiety
In some cases benzodiazepine intake may cause as much anxiety as it alleviates. This effect is similar to an effect produced by alcohol. Individuals with marked anxiety problems, such as phobias, often turn to alcohol to help them cope with situations they know will provoke anxiety. Whilst it may help in the short term, becoming alcohol dependent leads to withdrawal anxiety as the alcohol wears off. Similarly, intake of benzodiazepines, particularly of the shorter-acting benzodiazepines, may lead in susceptible individuals to an early development of withdrawal-based rebound anxiety. (See rebound insomnia in Section 6.)

Amnesia
The amnestic effects of benzodiazepines have been the basis for many complaints regarding their use. However, these amnestic effects can also be put to good use before an operation, for instance, as well as for dental procedures, endoscopy or other procedures that involve the passage of tubes or instruments into the body for investigative purposes.

Concerns surrounding procedures such as these led to the first clear recognition of the amnestic effects of benzodiazepines. Patients undergoing dental procedures and endoscopy claimed that they had been taken advantage of.[14,21] The investigation of these claims led to the recognition of a complicated picture. There was usually a clear relationship between events that had occurred and the complaint made. For example, in the case of dental procedures and endoscopy it was claimed that oral sex had taken place. Similarly, in procedures involving an individual having to squeeze a hand to pump up their vein before a blood sample was taken, it was claimed that the patient had been forced to masturbate the other person. In some cases accusations have been upheld; in others the judgement has been that the drowsy state the subject was in made them more suggestible.

Ordinarily, the amnestic effects of benzodiazepines are not noticed. Every so often, however, people taking benzodiazepines find that something dramatic happens. For example, a colleague of mine, after flying home from abroad and taking a short-acting benzodiazepine on the flight to promote sleep, went to his parents' house immediately after getting off the plane. He met his sister in the drive and talked with her at length. The following day, when he met her again, he had no recollection of their encounter the previous day.

The benzodiazepines produce an anterograde amnesia – events that occur after taking them may not be registered fully. This effect is similar to the anterograde amnesia produced by alcohol. Benzodiazepines may interact with both the anticholinergics and alcohol to make amnesia even more likely. The effects are comparable to the blackouts some people have on alcohol, which can occur after having had only one or two units of alcohol. Conversations that have taken place after this modest amount of alcohol may not be recalled the next day.

User issues—cont'd

Dementia
A flurry of studies have linked benzodiazepine use to later dementia.[22] The links are clear but not big. The first point is that all psychotropic drugs can lead to nerve cell loss and, as a result, earlier brain failure than would otherwise have happened. The indications from studies are that some but not all takers are at risk for reasons we do not understand. Beyond this, it is difficult to advise other than to say this is a risk that needs to be in the frame – as much for the takers of hypnotics as the takers of anxiolytics.

Dissociation
Occasionally the benzodiazepines may produce dissociative reactions. The most commonly described reactions are states of hyperactivity. It is often thought that these involve disinhibition – that the benzodiazepines have inhibited some inhibitory pathway on the brain. This seems unlikely. What seems more likely is that just as alcohol in minute amounts may in certain individuals produce quite marked dissociative reactions characterised by profound amnesia and explosive behaviour, so also the benzodiazepines in certain individuals who are particularly sensitive to them may have toxic effects leading to excitability and overactive or explosive behaviour. Benzodiazepines have also been reported to produce depersonalisation, derealisation and hallucinatory experiences. The frequency of these is unknown.

Depersonalisation, derealisation and dissociative experiences are most commonly a feature of anxiety. When they occur in this context, a benzodiazepine is the most reliable treatment.

User issues

Benzodiazepines and driving
Psychiatric illnesses of all sorts slightly increase the risks of a road traffic accident (RTA). The relative effects of dementia, anxiety or depression are not known. Neither has work been done to differentiate between the RTAs stemming from untreated illness and those that stem from individuals on treatment. It would seem highly likely that antidepressants, antipsychotics, anticonvulsants and benzodiazepines or other agents with sedative properties, or disinhibiting agents might contribute to RTAs.

Section 4 of the 1988 Road Traffic Act makes it a criminal offence for a person to drive under the influence of drugs, prescribed or otherwise. Present recommendations suggest that driving licences should not be issued to or renewed for individuals who regularly take psychotropic regimens that would hamper their ability to drive safely.[23] There are a number of problems here, one of which is the fact that there can be considerable interindividual variability in terms of how disabling a treatment is. Another concerns the locus of responsibility should an accident happen. At present the climate is shaping up that mental-health professionals are best advised to warn subjects taking

Continued

User issues—cont'd

benzodiazepines, other sedatives or antidepressants of the potential risks, of the need for them to avoid driving if they are experiencing difficulties and to record that they have issued such advice. In the case of individuals who drive large goods vehicles or passenger-carrying vehicles, the problems are clearly of a much more serious order and merit careful consideration. This is one of those situations where, in certain circumstances, the professional duties of confidentiality may be outweighed by other considerations.

BENZODIAZEPINE DEPENDENCE AND WITHDRAWAL

The significance of benzodiazepine dependence will be considered further in Chapter 23. This chapter overviews the clinical management of possible problems.

A significant number of people have problems with withdrawal from benzodiazepines. Others do not. The medical response to this issue has been terrible – writing off the problem as stemming solely from individuals who either have a personality problem or who are experiencing a recrudescence of the initial anxiety, which their benzodiazepines had suppressed for a period of time. This recourse to personality is unwarranted given the current state of the evidence. But it's the typical medical response to a problem – blaming antipsychotic-induced tardive dyskinesia or antidepressant-induced suicidality on the sufferer rather than the treatment.

The developments in our understanding of how benzodiazepines work, outlined above, shed some light on the question of why some individuals develop problems on these drugs. The nature of the benzodiazepine receptor and the dual action of endogenous compounds, such as the β-carbolines, on it opens up the possibility that one cause of problems following benzodiazepines may be that the receptors on which they work have been blocked for so long by these compounds that they become hypersensitive to the effects of the natural compounds in the brain that cause anxiety, insomnia, muscular tension and convulsions. Discontinuing drug treatment then leaves a hypersensitive receptor bombarded by anxiogenic compounds.

The degree to which the benzodiazepine receptors shift to a state of being sensitive to the natural compounds acting to produce anxiety in the brain is almost certainly genetically determined. There will therefore be a range of liabilities to shift. This range is, in turn, likely to cause some people to become more sensitive to withdrawal of these compounds and to become sensitive at a quicker rate than others.

If a large number of people are given the same benzodiazepine for the same period of time, different people will show differential rates at which rebound anxiety and rebound insomnia develop. Current research suggests that 20–25% of us are at risk of having marked sensitivity to benzodiazepine withdrawal. The corollary of this is that, for the remaining 75%, benzodiazepines are safer than they have been portrayed.

But there is another issue here, aside from withdrawal. Benzodiazepines appear to cause damage – in both the peripheral and central nervous system and some those who can take them without having a marked withdrawal problem may have other problems if they take them chronically.

In the sections on antidepressants and anticonvulsants, the risks of sensory neuropathies were outlined – burning hands and feet as well as mouths or genitals, along with a range of strange pain experiences, for instance, in response to altered temperature, or numbness. These effects are commonly reported by takers of benzodiazepines also. And it is likely that they represent damage that emerges once treatment is reduced or stopped just as tardive dyskinesia does. The good news is that whilst there is no clear remedy, it does seem like many of these are in principle treatable – it's just a matter of finding what helps.

Apart from physiological factors in the takers of benzodiazepines, there appear to be pharmacological factors to do with the drugs themselves that may produce sensitivity to withdrawal. It increasingly appears that benzodiazepine compounds that have a short half-life and that enter the brain rapidly are more likely to produce problems on withdrawal. Such compounds include alprazolam and lorazepam. The irony here is that the short-acting compounds were produced in the first instance to avoid the prolonged sedation that may be associated with benzodiazepines with a longer half-life such as diazepam or chlordiazepoxide.

SYMPTOMS OF BENZODIAZEPINE WITHDRAWAL

Box 10.2 lists the symptoms that are now accepted as features of the withdrawal syndrome associated with benzodiazepines, but which for a long time

BOX 10.2 Symptoms associated with benzodiazepine withdrawal

- Increased anxiety with all its physical symptoms
- Poor sleep
- Unsteady gait
- Numbness
- Muscle pains
- Feeling of things moving, as though on a boat
- Aggressive feelings
- Depression
- Weakness and tiredness
- Flu-like symptoms
- Hallucinations
- Paranoid ideas
- Seizures
- Confusion
- Depersonalisation or derealisation
- Paraesthesiae – a range of odd sensations including burning feet and hands
- Restlessness
- Nausea, abnormal taste and gastrointestinal cramps

were dismissed by sceptical medical practitioners as manifestations of a recrudescence of anxiety.

Withdrawal is most likely to occur if a person is taking a high dose of a short-acting benzodiazepine that is tapered abruptly. It also seems somewhat more likely if the individual was highly anxious before being put on benzodiazepines and if they have a previous history of neurosis, although this latter is controversial. Current recommendations are that an individual should consider themselves hooked or at serious risk if they cannot stop benzodiazepines for 2–3 days, whenever called upon to do so.

At present it is also recommended that benzodiazepines should not be prescribed for longer than 4 weeks. After that, prescribers should review the issues rather than simply repeat the prescription. As a result of these restrictions and replacement by the SSRIs, in some countries (UK) benzodiazepines are prescribed less frequently as a first-line treatment for anxiety, but in others (US) they are still widely prescribed.

Along with recent horror stories of medical negligence in creating physical dependence on benzodiazepines has gone a set of stories, less widely publicised, of doctors who, reacting with therapeutic Calvinism to the current climate, have withdrawn all benzodiazepines from all their patients regardless. This is often highly inappropriate, particularly in the case of older individuals who have been on the drugs for a decade or more with little or no ill effect.

WITHDRAWAL STRATEGIES

There is a recognised strategy for withdrawal management. If an individual has difficulty in withdrawing from a short-acting benzodiazepine, they should be switched to a compound with a long half-life, such as diazepam, as this is less likely to give rise to rebound phenomena.

Using the long half-life strategy, the usual regimen is to taper over 6 weeks or so, reducing one-quarter of the dose in the first week, one-quarter in the second week and one-eighth in each of the subsequent 4 weeks. The last dose level or two may need to be drawn out longer in some cases.

There have been attempts to find a compound that would attenuate benzodiazepine withdrawal. To date, none seems particularly effective. Clonidine, carbamazepine, antidepressants and beta-blockers have been used but with no convincing effects. The benzodiazepine antagonist, flumazenil, can both push individuals into withdrawal and dramatically shorten the length of time for which withdrawal is liable to last, but it doesn't seem to reduce the number of complaints of enduring post-withdrawal problems.

There is some dispute as to how long the withdrawal syndrome lasts. For most it appears to be effectively over in a matter of weeks, but others have symptoms recurring for months or years. Recent indications that SSRI 'withdrawal' may last months or more gives credence to claims regarding the duration of benzodiazepine problems, but these problems may stem from damage rather than withdrawal.

PSYCHOLOGICAL MANAGEMENT OF WITHDRAWAL

Whilst it is clear that dependence is not a matter of some neurotic flaw in the personality of the affected individual, an individual's psychology may play a part in the ease or otherwise with which they can withdraw from benzodiazepines. A phobia of withdrawal is accordingly something that can be predicted in certain individuals and, where it occurs, it can be managed psychologically as any other phobia might be managed.

There have now been a number of trials showing that a package involving education about the nature of panic and anxiety, training in slow diaphragmatic breathing, correction of maladaptive thinking about anxiety and repeated exposure to feared bodily sensations can make a significant difference for some – but not all – individuals.[24]

Anxiolysis and the serotonin system

11

CHAPTER CONTENTS

INTRODUCTION

Serotonin was first isolated in the intestine in 1933 and called enteramine. Ninety per cent of it is found in our gut. It was rediscovered in blood vessels in 1947 and found to cause them to constrict, which led to it being called serotonin. In 1949, it was established that the chemical structure of serotonin was 5-hydroxytryptamine (5HT). Both names, 5HT and serotonin, have remained in use. The name serotonin survives partly because SmithKline Beecham stumbled on the marketing appeal of the acronym SSRI (selective serotonin reuptake inhibitor) for paroxetine.

Shortly before serotonin was discovered in the brain, lysergic acid diethylamide (LSD) had been discovered. It became clear that there were structural similarities between serotonin and LSD. This led, at the beginning of the psychopharmacological era, to interest in the role that serotonin might play in mental illness.[25–27] However, serotonin disappeared from view, partly because of the emergence in 1965 of the catecholamine hypothesis for depression.

By the 1970s, it seemed that dopamine was the 'psychosis' neurotransmitter, noradrenaline the 'mood' neurotransmitter and acetylcholine the 'dementia' neurotransmitter (see Section 7). The one disorder left for serotonin was anxiety. Whilst this parcelling out of disorders appears simplistic, the SSRIs are in some way anxiolytic. Clomipramine, fluoxetine and paroxetine are useful for phobic and obsessional states as well as depression. This applies far less to antidepressants that do not inhibit serotonin reuptake.

With the development of the SSRIs, there was increasing interest in the serotonin system. This led during the 1980s to a sustained effort to characterise the receptors that serotonin acts on and to develop drugs specific to each of these.

SEROTONERGIC RECEPTORS AND DRUGS

Over 17 different types of serotonergic receptor have been described. For our purposes, the ones of interest are S1, S2 and S3 receptors. Drugs acting on serotonergic (S) receptors divide into agonists (drugs acting on a receptor) and antagonists (blocking the receptor) (Table 11.1). One of the key points to remember about the SSRIs is that they make more serotonin available at these receptors, and they are therefore either indirect serotonergic agonists or antagonists.

SSRIS

SSRIs as a group are more clearly anxiolytic than antidepressant. But when the SSRIs launched, the marketing imperatives dictated that they were marketed as antidepressants rather than tranquillisers. It was clear however that the companies would seek licences for anxiety states also, and this they did during the 1990s. Paroxetine, venlafaxine, sertraline and other SSRIs have been licensed for post-traumatic stress disorder (PTSD), obsessive–compulsive disorder (OCD), generalised anxiety disorder (GAD), social phobia and other anxiety states. What a licence means is not that clinicians are now able to

Table 11.1 ***Serotonergic system drugs***

	Agonist	Antagonist
S1a	Buspirone Flesinoxan Gepirone Ipsapirone flibanserin	Spiperone Propranolol
S2a	D-LSD	Ketanserin Mianserin Mirtazapine Trazodone Nefazodone All antipsychotics
S2b	mCPP	Ritanserin
S2c		Mianserin Mirtazapine Agomelatine
S3	Varenicline Ethanol	Ondansetron Granisetron

prescribe these drugs for patients who are anxious, but rather that companies have the chance to market anxiety, and they did this to the tune of hundreds of millions of dollars per year. This marketing has come complete with references to the chemical imbalance that is supposedly the cause of GAD or social phobia. What chemical imbalance – lowered serotonin levels. There are also references to non-habit-forming paroxetine or to the fact that anxiety can be treated with benzodiazepines or SSRIs, but the benzodiazepines cause dependence. The implication is that SSRIs do not cause dependence. But SSRIs cause a severe dependence just as much as benzodiazepines do.

The side effects and interactions of the SSRIs listed in Chapter 5 are the same for both anxiety and depression. Dependence on SSRIs is dealt with in Chapter 23.

S1 AGONISTS

Buspirone, an S1 agonist, was marketed under the trade name Buspar in the mid-1980s as an anxiolytic. Given the degree of concern there had been about the use of benzodiazepines to treat anxiety, it seemed a safe bet that a non-benzodiazepine anxiolytic, an anxiolytic that did not produce dependence, would sweep the market. Buspirone flopped.

There seems to be three reasons for this. First, buspirone does not give the same pleasant feeling that the benzodiazepines produce. Patients didn't 'go for it'. Second, it does not work immediately. The benefit can take anywhere from 2 to 4 weeks to appear, which is not much help for someone who is acutely anxiety. Finally, the reaction to claims that it is not dependence producing were: 'Oh yes, we've heard that one before…'.

In the treatment of anxiety, buspirone is used in doses from 5 mg three times a day to 30–60 mg daily. The side effects are those of the SSRIs. The problems are worse if it is combined with other drugs active on the serotonin system, such as SSRIs, or with antipsychotics. The use of drugs active on the serotonin system in combination with a variety of other psychotropics also may lead to the development of a 'serotonin syndrome' (see Chapter 5).

Other S1 agonists followed buspirone, including ipsapirone, flexinoxan and flibanserin. These all show efficacy in screening tests for anxiolytics. At one point it seemed like some of them might be marketed as a new class of compound – serenics. Instead, all three were developed for depression but failed to make it as antidepressants. Buspirone was also repackaged as an antidepressant. Why? And what does the failure mean?

There is some clinical trial evidence in support of this strategy, but the real reason appears to be that drug treatment of anxiety had a bad name in the wake of the benzodiazepines. For this reason, the word tranquilliser is banned. General practitioners and others are happier handing out antidepressants or anxiolytics, which they think are not habit forming.

There is, in fact, little basis to distinguish between S1 agonists and SSRIs. If the SSRIs work, it must be through one of the serotonergic receptors. S1 agonists are essentially SSRIs, with less serotonin around to act indiscriminately on a range of other receptors. Just like the SSRIs, S1 agonists take 2–4 weeks to take effect. This is unlike benzodiazepines and more like an 'antidepressant'. Are the S1 agonists then antidepressants? Or are the SSRIs anxiolytics that happen to be effective in milder depressions? Is the marketing of both of these groups of drugs[8] as antidepressants a clever or perhaps a cynical marketing exercise?

This returns us to the question of what do the SSRIs do? The SSRIs are beneficial in milder depressions, OCD, panic disorder, social phobia, GAD and PTSD. The easiest way to explain this broad effectiveness is to argue that SSRIs have a common serenic effect across these conditions. There is, in fact, good physiological evidence to indicate that SSRIs damp down fight-or-flight systems in the brain, making the individual less responsive to either internal or external signals of threat. Clinically it is very clear that when SSRIs work they make the taker more mellow, docile and serene. In some cases they do this to a greater extent than is desired, leading to complaints of emotional blunting or numbness.[28] An action such as this would explain why SSRIs are of benefit in a broad range of anxious states and beneficial only in anxious or primary care depressions and not in hospital or melancholic depressions.

The fact that the S1 agonists have failed as antidepressants also suggests that the SSRIs may be better viewed as having an anxiolytic effect rather than being antidepressants. The companies market the same mythical chemical imbalance to account for the benefit of the drugs whether they are advertised as antidepressants or anxiolytics. This myth worked much better for the SSRIs, which can be seen as restoring something to normal more than it did for the S1 agonists.

Migraine

Before leaving the S1 receptor, some mention can be made of the triptans, of which sumatriptan was the first launched. These drugs are used for the treatment of migraine. Serotonin is released into the bloodstream during a migraine attack. The previous treatments for migraine came from the fungus ergot, such as dihydroergotamine, which acts weakly on most serotonin receptors as well as on many non-serotonin receptors.

The conventional wisdom is that by acting on the S1 receptor on arteries leading to the brain, the triptans constrict cerebral arteries and thereby prevent the alternating constriction and dilatation of arteries that gives rise to the throbbing headache of migraine. One logical extension of this hypothesis is that other drugs active on the serotonin system, including the SSRIs, should have some potential either to alleviate or to aggravate migrainous attacks. In fact, however, SSRIs are also used to treat migraine, raising the possibility that just as the SSRIs blunt emotions, the triptans in fact work by blunting the perceptions of migrainous pain rather than by taking away its cause. In common with the effects of SSRIs for anxiety and depression, there is also some evidence from the treatment of migraine that whilst the triptans can be effective in relieving a headache that has just started, in a number of patients their use in fact leads to a greater frequency of headaches.

S2 AND S3 ANTAGONISTS

LSD and mescaline produce their effects by binding to the S2 receptor. These effects can be blocked in animals by ketanserin, an S2 antagonist. All antipsychotics, in addition to having common actions on D2 receptors, also block S2 receptors. Surprisingly, neither ketanserin nor any other S2 antagonists produce benefits in psychoses.

The presence in Table 11.1 of mianserin, mirtazapine, nefazodone and trazodone, and agomelatine, which have all been marketed as antidepressants, is of interest. Mianserin, mirtazapine and trazodone also have significant effects on adrenergic receptors, but this is much less so with agomelatine. mCPP, a compound related to trazodone, is an agonist for the S2b receptor and is potently anxiogenic. Also of interest is that trazodone and cyproheptadine and nefazodone, which are S2 antagonists, have aphrodisiac properties (see Section 8).

It seems likely that S2 antagonism also produces sedation. Compared with other antipsychotics, clozapine and chlorpromazine are sedative. Trazodone and mirtazapine, which are S2 antagonists, are also among the most sedative antidepressants.

S2c antagonism is thought to be a source of weight gain. The weight-gaining properties of antipsychotics such as chlorpromazine and clozapine, which act more potently at the S2c receptor, may stem from this source. Similarly, mirtazapine is particularly likely to cause weight gain. It remains somewhat unclear, however, just what role pure S2 drugs have.

S3 antagonism led to drugs like ondansetron and granisetron, which have been used for nausea. But recently another action has emerged. It seems clear that a number of people taking SSRIs become 'alcoholic'. They start craving alcohol and drinking compulsively.[29] Stopping the SSRI leads the alcoholism to clear up as does switching to a S3 antagonist like mirtazapine. A number of companies are developing S3 antagonist drugs for just this purpose at the moment.

SEROTONIN AND ANXIOLYSIS

WHERE THE DRUGS GO

It seems clear that serotonergic drugs are anxiolytic. How? One option lies in the overlap between the serotonin and dopamine systems. Both S3 and D2 antagonists are anti-emetic. D2 antagonists, SSRIs and S1 agonists all produce akathisia and dyskinesias. More directly, it has been shown that S3 antagonists modulate dopamine release. One possibility, therefore, is that many of these compounds that are active on the serotonin system are, as it were, atypical neuroleptics. That is, they produce the benefits of an antipsychotic without the same side effects.

The benefit of clomipramine and SSRIs in OCD is rather like the benefit produced by some antipsychotics – they produce a state of indifference to intrusive thoughts and imagery. The effect of antipsychotics however appears to come on far more rapidly than that induced by clomipramine or SSRIs.

On the other hand, some people can have both groups of drugs at the same time and distinguish between the 'indifference' caused by each. Furthermore, where antipsychotics help in schizophrenic disorders, SSRIs and tricyclics with clear actions on the serotonin system can often trigger psychotic decompensation.

There is a good case here for saying that the best scientific way forwards with this question would be to enlist the takers of these various drugs to attempt to determine whether the effects of antipsychotics and the effects of serotonergic drugs are similar, and if not similar, in what way do they differ? This, however, is not the way in which the modern pharmaceutical industry works. Uncontrolled observations by users or clinicians are not welcome. From the industry's point of view, any recognition of similarities of this type would not help the marketing process, which wants to keep these drugs in separate boxes.

Apart from the interaction between the serotonin and dopamine systems, there is also an interaction between the serotonin system and the γ-aminobutyric acid (GABA) system on which benzodiazepines work. Thus, it may be that benzodiazepines in part exert their anxiolytic action through effects on the serotonin system. Whilst this is theoretically possible, it seems that the benzodiazepines and the drugs active on the serotonin system bring about very different kinds of anxiolysis.

It is difficult to be more specific than this. As is the case with most drugs that have effects on behaviour, we know a lot about what receptors these drugs work on and how quickly they get there but very little about what the drugs actually do to those who take them, what it feels like to have them and exactly what aspects of anxiety respond to particular anxiolytics. We know a lot about where drugs go in the brain but very little about how they work.

This is surprising because, on the face of it, these should be the easiest of all data to collect. It reflects the fact that we simply have not been in the habit of sitting down and listening to the reports of those who take the pills, which is an unfortunate and even dangerous development.

Beta-blockers and anxiety

12

CHAPTER CONTENTS

INTRODUCTION

During the 1990s, with concern over benzodiazepine use, there was interest in the use of beta-blockers to treat anxiety. The principal drugs in this group are shown in Table 12.1.

Beta-blockers are used mainly in the treatment of hypertension, angina and cardiac arrhythmias. The rationale for their use in psychiatry is that they block the peripheral manifestations of anxiety, such as increased heart rate or shaking in the hands. Signs such as these are the cues we all use to judge how anxious we are. When these effects of anxiety are controlled, it seems that two sets of feedback loops may be interrupted. Part of getting anxious involves getting anxious at signs that one is getting anxious, such as increased heart rate and shaky hands. These manifestations of anxiety can lead to worries in their own right, for example the concert performer who may worry about both the audience and the effects of a shaky hand on the violin bow. Similarly, public speakers may have their nervousness made worse by the effects of a tremulous voice or a dry mouth in the act of speaking. Controlling effects such as heart rate, voice timbre and hand steadiness, therefore, can ease anxiety by removing the cues by which we all judge just how anxious we are.

PERFORMANCE-RELATED ANXIETY

The role of beta-blockers in anxiety was highlighted by their use by musicians experiencing stage fright, who find that by using them they are able to cope with being on stage and to give more assured performances. Up to one-third of orchestral musicians have been reported to use beta-blockers to steady their

Table 12.1 *Beta-blockers used for psychiatric illnesses*

Generic drug name	UK trade name	US trade name
Propranolol	Inderal/Beta-Prograne	Inderal
Atenolol	Tenormin	Tenormin

hands or control palpitations. They were also used by snooker players to reduce the amount of shake in a cue arm, allowing the player to hit the ball more surely.[21]

As little as 10 mg of propranolol per day may be all that is needed to block the manifestations of stage fright of this type. Doses greater than 40 mg are rarely needed.

GENERALISED ANXIETY DISORDER (GAD)

Because of concerns about benzodiazepines, primary-care doctors often prescribe beta-blockers for many of their more diffusely anxious patients. The rationale for this is much more tenuous than using these drugs for stage fright. In stage fright, treatment is tied to specific situations, but this is not the case in GAD and, as a consequence, much larger doses of beta-blockers have tended to be used and for longer periods of time.

The standard dose for propranolol used for GAD has been 20 mg four times a day, or 80 mg of longer-acting preparations. There have been trials on propranolol, oxprenolol, sotalol and practolol for GAD. Practolol has since been withdrawn from widespread use. Sotalol and oxprenolol had no clear anxiolytic effects. Other beta-blockers such as labetalol, metoprolol, timolol, pindolol, nadolol and atenolol have not been investigated for anxiolytic effects.

Propranolol, however, came out as being significantly anxiolytic without causing the sedative effects found with benzodiazepines. It brings about improvements in palpitations, sweating, diarrhoea and tremor. But propranolol has prominent effects on the serotonin system (see Chapter 10). Given that other beta-blockers are not effective in GAD, it seems quite possible that it is propranolol's effect on the serotonin system that is helpful.

PANIC ATTACKS: A PUZZLE?

Beta-blockers can be helpful in individuals who have prominent peripheral manifestations of anxiety – increased heart rate, etc. Surprisingly, however, there are no reports of these drugs being beneficial in panic attacks, in which physical symptoms of disabling intensity predominate.

TREMOR

The beta-blockers are also of use for lithium-induced tremor (see Chapter 7) and for a number of neuroleptic-induced dyskinesias (see Chapter 3).

AKATHISIA AND RESTLESSNESS

Propranolol, but not other beta-blockers, may also be of benefit in states of akathisia unresponsive to anticholinergic compounds (see Chapter 3 and Chapter 5). It also seems to be of some benefit in selective serotonin reuptake inhibitor (SSRI)-induced akathisia or dyskinesia.

PRAZOSIN AND POST-TRAUMATIC STRESS DISORDER (PTSD)

Prazosin is an alpha-blocker that also lowers blood pressure. It has crept into use as a treatment for the nightmares of PTSD. There may be some benefits but this is unclear. The chances are if used for this purpose it will be added to a cocktail of other drugs, and this is unsafe.

User issues

Side effects of beta-blockers

- All beta-blockers can cause shortness of breath. They should therefore be used with caution in anyone who has a history of wheezing or asthma.
- Beta-blockers can reduce circulation of blood to the extremities. In cold weather this may lead to painful and cold fingers, which of course may in their own right interfere with performances requiring dexterity, such as playing music.
- Beta-blockers also reduce the circulation of blood to muscles, and on this basis may need to be used with caution for performance-related anxiety. They may be unhelpful for singers because they may cause wheezing or shortness of breath and unhelpful to dancers or athletes because they reduce blood flow to muscles that may be needed for use. They may also inhibit performance by dropping blood pressure, leading to fainting.
- Some individuals have difficulties with sleep and nightmares on beta-blockers, especially propranolol. The reason for this is uncertain.
- Tiredness and lassitude are sometimes reported. This may be allied to a clear feeling of muscle weakness on exertion. There is no clear sedative effect of these compounds, however, and no indication that they interfere with ability to drive, for instance.
- Poor concentration and memory disturbances have also been reported. Propranolol does seem to reduce short-term memory span, even in healthy control subjects. This is different to the effects of benzodiazepines on memory, which involve not being able to recall things afterwards. Beta-blockers involve not being able to take in as much as usual at any one time.
- Hallucinations. In common with many other centrally acting compounds, the beta-blockers seem capable of producing dissociative effects, including hallucinations and confusion.
- In high doses, beta-blockers may cause nausea and vomiting, diarrhoea, dry eyes and skin rashes, but such doses should never be needed for the control of anxiety.
- Beta-blockers interact with many other drugs used for heart disease or hypertension.
- Beta-blockers cause fainting because of lowered blood pressure and nasal congestion.

REFERENCES

1. Marks IM. Living with fear. London: McGraw-Hill; 1978.
2. Klein DF, Healy D. Reaction patterns to psychotropic drugs and the discovery of panic disorder. In: Healy D, editor. The psychopharmacologists. London: Chapman & Hall; 1996. p. 329–51.
3. McNally RJ. Psychological approaches to panic disorder. Psychol Bull 1990;108:403–19.
4. Healy D. Social phobia in primary care. Prim Care Psychiatry 1995;1:31–8.
5. Moynihan R, Cassels A. Selling sickness. New York: Nation Books; 2006.
6. Rapoport J. The boy who couldn't stop washing. London: Fontana; 1990.
7. Beaumont G, Healy D. The place of clomipramine in psychopharmacology. In: Healy D, editor. The psychopharmacologists. London: Chapman & Hall; 1996. p. 309–28.
8. Healy D. The marketing of 5HT: depression or anxiety? Br J Psychiatry 1991;158:737–42.
9. Lucire Y. Constructing RSI: belief and desire. Sydney: University of New South Wales Press; 2003.
10. Healy D. Images of trauma: from hysteria to post-traumatic stress disorder. London: Faber and Faber; 1993.
11. Warwick HMC, Salkovskis PM. Hypochondriasis in cognitive therapy in clinical practice. In: Scott J, Williams JMG, Beck AT, editors. An illustrative casebook. London: Routledge; 1990. p. 78–102.
12. Smail D. Illusion and reality: the meaning of anxiety. London: Dent; 1984.
13. Pearson P. A history of anxiety. yours and mine. New York: Bloomsbury Books; 2008.
14. Healy D. Catatonia from Kahlbaum to DSM 5. Aust N Z J Psychiatry 2013;47:412–16.
15. Hindmarch I, Beaumont G, Brandon S, et al. Benzodiazepines: current concepts. Chichester: John Wiley; 1990.
16. Tone A. The age of anxiety: a history of America's turbulent affair with tranquilizers. New York: Basic Books; 2008.
17. Herzberg D. Happy Pills in America. Baltimore: Johns Hopkins University Press; 2008.
18. Bury M, Gabe J. A sociological view of tranquilliser dependence: challenges and responses. In: Hindmarch I, Beaumont G, Brandon S, et al., editors. Benzodiazepines: current concepts. Chichester: John Wiley; 1990. p. 211–26.
19. Fink M, Abrams R. Catatonia. Oxford: Oxford University Press; 2003.
20. Pilowsky L, Ring H, Shine PJ. Rapid tranquillisation. Br J Psychiatry 1992;160:831–5.
21. Wheatley D. The anxiolytic jungle; where next? Chichester: John Wiley; 1990.
22. Gage SB, Moride Y, Ducruet T, et al. Benzodiazepine use and risk of Alzheimer's disease: case control study. BMJ 2014;349:g5205.
23. Royal College of Psychiatrists. Psychiatric standards of fitness to drive large goods vehicles and passenger carrying vehicles. Psychiatr Bull 1993;17:631–2.
24. Barlow DH, Craske MG. Mastery of your anxiety and panic. Albany, NY: Graywind; 2007.
25. Carlsson A, Healy D. Early brain research in psychopharmacology: the impact on basic and clinical neuroscience. In: Healy D, editor. The psychopharmacologists. London: Chapman & Hall; 1996. p. 51–80.
26. Healy D. The antidepressant era. Cambridge, MA: Harvard University Press; 1998.
27. Healy D. Let them eat Prozac. New York: New York University Press; 2004.
28. Price J, Cole V, Goodwin GM. Emotional side-effects of selective serotonin reuptake inhibitors: qualitative study. Br J Psychiatry 2009;195:211–17.
29. Brookwell L, Hogan C, Mangin D, et al. One hundred cases of alcoholism triggered by serotonin reuptake inhibitor intake. Int J Risk Saf Med 2014;26:99–107.

SECTION 6
MANAGEMENT OF SLEEP DISORDERS AND INSOMNIA

SECTION CONTENTS

Sleep disorders and insomnia

13

CHAPTER CONTENTS

INTRODUCTION

Strictly speaking, insomnia is a complaint rather than a sleep disorder. The management of insomnia is not the management of people who have sleeplessness. Rather it is the management of people who complain about sleeplessness. In fact, the sleep of those who complain about insomnia differs little from that of those who do not complain. In both groups there are several people who have little sleep or poor-quality sleep. In both groups there are individuals who appear on objective tests, such as sleep electroencephalography, to have excellent sleep. Surveys suggest that about one in five individuals in the general population feel their sleep is not as satisfying as it should be.[1] The management of this state of affairs is clearly complex.

There is therefore a fault-line down this section between the management of sleep disorders and the management of insomnia. In some instances a pharmacological management of sleeplessness will be appropriate. In others the management of a complaint may be called for. In yet others a judicious use of both pharmacological and psychological approaches is required.

THE SLEEP DISORDERS

An initial complaint of insomnia may refer to a number of different things, as shown in Box 13.1.

A range of physical problems causing coughs, itches, pain, restlessness, frequency of urination and breathlessness can contribute to sleep disturbances. These may include cancer, infection, trapped nerves, depression, drug reactions and many others. These conditions need diagnosis and the proper treatment for whatever condition is revealed.

BOX 13.1 Aspects of insomnia

- An inability to get to sleep
- An inability to stay asleep
- Waking too early
- Unsatisfying sleep
- Tiredness during the day, which individuals assume is caused by inadequate sleep the previous night

One disorder that contributes to this list deserves special notice: obstructive sleep apnoea. This is commonest in overweight middle-aged men with large necks. It may affect up to 3% of men. It involves airway collapse on inspiration. This typically happens when sleeping at night lying on the back. Airway collapse stops any breathing until the respiratory drive becomes so intense that the airway is forced open – usually with a loud snort. The effort is so intense that the individual usually has their sleep disturbed and hence is tired the next day. The snort is so dramatic and loud that bed partners are often woken. The diagnosis is therefore often made by interviewing a partner, who complains about snoring. They will often have noticed their partner appears to stop breathing for anything from 10 to 60 seconds. The significance of this condition is that poor sleep and fatigue the next day may lead to requests for something to improve sleep – but treatment with hypnotics may be fatal. The condition can be treated successfully with devices delivering continuous positive airways pressure (CPAP).

There are two other notable but uncommon conditions, which are partly physical and partly social: advanced sleep-phase insomnia and delayed sleep-phase insomnia. In advanced sleep-phase insomnia, individuals fall asleep too early in the evening and wake too early, whilst in delayed sleep-phase insomnia, they fall asleep too late and are then unable to get up the next day. These disorders stem from the functioning of the circadian clock. Essentially we all tend constitutionally to be either 'larks' (waking early and at our best early in the day) or 'owls' (at our best later in the day or in the evening). Advanced and delayed sleep-phase disorders are exaggerations of these tendencies that may require specialist help to correct.

The management of delayed sleep-phase insomnia involves getting the individual to go to bed even later by 3–4 hours, every night for 5–7 nights until their sleep-onset time has come back to normal. The rationale behind this – as anyone who enjoys a sleep in at the weekend knows – is that it is easier for the circadian clock to drift backwards rather than for it to be advanced. This strategy is more successful than efforts to medicate the person to sleep at the correct time.[2]

THE PARASOMNIAS

Alongside these sleep disorders, there is a group of disturbances called the parasomnias. These involve disturbance of arousal-sleep maintenance mechanisms that lead to behaviours associated with (para) sleep. The most common parasomnias are the motor parasomnias, which include sleepwalking, bruxism (tooth grinding), night terrors and restless leg syndrome. These different conditions run in families. The behaviours usually have their onset in association with the deeper stages of non-rapid eye movement (non-REM) sleep. Therefore, they typically start around 2 hours after the onset of sleep, unlike sleep apnoea, which starts immediately after falling asleep.

There has been a very active marketing (disease mongering) of one parasomnia – restless leg syndrome. This may appear first as a distinctly unsettling pre-sleep impatience or twitchiness of the legs. This is a familial condition. Until recently it was most likely to be treated with clonazepam, relatively successfully. In recent years, GlaxoSmithKline have released ropinirole, a drug otherwise used for Parkinson's disease, as a new agent for the condition, and with its launch there have been vigorous efforts to persuade clinicians that this condition is widespread and is in great need of treatment.[3] Ropinirole can lead to compulsive gambling, prostitution and other risky behaviours – a high cost to pay.

NARCOLEPSY

As with the parasomnias, narcolepsy involves a disturbance of arousal mechanisms, but where the parasomnias lead to behaviour in someone who is deeply asleep, narcolepsy involves an abrupt onset of sleep in an individual who is wide awake. This starts usually around the age of 19–20 years. The primary feature of the condition involves falling asleep in company.

Linked into narcolepsy is a spectrum of other problems including catalepsy, sleep paralysis and hypnogogic hallucinations. Catalepsy involves episodes of a temporary paralysis of the mouth, limbs and sometimes the whole body so that you slump to the floor in what appears to be a fit. It is often triggered by strong emotion. On laughing or crying, the individual may suddenly collapse. The problem can be triggered by a variety of drugs. If troublesome, this symptom, which may occur without narcolepsy, often responds to selective serotonin reuptake inhibitors (SSRIs).

Sleep paralysis refers to waking up to find oneself unable to move – even to speak. The condition usually lasts for only a few minutes but may be sufficiently alarming to lead people to make a 'buried will' out of fear of mistakenly being thought to be dead and ending up being buried alive. Finally, individuals with narcolepsy may have intense visual or auditory hallucinations on falling asleep or waking up. These may sometimes lead to a referral to a psychiatrist with a query as to whether the condition might not be an early schizophrenia.

The treatment of narcolepsy is with stimulants (see Chapter 8) – methylphenidate, dexamphetamine, modafinil and sometimes selegiline.

INSOMNIA

Aside from the transient causes of sleep disturbance such as jet lag, shift work or the physical causes of sleeplessness, poor sleep and/or a complaint of poor sleep most commonly arise:

- as a consequence of an emotional shock;
- as part of an anxiety state;

- spontaneously;
- initially either spontaneously or after a shock or as part of an anxiety state, leading to a habitual inability to fall asleep properly and increasing frustration or anxiety;
- as a symptom of depression (see Chapter 4). Depression typically causes early morning wakening with an inability to fall asleep again. It may also cause repeated awakening during the night. The treatment is an antidepressant, as the usual benzodiazepine hypnotics may be relatively ineffective.

The proper management of a complaint of insomnia will eliminate physical causes of poor sleep as well as recognise and treat any depressive disorder or anxiety state. However, there will still be a group of individuals who complain of poor sleep. This group is particularly likely to expect drug treatment to solve the problem, but the role of pharmacotherapy here is as uncertain as it is in the management of anxiety states such as hypochondriasis.

The great problem is that current evidence suggests that many people in this group have sleep that is no worse than that of the rest of the population. Complainers are often slightly older, in which case the complaint will be justified to the extent that sleep depth does decline with age and naps during the day may lead to less than the former 6–8 hours of sleep at night. The problem, however, is that others who are ageing do not complain.

In the non-complaining population there are individuals who, for no apparent reason, at some point during their lives find themselves unable to sleep for more than only 2–3 hours. This may be highly distressing as they are left wandering the house whilst everyone else is sleeping peacefully. Often the only remedial treatment that can be undertaken in such cases is to minimise the frustration that the problem causes, for example by finding something constructive to do.

In the case of complainers, the problem seems in many respects similar to that of health anxiety (see Chapter 9), with a specific focus on sleep. As in health anxiety, individuals become concerned about a symptom, which is made worse by noticing it. The problem may start during a period of stress, which in its own right will cause sleep quality to decrease. All of us faced with stress have a tendency to focus away from the stressor and on to something else; this is called displacement. Focusing on sleep (or stomach problems) means that individuals end up thinking or feeling that everything would be okay if only their sleep (or their bowels) were okay. This is likely to become a chronic rather than just a passing problem if the individual has a history of sleep problems, a family history of sleep problems or very fixed ideas about sleep.

Unhelpful ideas about sleep may include the idea that it is necessary to get 8 hours' sleep a night or else health will suffer. This is similar to the idea that it is necessary to have a bowel motion every day. Temporary constipation is clearly going to be more worrying to people who have fixed ideas about regular bowel motions, and such ideas in turn are more likely in someone who comes from a home where there were such ideas or where there were bowel problems of one sort or another.

Another unhelpful idea is the notion that sleep is something that should be under conscious control. There is a paradox here in that we all, to some extent, have the illusion that we control our sleep, but attempts to sort out sleeplessness by re-exerting control are likely to fail.

The complaint of insomnia may cover a number of different conditions that are important to distinguish as the treatment for each differs (see Chapter 14):[4]

- For some people, the primary concern is with the after-effects of poor sleep on how they are likely to concentrate and operate in general the next day.
- For others, the concern is with the problem of falling asleep. These people have a sleep-related performance anxiety.
- For yet others, the problem seems to be one of finding their mind more active just as soon as their head hits the pillow, and this activity then interferes with sleep.
- A fourth group has difficulty in staying asleep. They wake up and are bothered by their awakenings more than others. We all awake more often during the night than we suspect, but it seems that we are in the main unaware of such episodes or even amnesic for them.
- Finally, there is a group that is simply dissatisfied with the quality of their sleep.

One further problem that needs to be mentioned is the question of perception. Individuals with insomnia appear to overestimate the amount of time it takes them to fall asleep and the frequency with which they wake up during the night. Hypnotics may make this perceptual difficulty worse.[5] It seems that individuals on sleeping pills underestimate the time it takes to fall asleep and have amnesia for their awakenings during the night. This compounds the problem of how adequate sleep is perceived to be on withdrawal of sleeping pills. On withdrawal, there appears to a rebound overestimate of how long it takes to fall asleep and a hyper-awareness of any awakenings that occur during the night.

Non-pharmacological management of insomnia

14

CHAPTER CONTENTS

There are a number of steps to take in the management of insomnia before turning to hypnotics.

CAFFEINE

A first step is to eliminate all caffeine-containing drinks, such as tea, coffee and colas, even if taking tea or coffee late in the evening has not been the cause of the problem. (See routines below.)

ENVIRONMENTAL FACTORS

It is important to ensure quiet surroundings. This is a particular problem for shiftworkers, especially where someone wants to burn the candle at both ends or resents having to be on shift work. Further shift work-related difficulties are outlined under body awareness below.

RELAXATION

Relaxation exercises, particularly progressive muscular relaxation, are useful, but they are not particularly sleep inducing in the short term. They also require considerable patience and regular practice to master, as a great part of how they work depends on building up associations between relaxation and sleep. With regular practice, subjects find they drift off halfway through their exercises. Cassette tapes or relaxation programmes promising sleep, however, rarely mention the fact that considerable hard work and patience are required. The failure of these methods to deliver a short-term result leads many to feel frustrated and to abandon what is a useful skill.

BODY AWARENESS

There is a regular cycle, operative in all of us, called the basic rest–activity cycle.[2] This produces alternating peaks and troughs in arousal at regular intervals. This rhythm can be seen most clearly in infants, who wake and sleep on a 3- to 4-hour cycle. In later life, this cycle continues so that we have our mid-morning and mid-afternoon dips. The same cycle also underlies the stages of sleep. In normal sleep, we progress through a series of stages of sleep called stages 1, 2, 3 and 4 of non-REM sleep and then REM sleep. In this process, we sink deeper into sleep and come back to the surface before sinking again, several times during the night.

What often happens in insomnia is that an individual goes to bed and finds that they seem to become more awake as they lie there. This is no illusion. It is a correct perception of what is happening. Owing to difficulties in getting to sleep, the person may have waited until they are exhausted and gone to bed, thinking that they have thereby given themselves the best chance for falling asleep. But in fact, they are just about to 'turn the corner' and head into an upswing in the arousal curve, which will make it very difficult to fall asleep. What is needed in such instances is for the individual to get out of bed before becoming too worked up about not being able to drift off. They should go downstairs, have a small snack or hot drink, read the newspaper or listen to something soothing until they feel the first hints of a downward swing. What they should not do is to wait until fatigue sets in.

A regular sleeping pattern makes this easier to achieve because the rest-activity cycle switches around to track cues from the environment indicating likely sleep-onset times and rising times. Switching typically takes several days to a week or two depending on how great the change is from the former routine. The resolution of jet lag is based on just such switching. Our sleep rhythms are tied in to important processes such as the temperature rhythm. Normally as we fall asleep, our body clock programmes a drop in temperature, and falling asleep is associated with this. As body temperature rises in the early morning, there is an associated gearing up of physiological functions in preparation for the day ahead. These lead to our waking up. It becomes increasingly difficult to get off to sleep in the face of this rise, and this underlies the problems that shift workers have trying to sleep during the day.

The significance of this is that, with practice, it is possible to learn to read our bodily cues quite accurately. A complication of the treatment of insomnia with alcohol or drugs is that these agents mask the bodily cues we might be better off in the longer term learning to read. Having said this, on occasion our lifestyles get out of kilter with our basic rest–activity cycles, at which times the inappropriate alerting effects of the rest–activity cycle can be usefully over-ridden by alcohol or hypnotics. This should be necessary only on a short-term basis, as the cycle can be expected to realign itself rapidly to a new routine.

STIMULUS-CONTROL TREATMENTS

This approach grew out of learning theory, which believes that behaviour is determined or at least shaped by associations. According to this, treatment should aim to build up associations between behaviours and sleep and to reduce behaviours associated with being awake. This leads to advice such as never to do work in the bedroom, remove the television from the bedroom or not to read in bed. Do nothing except sleep. (Leaving sexual activities in is not seen as a problem, although in theory it should be.) This approach may often be helpful, although there are good grounds to believe that learning theory has little or nothing to do with automatic behaviours such as sleep or sex. Another explanation why this approach works may simply be that it gives some people the impression of control and this allays their anxiety and permits sleep.

ROUTINES

A number of the above techniques interface with the generation or maintenance of routines. Routines are probably the single most potent contributor to sleep. This becomes clear in the case of individuals who routinely drink a cup of strong black coffee just before going to bed and who, far from having problems falling asleep on it, would have much greater problems if they were denied their coffee. In this case coffee has become part of the bedtime routine. In the case of many people on continuous treatment with a hypnotic, the pills have stopped working physiologically and are now working because they have been incorporated in a successful routine. It is worth noting that essentially the same pills may be used during the day for anxiolytic purposes, but in these circumstances people do not fall asleep with them.

PARADOXICAL INTENTION

This involves telling the individual to try to stay awake as long as possible. This may be particularly useful in those who have a performance anxiety where sleep is concerned. This technique picks up on the paradox inherent in sleep, which is that we have the impression we control it but actually have very little control one way or the other. This leads to a range of paradoxes. For example, giving good advice, such as do not take your worries to bed, is likely to be unhelpful, as it will only lead to the individual worrying about not worrying. This is an instance of the pink elephant principle, whereby telling someone to avoid thinking about pink elephants causes them immediately to think of almost nothing but pink elephants.

FORWARD PLANNING

This technique advocates spending some time during the evening in reviewing the day and settling or at least noting worries. These may be reviewed and then symbolically filed or binned. The method appears to work, especially for people who have difficulties falling asleep. This technique is one that most cultures seem to have discovered. The Guatemalan Indians, for instance, used Troubledolls for the purpose – hanging a separate worry on each of a number of dolls – and the German philosopher Immanuel Kant did something very similar.

USE OF MANTRAS AND YOGIC BREATHING EXERCISES

A technique common to transcendental meditation exercises involves the creation of a personal mantra. This is a word or set of words that are chanted or thought about. Alternatively, a breathing technique may be used. There are good grounds in current psychological theory to believe that such approaches induce sleep.[6] In brief, these approaches, which are variations of the age-old remedy of counting sheep, act to suppress the intrusion into consciousness of thoughts that might be alerting. Current evidence suggests that this type of procedure works best when the problem is one of waking up during the night with subsequent difficulties in getting back to sleep. Just as with relaxation exercises, transcendental meditation and yoga techniques are deceptively simple. Their mastery, however, requires weeks or even months of regular practice. They are not a quick fix for insomnia.

Hypnotics

15

CHAPTER CONTENTS

INTRODUCTION

The place for hypnotics in the treatment of sleeplessness and insomnia outlined in Chapters 13 and 14 is close to the place that alcohol has occupied for centuries. Most of us, every so often, if we are anxious or have a lot of things on our mind, will have resorted to alcohol to knock ourselves out. It does this effectively on an episodic basis. There are drawbacks to regular alcohol, however. One is that it produces a rebound insomnia: it knocks you out but also wakes you up several hours later as the effects wear off. It may also wake you up to pass urine or because of dehydration.

Hypnotics do roughly the same thing, with similar benefits and side effects. Judiciously used, they are wonderful. Taken in the early stages of a problem, they may abort the later development of habitual or anxiety-based insomnia. Taken too regularly or chronically, they produce their own problems.

The place for the hypnotics lies in the management of sleeplessness rather than in the management of insomnia. Where there is genuine sleeplessness stemming from jet lag or an underlying physical condition or problems with

Table 15.1 *Common benzodiazepine and Z hypnotics*

Generic drug name	UK trade name	US trade name
Nitrazepam	Mogadon	
Flurazepam	Dalmane	Dalmane
Temazepam	Normison	
Loprazolam	Dormonoct	
Lormetazepam	Noctamid	
Triazolam	–	Halcion
Z hypnotics		
Zaleplon	Sonata	Sonata
Zolpidem	Stilnoct	Ambien
Zopiclone	Zimovane	
Eszopiclone		Lunesta

falling asleep in what may be uncomfortable circumstances or situations of stress, a hypnotic may be of benefit. The presumption in these cases is that there is a transient sleeplessness that is being managed until normality returns. Where a chronic physical condition regularly compromises sleep, hypnotics can be used chronically without causing dependence. The management of acute or chronic sleeplessness is important as, although the sedative effects of hypnotics may pose risks to driving for example, the fatigue consequent on sleeplessness can lead to accidents. The management of sleeplessness is too often trivialised.

Current hypnotics include a number of benzodiazepine and related compounds (Table 15.1), which act at different sites on the γ-aminobutyric acid (GABA) receptor. These bind to a 'benzodiazepine' receptor on the GABA receptor and thereby modulate the action of GABA. At present, distinctions are drawn between benzodiazepine BZ1, BZ2 and BZ3 receptors. The BZ1 receptor leads to sedative effects, the BZ2 to myorelaxant and anticonvulsant effects, and BZ3 to anxiolytic effects. Older benzodiazepines supposedly bind to all three types and are, therefore, sedative, anxiolytic, muscle relaxant and anticonvulsant. It is claimed that newer agents bind primarily to the BZ1 site and are accordingly just hypnotic, but statements like this contain a good deal of biomythology as marketing copy.

COMMON HYPNOTICS

Any of the benzodiazepines listed in Chapter 10, such as diazepam, may be used in addition to the hypnotics given in Table 15.1.

BENZODIAZEPINE HYPNOTICS

The benzodiazepine hypnotics are essentially the same as the benzodiazepine anxiolytics. Calling one compound an anxiolytic and another a hypnotic is a marketing convenience, although a compound is likely to have greater potential as a hypnotic if it penetrates the brain quickly. It was this that underlay the success of temazepam gels. Temazepam as a conventional tablet is less effective, but the gels proved too open to abuse.

Z HYPNOTICS

The Z hypnotics are so-called primarily because the names of all drugs in the group begin with Z, and this is a convenient way to suggest these drugs are not benzodiazepines. This distinction from benzodiazepines is misleading, in particular in so far as it suggests these drugs will be safer than benzodiazepines.

These drugs are short-acting to avoid dependence and withdrawal problems, but making drugs like this short acting opens up a range of other problems. The speed of onset and offset precipitates a range of behavioural problems not found with the longer-acting benzodiazepines.

The result is the Z-hypnotics are linked to a range of abnormal behaviours, including catatonic features and hallucinatory or psychotic phenomena.

The capacity of benzodiazepine and related drugs to cause dysphoria is more clear with these drugs, which have large numbers of reports of depression, suicidality, aggression and violence.

On these drugs, there are even more reports of sleep-related events – sleep eating, sleep walking, sleep driving, sleep sex and automatisms.

Other prominent problems are amnesia, binge eating and weight gain, cardiac arrests and QT interval chances, and a range of paraesthesiae including burning mouth, hands or feet. Confusion is not uncommon, and this can lead to falls in the elderly.

ZOPICLONE

This cyclopyrrolone was marketed as the first Z-hypnotic or non-benzodiazepine hypnotic, giving more natural sleep as well as freedom from hangover effects and risk of dependence. It binds to BZ1 receptors. It produces hangover effects and dependence. No hypnotic gives natural sleep.

It has a short half-life, which means that in older individuals, for instance, who are slower to excrete drugs, this, zolpidem and zaleplon are the only hypnotics not likely to accumulate. For this reason, these drugs have some features that may make them better than some longer-acting benzodiazepine hypnotics in the elderly. Among the side effects reported with zopiclone are a metallic taste, heartburn, broken sleep, rebound insomnia and poor sleep on withdrawal.

ZOLPIDEM

This imidazopyridine also binds BZ1 receptors. Claims that zolpidem leads to more natural sleep and less dependence or rebound insomnia than benzodiazepine hypnotics need to be treated with scepticism. Side effects include drowsiness, fatigue, depression, broken sleep, falls and amnesia.

ZALEPLON

This is another post-benzodiazepine hypnotic that acts on BZ1 receptors. As with zopiclone and zolpidem, it has a short half-life. Short half-lives were introduced to minimise hangover effects the next day, but these agents seem more likely to cause amnesia and dissociation than longer-acting agents and paradoxically can continue to cause problems after they have been excreted.

User issues

Side effects of hypnotic drugs

The side effects of the hypnotics resemble those of benzodiazepine tranquillisers, outlined in Chapter 10, with the following additional problems.

Tolerance

Within 2–4 weeks of continuous use, tolerance is likely to develop to hypnotics. This means that they will not be as sedating. Nevertheless, continuing with a hypnotic beyond 2–4 weeks may be helpful for two reasons. First, although no longer as sedative, the same drug may continue to be anxiolytic. Second, as mentioned in the last chapter, the psychological effect of getting into the habit of falling asleep on these drugs may also help to promote sleep even after the sedative effect of the drug has worn off.

Rebound insomnia

This effect probably relates to the development of tolerance, as instanced by the example of taking coffee before going to bed. Once the habit is created of sleeping on hypnotics, their absence may make sleep difficult until new habits are established. Rebound insomnia may be demonstrated within 2 weeks of continuous hypnotic ingestion. In practice, what this means is that individuals who stop a sleeping pill may lie awake for several nights afterwards, which of course confirms their worst fears – that they need the pills. Or whilst still on the medication the effects may wear off earlier in the night leading to broken sleep as outlined below.

Broken sleep

Just as with alcohol, modern hypnotics induce sleep but may also cause an awakening from sleep as their effects wear off. This is particularly likely to be the case with the shorter-acting compounds: temazepam, lormetazepam, zolpidem and zopiclone.

Hangover

Hypnotics with shorter half-lives were synthesised to avoid the hangover effects produced by older benzodiazepines, such as nitrazepam or flurazepam. This was a state of muzziness, with slowing of cognitive functioning and impaired reaction times, the morning after the night before. In occasional individuals, this can last for most of the next day. This problem usually reduces in severity as

User issues—cont'd

tolerance develops. In controlled clinical trials, the shorter-acting compounds appeared to eliminate this problem. However, in real life, they may also cause a similar problem if people resort to having another short-acting sleeping pill on waking up at 3 or 4 a.m.

Often, sometimes for the benefit of carers, the dose of a hypnotic will be pushed up in an elderly individual, in which case traces of even a short-acting drug will begin to build up in the system just as if the subject had been put on a compound with a longer half-life. If the original dose fails to work – and in the elderly the dose should be lower than for younger subjects – management strategies should involve something other than increasing the dose of the medication.

Inappropriate sedation

Packages of hypnotics usually state that driving or operating machinery after taking a hypnotic may be hazardous. In practice, if the individual does not feel unduly affected, they are likely to take a risk and drive or work. It is difficult to calculate what the effects on the economy might be if everyone on any psychotropic drug were to refrain from driving or operating machinery. The problem is that some people will be more impaired than they are aware of, and there is an increasing body of evidence that a significant number of accidents happen to individuals who are taking psychotropic medication.

Dementia

Recent studies have linked benzodiazepine use to dementia.[7] The links are clear but not big. The first point is that all psychotropic drugs can lead to nerve cell loss and, as a result, earlier brain failure than would otherwise have happened. The indications from studies are that some but not all takers are at risk for reasons we do not understand. Beyond this, it is difficult to advise other than to say this is a risk that needs to be in the frame. It may be more of an issue for anyone chronically taking hypnotics than for those taking short-term anxiolytics.

Other

All the other side effects of benzodiazepines listed in Chapter 10 apply to the hypnotics. Amnesia is less of a problem, as the person sleeps it off. When taken in large amounts either intravenously or orally, one of the notable side effects of temazepam abuse has been a profound amnesia. Abusers who present at clinics often appear to have no recollection of visits they may have made to the same clinic several days before.

In contrast to amnesia, dissociation may be a greater problem when these compounds are used as hypnotics, precisely because the confused overactivity that results may be more at odds with the tranquil sleep that is being sought than it would have been with anxiety if the pills had been given during the day. Dissociation is more likely with the elderly but, as with antidepressants or neuroleptics, a range of problems – from confusion to hallucinations – is possible.

User issues

Dependence

The use of the benzodiazepines as hypnotics raises the issue of dependence. However, the risks of dependence stem not just from the pills but from the marketing that distinguishes hypnotics from anxiolytics. When the benzodiazepines were used more widely as anxiolytics, it was common to find individuals on a benzodiazepine, such as lorazepam or diazepam, by day and a benzodiazepine at night. Such combinations promote a more rapid production of tolerance, a greater likelihood of dependence and a more general scrambling or overriding of the body prompts that might help an individual manage insomnia or anxiety. The prescription of benzodiazepine anxiolytics has risen again recently, making it more likely that the Z hypnotics will be implicated in the production of dependence.

Where individuals have been taking hypnotics for years, forcing them to discontinue may be cruel. For some subjects, chronic hypnotic intake, provided there is no concurrent daytime use of benzodiazepines, may cause dependence but not problems. Taken once at night, rather than regularly over the 24-hour period, the drug may not build up in the system. At the correct dose, there may be little more harm in taking hypnotics for such individuals than in taking Ovaltine or a nightcap. The harm is more likely to come from the levels to which the dose of the drug has been pushed by prescribers than from the intrinsic properties of the drug. At high doses, all hypnotics, long and short acting, can cause sedation the next day, confusion, amnesia and possibly ataxia.

Nevertheless, guidelines for the use of hypnotics now suggest limiting their use to something like 10 pills per month.[8] Many takers are likely to find increasing pressure on them to stop their continuous use of these compounds. Where discontinuation is indicated or desired, a regimen like that for the withdrawal of benzodiazepine anxiolytics is indicated (see Chapter 10), with supplementary education about sleep hygiene and the misperceptions the person is likely to experience on halting a hypnotic after some months or years of intake.

Sedatives

16

CHAPTER CONTENTS

Before the benzodiazepines, anxiety and sleep problems were treated with sedatives. The emergence of the benzodiazepines led to distinctions between anxiolysis and sedation and to the discovery of the idea of an anxiolytic. It also led to distinctions between sedatives and hypnotics. The hypnotics were supposed to induce a truer sleep than older sedatives did. Concerns about the overprescription of benzodiazepines in the 1980s led prescribers to look at alternative agents. This has meant either a return to older sedatives, such as the barbiturates or chloral agents, or the use of antidepressants or antipsychotics with a sedative profile, or more recently the use of melatonin or related compounds. There are a number of problems with any of these options.

MELATONIN AND ITS ANALOGUES

It has been known for decades that the circadian system in the brain is regulated by the hormone melatonin.[2] This naturally occurring agent has been used for conditions like jet-lag without great evidence that its use speeds up the resolution of jet-lag. But its use has been helpful in jet-lag because in larger doses, melatonin is sedative. This led to its use in many countries as an over-the-counter sleeping pill. In the doses used the effects have very little to do with modulation of the circadian system, although the sales pitch emphasises how natural melatonin is compared to other hypnotics. The doses are much higher than would occur naturally.

Table 16.1 *Melatonin compounds*

Generic drug name	UK trade names	US trade names
Melatonin	Melatonin	Melatonin
Ramelteon	Rozerem	Ramelteon
Agomelatine	Valdoxan	n/a

From over-the-counter use, melatonin spread to child psychiatry where it was used for years as a supposedly gentle sleeping pill – something to use where child psychiatrists would be reluctant to give a benzodiazepine.

From a company point of view, though, melatonin has been a problem. As a natural product, it cannot be patented, and many companies can produce versions of it. This led companies to produce versions of it that differ from the natural product and that could be patented. This led to the marketing of ramelteon (Rozerem) as a hypnotic and agomelatine (Valdoxan) as an antidepressant (Table 16.1).

In general these produce more side effects than melatonin, especially sedation, weight gain and suicidality.

CHLORAL COMPOUNDS

Chloral compounds (Table 16.2) were first produced in 1869.[9] Their sedative effects were quickly recognised. A number of factors militated against their widespread use. One was the difficulty in making them in other than foul-tasting liquid formats. The subsequent discovery of the barbiturates around 1900 led to a decline in their use.

The chloral compounds are now produced in tablet and liquid form. They are popular with some prescribers as they do not appear to give the buzz sometimes obtained from benzodiazepines and are, therefore, considered by some less likely to be abused. For this reason, they are used in some hospitals as the sedative of choice for illicit-drug users. They are also popular with hospital pharmacies in that they cost pennies rather than pounds. A chloral prescription may cost the pharmacy as little as 5p per week.

Chloral compounds, however, cause dependence as well as gastric irritation, heartburn and rashes. They are hazardous in overdose. These compounds are contraindicated where there is a coexisting disorder of almost any sort – cardiac, renal or gastric.

The trend to prescribe any hypnotic other than a benzodiazepine, owing to the fear of creating dependence, ignores the fact that the benzodiazepines came to prominence because they were safer than older compounds. In particular, they are less likely to cause problems such as heartburn, so that people taking chloral hypnotics are often also put on treatments for heartburn or ulcers that are more expensive than any new psychiatric drugs

Table 16.2 *Chloral compounds*

Generic drug name	UK trade name	US trade name
Chloral hydrate	Noctec/Welldorm elixir	Somnote
Chloral betaine	Welldorm tablets	n/a
Triclofos sodium	–	

and that have side effects of their own, so no savings are in fact made and no benefits gained.

BARBITURATES AND RELATED COMPOUNDS

The first barbiturate compounds were produced in the 1860s, but the discovery of their useful sedative properties stems from 1900. They were the first group of psychotropic drugs to be marketed systematically. Since then, there have been a great number of barbiturate compounds. They are widely used in anaesthesia and for the control of epilepsy, with fewer complications than their fearsome reputation in psychiatry might suggest. Until the mid-1960s the barbiturates and related compounds, such as glutethimide, were the standard hypnotics (Table 16.3). Concern about their dependence-producing potential, their dangers in overdose and the fact that these drugs interacted with a large number of other psychiatric drugs led to their abandonment with the emergence of the benzodiazepines. But, essentially, the barbiturates and benzodiazepines both work on the same γ-aminobutyric acid (GABA) receptor complex.

It is rare to find any barbiturate prescribed now as a hypnotic. Barbiturates have some use as general sedatives in states of acute agitation. They combine well with antipsychotics in the short term, allowing lower doses of each to be used. They may also be used for abreaction.

User issues

Unwanted effects of barbiturates

Their use as sedatives for the management of acute agitation is one thing, but chronic use as hypnotics is quite another. The barbiturates induce the liver enzymes that metabolise other drugs and, accordingly, the plasma levels of co-administered contraceptives, antibiotics, antidepressants, steroids, anti-asthmatic and anti-arrhythmic compounds may fall. If taken in overdose, barbiturates are fatal where the benzodiazepines are not. Even the shorter-acting compounds of the group listed in Table 16.3 are liable to cause hangover effects the next day. Less commonly they may produce dissociative reactions, unsteadiness of gait, blurred or double vision and skin reactions.

Table 16.3 *Barbiturates and related drugs*

Generic drug name	UK trade name	US trade name
Amylobarbitone	Amytal/Sodium Amytal	
Butobarbitone	Soneryl	
Quinalbarbitone sodium	Seconal Sodium	
Quinalbarbitone	Tuinal amylobarbitone	
Glutethimide	Doriden	

CHLORMETHIAZOLE

Marketed as Heminevrin, this is one of the most widely used hypnotics. It is also used in alcohol withdrawal. It is either loved or hated. It is liked by prescribers in that it works and does not produce hangover effects because of its short half-life. This makes it suitable in the elderly, for whom it is often used. It is also popular with consumers because for a considerable proportion of takers its effects are distinctly pleasant, giving it a greater street value than benzodiazepines, for instance.

Chlormethiazole is unsettling to many psychopharmacologists because it is a drug that defies conventional classification, distrusted by some prescribers because it is over-liked and has a high dependence potential, and disliked by companies because it is off-patent and cheap. In terms of side effects, it can also produce nasal congestion, nasal irritation and heartburn.

SEDATIVE ANTIDEPRESSANTS AND ANTIPSYCHOTICS

Given concerns about both benzodiazepines and barbiturates, many clinicians switched to sedative antidepressants (trimipramine, trazodone or mirtazapine) or antipsychotics (levomepromazine, olanzapine or quetiapine).

The sedative antipsychotics are only sedative for some, and they produce side effects, a number of which may be very worrying if the person is unaware of what to expect. If the taker is unaware of the possible emergence of tardive dyskinesia, heart rhythm or other problems, one imagines that prescribers would be on very shaky grounds. Quetiapine and mirtazapine have reputations of being difficult to stop.

Against that, there is a certain logic to the prescription of these agents. A common feature of all the agents used is S2 antagonism. Drugs that act on S2 receptors can increase the amount of slow-wave sleep. In some cases this will happen without any obvious sedation. In other patients, because of other effects of these drugs, there may be clear sedation. There may be some place for such agents in chronic sleep disorders, but they have little use in the management of acute sleeplessness. In the case of electroencephalographic evidence of deficient stage 4 or stage 3 sleep, such compounds may be quite appropriate.

ANTIHISTAMINES

A number of antihistamines, especially promethazine (Phenergan/Avomine) and trimeprazine (Vallergan), are also used as sedatives, mainly for children. They often 'work', although their use arguably should be discouraged for this purpose as they may have marked hangover effects on the child the next day, which may potentially lead to accidents and/or poor performance at school, besides having many of the hazards of the selective serotonin reuptake inhibitors (SSRIs) (see Chapter 5).

REFERENCES

1. Espie C. The psychological treatment of insomnia. Chichester: John Wiley; 1991.
2. Waterhouse JM, Minors DS, Waterhouse ME. Your body clock: how to live with it, not against it. Oxford: Oxford University Press; 1990.
3. Woloshin S, Schwartz LM. Giving legs to restless legs: a case study of how the media helps make people sick. PLoS Med 3:e170. doi:10.1371/journal.pmed.0030170.
4. Coyle K, Watts FN. The factorial structure of sleep dissatisfaction. Behav Res Ther 1991;29:513–20.
5. Schneider-Helmert D. Why low-dose benzodiazepine-dependent insomniacs can't escape their sleeping pills. Acta Psychiatr Scand 1988;78:706–11.
6. Levey AB, Aldaz JA, Watts FN, et al. Articulatory suppression and the treatment of insomnia. Behav Res Ther 1991;29:85–9.
7. Gage SB, Moride Y, Ducruet T, et al. Benzodiazepine use and risk of Alzheimer's disease: case control study. BMJ 2014;349:g5205.
8. Lader M, Healy D, Beaumont G, et al. The medical management of insomnia in general practice. Royal Society of Medicine Round Table Series no. 28. London: Royal Society of Medicine Publications; 1992.
9. Healy D. The creation of psychopharmacology. Cambridge, MA: Harvard University Press; 2002.

SECTION 7
MANAGEMENT OF COGNITIVE IMPAIRMENT

SECTION CONTENTS

Cognitive enhancement and the dementias

17

CHAPTER CONTENTS

INTRODUCTION

While the 1990s saw the first systematic attempts to enhance cognitive performance, whether in normal subjects of all ages or in individuals who suffered from either strokes or a dementing process, drugs such as the stimulants have been used for cognitive enhancement for decades. The term cognitive enhancer now refers to the action of a drug that in some way improves cognitive performance, with memory being the performance most commonly looked at. An older term for this group of drugs was the nootropics. A looser term is smart drugs.

The initial goal was to find drugs to treat or ameliorate dementia. More recently efforts have broadened out to include drugs that might limit the consequences of having a stroke or might be neuroprotective or drugs that might reverse age-associated decline in memory. It is quite probable that drugs that are cognitively enhancing will not in any meaningful way treat or reverse any of the dementing processes. Conversely, agents that bring a dementing process to a halt are unlikely otherwise to be cognitive enhancers. There is accordingly a fault-line down this section with the treatment of dementia on the one side and on the other cognitive enhancement.

The larger pharmaceutical companies have in recent years moved out of the anxiolytic, antidepressant and antipsychotic fields and into neuroprotection and cognitive enhancement.[1] As with all other agents considered in this book, any treatments that come out of such research should be looked at closely by all areas of clinical practice because there is no such thing as a drug working on the brain that affects only one set of behaviours. The example of the antidepressants and sexual functioning is worth bearing in mind here (see Section 8). It is not inconceivable that a new generation of neuroprotective agents will be as useful in the management of schizophrenia as they may be for dementia. The people best placed to discover this will be those on treatment and those most closely involved in their care.

THE DEMENTIAS

Part of the problem in finding drugs effective for dementia lies in our ideas about what constitutes dementia. It had been traditional to distinguish between Alzheimer's dementia, or senile dementia of the Alzheimer type (SDAT), and multi-infarct dementia (MID), which is theoretically caused by small strokes that insidiously pick off brain tissue to the point where an individual's cognitive function is compromised.

STAGE 1

MID was originally thought to account for most dementias, and accordingly early treatment attempts concentrated on MID. The initial hypothesis was that these multiple small strokes were being caused by hardening of the arteries, sometimes called arteriosclerosis and sometimes atherosclerosis (although these terms refer to two different disorders), which impaired blood supply to the brain. The logical treatment, therefore, was to attempt to dilate the blood vessels. This led to the use of a number of vasodilating drugs such as hydralazine and hydergine. It is now quite rare for such drugs to be used for this purpose. The hypothesis has fallen out of favour even though there is some evidence the drugs may be of some benefit – for whatever reason – and increasing evidence that small-vessel disease in our brains may affect many of us as we age leading to rigidity of both posture and personality – what Shakespeare called crabbed age.

STAGE 2

More recent attempts to treat the dementias have proceeded on the basis that Alzheimer's disease is the commonest form of dementia. For many years, the term Alzheimer's dementia was reserved for dementias that came on before the age of 65 years, otherwise called presenile dementia. Alzheimer's-like dementia that came on after the age of 65 years was called senile dementia. All these dementias are now called SDAT, which is thought to be the commonest form of dementia.

In terms of treatment, the early focus was on dysfunction of cholinergic pathways in the brain. There are both historical and clinical reasons for this focus. Historically, in the 1960s, there were only four known neurotransmitters: noradrenaline, serotonin, dopamine and acetylcholine (ACh). Noradrenaline became linked to depression and mood disorders. Dopamine was known to be involved in Parkinson's disease but, through the antipsychotics, it also became linked to schizophrenia. Serotonin was associated with either depression or anxiety. This left ACh without a function. It seemed convenient to parcel it out to the dementias.

In addition, anticholinergic drugs can cause amnesia and confusion (see Chapter 3). However, drugs acting on the γ-aminobutyric acid (GABA) system, such as the benzodiazepines, caused even more obvious memory disturbances without being linked to dementia.

STAGE 3

Other dementias have since been emphasised. One is senile dementia of the Lewy body type (SDLT).[2] This is a mixed cortical and subcortical dementia, more likely to show motor abnormalities than Alzheimer's disease and to be characterised by prominent visual hallucinations or confusion. It appears to be related to Parkinson's disease, in that the Lewy bodies of SDLT are inclusion bodies that are also found in the brain cells of patients with Parkinson's disease. Unlike SDAT, which tends to begin insidiously and progress relentlessly, although slowly, SDLT may present dramatically and follow an episodic course. The first presentation may be episodic confusion. At times the person may seem almost delirious but, on later testing, may perform almost normally. The confusional episodes and disturbed behaviour may lead to the use of an antipsychotic, but in Lewy body dementia antipsychotics may dramatically worsen the clinical picture. Owing probably to its relationship to Parkinson's disease, patients with SDLT are more likely to have extrapyramidal symptoms even without neuroleptics. Faints and falls are common with SDLT.

A distinction has also been drawn between cortical and subcortical dementias. The cortex of the brain is the area responsible for higher cognitive functions such as speaking, reading, planning and executing actions. In the cortical dementias, memory is usually the function most noticeably affected, but sufferers also have problems with planning even simple functions such as dressing, reading, drawing or any complex tasks. Alzheimer's disease and MID are cortical dementias.

The subcortical parts to the brain involve midbrain and brainstem structures. When these are affected, the results may be a slowing of mental activity rather than its destruction (see below).

Current estimates about the relative proportion of the various dementias are:

- Alzheimer's dementia (SDAT) is now thought to comprise more than 40% of the dementias.
- The contribution of MID has shrunk to somewhere around 20% of the dementias.
- SDLT may account for 10–20% of the dementias.
- Frontal lobe dementia comprises 5–10% of the dementias. This condition used to be called Pick's disease. The involvement of the frontal lobes means disinhibited, silly or odd behaviour rather than memory difficulties are the first things noticed clinically.
- Subcortical dementia. All of the above disorders are cortical dementias. The subcortical areas of the brain may be affected by strokes and other diseases, such as Parkinson's disease, Huntington's disease, Wilson's disease, tumours, infections and trauma. If affected, the net result may be a slowing of cognitive functioning rather than an outright loss. Answering even simple questions, however, may be so slow that the questioner may assume that the affected individual has a profound memory problem. The importance of distinguishing this group of dementias from the others is that treatment may make a considerable difference to the picture.

Cognitive enhancement and neuroprotection

18

CHAPTER CONTENTS

INTRODUCTION

Psychiatric journals from the 1950s are full of adverts for treatments for dementia with stimulants such dexamphetamine or methylphenidate and a group of related compounds that were called analeptics rather than stimulants.[5] These included pipradole and metrazol.

Since the 1970s, the discussion has centred on the cholinomimetic drugs. There is no evidence that damage to the cholinergic pathway is the central deficit in Alzheimer's dementia. Indeed, many other neurotransmitters are affected in both Alzheimer's and other dementias. Given the interactions between various neurotransmitter systems, it is almost impossible to manipulate one neurotransmitter without affecting the others, and hence cholinergic drugs were never likely to be specifically helpful for dementia.

In addition, current research suggests that many cortical dementias may in part involve cell-protective mechanisms that have been thrown out of gear. Normally, there is a range of mechanisms within cells aimed at neutralising toxins of various sorts and in generally sculpting the nervous system.[3] These frequently involve the binding of a protein to the toxin, which labels it so that the cell's own degradative processes destroy the offending agent. In the dementias, such mechanisms appear to have been stimulated to the point where large amounts of these cell-protective proteins are produced – to the point that they themselves poison the cell. Whether the stimulus to this production is genetic, viral, toxic or some combination of these and other factors is uncertain. It may even represent a feature of normal ageing, with some people programmed to age quicker than others. The treatment options are to find compounds that will either switch off the process or else compensate for it or perhaps compounds that suppress inflammatory responses in general.

Historically, however, the aim of dementia treatment has always been one of giving a boost to the cholinergic system. Early efforts to do this clinically included the following:

- Choline. This is a precursor of the neurotransmitter acetylcholine (ACh). The rationale has been that, by increasing supplies of choline in the body, the brain might synthesise more ACh. Early studies reported some success, but this was not confirmed. Choline is also present in the essential fatty acid lecithin. For this reason, lecithin supplements have also been recommended in dementia.
- Piracetam/oxiracetam/aniracetam/pramiracetam/levetiracetam. In animal studies these nootropic drugs release ACh in the brain. They appear to be mildly stimulant in humans but ineffective in dementia. Levetiracetam (Keppra) is an anticonvulsant.
- Cholinesterase inhibitors block the breakdown of ACh. The first drug of this type was physostigmine. But this has an extremely short half-life, and doses that bring about improved performances in one person produce deterioration in others. Tetrahydroaminoacridine (THA) (tacrine) is a longer-acting cholinesterase inhibitor that was licensed for Alzheimer's disease in the USA. The benefits, if present, are slender set against significant liver toxicity.
- Angiotensin-converting enzyme (ACE) inhibitors. The best-known ACE inhibitors, captopril, enalapril and lisinopril, are used in the treatment of hypertension and cardiac failure. They also release ACh in the brain. The marketing of ACE inhibitors for hypertension emphasises that these drugs both lower blood pressure and provide some sort of 'zest for life'. There appears to be some stimulant quality to these compounds. In studies with aged rats, ACE inhibitors appeared to improve performance in some behavioural tasks back to the performance level shown by young rats. None of these drugs have been developed further.

SECOND-GENERATION CHOLINOMIMETICS

A second generation of agents acting on the cholinergic system has proven more successful, but the use of these agents has been controversial because of their cost. Critics claim that the clinical trials provide barely perceptible benefits in dementia and that the widespread use of such agents, given the modest benefits set against the high costs, would be crippling financially.

Modest clinical trial effects like this may stem from two sources. The drugs may not work, or they may work reasonably well in some but not at all in others. Average effects can underestimate the benefits in some patients. In dementia, some clinicians claim the latter option is the correct one. If so, there is no reason to believe that the cognitive-stimulating effects such drugs produce will be of benefit only in clear dementia. There might be a potential for patients with difficulty following head injury, for instance, to respond. Opinions are split. The French pharmacovigilance journal *Prescrire* lists all of these drugs as drugs not to be given.

DONEPEZIL (ARICEPT)

The claims are that this cholinesterase inhibitor in 5–10 mg doses can produce cognitive benefits in patients with mild-to-moderate dementia, that it sustains functional ability and delays the emergence of behavioural symptoms. (Similar claims have been made for rivastigmine and galantamine.) Donepezil's main selling point is that it comes in a single dose.

RIVASTIGMINE (EXELON)

This cholinesterase inhibitor is used in doses of 3–12 mg per day. It has a similar profile of side effects and precautions as donepezil.

GALANTAMINE (REMINYL)

Galantamine is also a cholinesterase inhibitor, used in doses of 16–32 mg per day, with a similar profile of side effects and precautions as donepezil and rivastigmine. Its selling point is that it also has direct effects on cholinergic receptors in addition to enhancing ACh, but it is not known whether this produces a real clinical benefit or simply a piece of mythology.

> **User issues**
>
> **Side effects of cholinesterase inhibitors**
> The common side effects include diarrhoea, muscle cramps, fatigue, nausea, insomnia, aggression, confusion and psychosis. The commonest effects are on the heart, leading to arrhythmia and QT interval problems. This is a real hazard in the elderly, especially if combined with other drugs that lead to QT interval changes.
>
> Overdosage produces nausea, vomiting, diarrhoea, confusion, convulsions, and cardiac and respiratory depression. This can be treated with atropine.
>
> At present there may be other effects of these drugs that are side effects in one setting but useful in others waiting to be discovered.

CHOLINOMIMETICS IN OTHER THERAPEUTIC AREAS

In addition to providing a possible benefit in Alzheimer's dementia, clinicians and patients have tried drugs like the cholinesterase inhibitors in other areas. At present there is evidence for benefits in the cognitive failures associated with multiple sclerosis, Parkinson's disease and Huntington's chorea. Claims have also been made for benefits in minimal cognitive or age-associated memory impairment.

In addition, there are reported benefits for these agents in the treatment of cognitive decline in schizophrenia and depression. The drugs have also been used to minimise any electroconvulsive therapy-linked memory loss.

There are reports of benefits in tardive dyskinesia,[6] Tourette's syndrome and attention deficit/hyperactivity disorder (ADHD). But of perhaps even greater interest are reports of benefits in autism and Asperger's syndrome.[7]

MEMANTINE (EVISTA)

Unlike other drugs for dementia, memantine works on the glutamate system, through the N-methyl-D-aspartate (NMDA) receptor. Glutamate is the commonest excitatory neurotransmitter in the brain, and there has been considerable evidence for some time that acting on these systems might produce memory-enhancing effects, although the discovery of the benefits of memantine was by accident as was the fact that it had actions on the glutamate system.

Memantine began life in the 1970s as a glucose-lowering drug, which it was hoped would be a treatment for adult-onset diabetes. It failed for this purpose but drafted into use in Germany as a geriatric tonic (Akatinol). Impressions developed that it seemed to be best in the presence of neurodegenerative disease, which led to trials in Alzheimer's disease.

Memantine blocks magnesium-linked voltage channels, and this ultimately blocks the entrance of calcium to cells. Once in the cell, calcium must be pumped out again by an energy-intensive process, as high levels lead to cell death.

User issues

Side effects of memantine
The side-effect profile includes balance problems, cardiac failure, depression, suicidality, psychosis, hallucinations, confusion, breathlessness, embolism, sedation and dizziness.

MANAGEMENT OF MULTI-INFARCT DEMENTIA

There are great efforts being put into managing the brain damage caused by strokes. The greatest destruction of brain tissue does not happen when the stroke begins, but rather happens over the course of several hours to 1–2 days later. The initial stroke may only affect a very small group of nerves, but these release a neurotransmitter called glutamate. Glutamate increases the permeability of adjacent nerve cells, which absorb both sodium and chloride, causing water to enter the cell, leading it to swell and burst.

This process does not happen if there is a low level of calcium in the medium surrounding the cells. Furthermore, the absorption of sodium and chloride also leads to a greater than usual entry of calcium into the cell, and this causes the activation of a number of enzymes that break down proteins and fats within the cell. If this entry can be blocked, the chances for cell survival are greatly increased. In essence, therefore, the toxicity of a stroke appears in a large part to be a question of calcium toxicity.

Efforts therefore focus on trying to prevent calcium entry into nerve cells in the period immediately after the stroke. This can be done in two ways. One is to block NMDA receptors, which are one of the receptors on which glutamate acts and that form one of the principal means of calcium entry. NMDA receptors can be blocked by anaesthetic agents such as ketamine, dextrorphan and a variety of barbiturate-related compounds. The other is to block voltage-operated calcium channels, with calcium channel blockers, such as verapamil, nifedipine and diltiazem.

MANAGEMENT OF SUBCORTICAL DEMENTIAS

The subcortical dementias are the most treatable of the dementias. Sometimes, if the precise nature of the disturbance can be diagnosed, the condition can be cured entirely; this is the case for benign subcortical tumours and hydrocephalus. If an underlying disorder cannot be identified and corrected, treatment with psychostimulants or with cholinomimetics, such as the ACE inhibitors, is worth trying and is more likely to yield improvements than in the case of the cortical dementias.

NEUROPROTECTION

The initial focus of interest in neuroprotection centred on Parkinson's disease and stemmed from several discoveries. One was that a severe Parkinson's disease-like state could be precipitated by the designer drug MPTP (1-methyl-4-phenyl-1,2,3,6-tetrahydropyridine). This is oxidised in the brain to 1-methyl-4-phenylpyridinium (MPP) by monoamine oxidase B (MAO-B), and MPP destroys the substantia nigra cells containing dopamine. This raised the possibility that MAO-B inhibitors, such as deprenyl (selegiline), might protect against the toxicity of MPTP and perhaps also protect against some unknown toxin that is responsible for the naturally occurring form of Parkinson's disease. A large study comparing deprenyl with other treatments (Deprenyl and Tocopherol Antioxidative Therapy of Parkinsonism, or DATATOP) suggested that it did slow the progression of the disease.[8]

Whether deprenyl helps by this means or some other is less clear. There is some evidence now to suggest that deprenyl and related compounds can inhibit apoptosis – the process of programmed cell death that seems to be activated in cells in response to a variety of stimuli, one of which appears to be toxin overload.

Another possibility is that deprenyl might reduce the production of what are called free radicals. These are derivatives of oxygen, which, if they arise within the body, inhibit a range of enzymes, the polymerisation of proteins and the reading of deoxyribonucleic acid (DNA). The oxidation of dopamine by MAO can increase free radical production, and there is some evidence of such processes at work in Parkinson's disease. Deprenyl can block a number of the enzymatic processes that might lead to increases in the levels of free radicals. Antioxidants, such as tocopherol or vitamin C, are often promoted in health food shops as the natural way to reduce free radicals, but whilst these agents may reduce free-radical formation in parts of the body, it is not clear that they get into the parts of the brain necessary for effective action in the degenerative disorders.[9]

However, more intriguingly, it appears that deprenyl, in addition to acting on MAO, also acts on a series of other monoamine mechanisms responsible for the release of noradrenaline, dopamine and serotonin. In laboratory animal experiments, there is evidence that boosting the release of amine neurotransmitters through these monoamine release-enhancing mechanisms promotes longevity. The argument put forwards by Josef Knoll, the discoverer of both deprenyl and monoamine release-enhancing mechanisms, is that the functioning of monoamine systems is intrinsically bound up with longevity and pushing these systems to a higher level of physiological functioning can prevent the appearance of disorders associated with senescence. As with any other physiological system, he argues that variation between individuals is to be expected, so that some age quickly and some more slowly. On this basis, Parkinson's and Alzheimer's diseases would stem from the early ageing that, would be expected in some people; the trick is not so much to treat a discrete disease as to postpone ageing.[8]

The dose of deprenyl required to achieve these effects, according to Knoll, is only 1 mg per day, compared with the 10 mg dose usually employed for monoamine inhibition. A range of agents aimed at stimulating monoamine release mechanisms that have no effects on MAO are at present being developed by Knoll and his collaborators.

There have been other efforts to prevent dementia. These follow results from epidemiological studies that have claimed that people taking aspirin or statins are less likely to dement than comparable groups not taking these drugs. In both cases, the anti-inflammatory effects of these drugs have been proposed as the key beneficial effect. These studies have never been confirmed. Even if these drugs help some, others may be harmed; the human body is not designed to take drugs chronically. Far from having cognitive benefits, the statins seem capable of producing states of global amnesia that, for the most part, are likely to be transient but may not be in all cases.[10]

COGNITIVE ENHANCEMENT AND THE POLITICS OF DIAGNOSIS

In addition to finding drugs that might be useful for dementia, manufacturers have their eyes on an even larger market. As mentioned, there are two ways to tackle dementia. One is to find a drug that would prevent, halt or reverse the illness. The other is to find compounds that might enhance cognitive function. The rationale behind the latter approach is that if the function of remaining brain tissues can be maximised, then the quality of life of individuals who have dementia will be improved.

However, if drugs can be found that have these benefits for individuals with Alzheimer's disease, why not give them to the population at large? Efforts to keep this issue within a medical framework have led to the popularity of the idea of age-associated memory impairment (AAMI).

AAMI is a state that is proposed to affect a great number of us once we get over the age of 50 years.[11] Many individuals over the age of 50 complain of changes in their memory, but formal testing with the usual tests for dementing disorders rarely picks up anything of note. At present, therefore, it is not clear just what exactly AAMI consists of, except that it is thought of as being part of normal ageing rather than as being related to dementia. The notion has developed, however, that there is such a condition and that cognitive enhancers may help it. In general, in younger populations it has been difficult to demonstrate that any drugs enhance cognitive function. Any results that have been positive have tended to come from older populations.

This seemingly minor point raises an issue about the politics of diagnosis. In general, cognitive-enhancing agents, when used in animal populations, offer benefits to less able or aged animals compared with younger more able animals. In our society, discrimination on the basis of sex, age, race or religion is unlawful, but discrimination on the basis of intelligence remains legitimate. Clever children go to college and are subsidised to do so. They end up with the better-paying and more prestigious jobs. This advantage, however, stands to be eroded by cognitive enhancers, unless, for instance, the use of these drugs is confined to diseases such as AAMI.[12] The political influence of current prescription-only arrangements and disease models to channel developments in particular directions can be seen clearly in the case of the possible restriction of cognitive-enhancing drugs to AAMI.

SMART DRUGS

Despite this, there has been a widespread interest at ground level in the idea of using cognitive enhancers. This has led to the notion of 'smart drugs'.[13] In the USA in particular, individuals have experimented with a wide range of compounds in an attempt to boost their cognitive performance and give themselves a competitive edge.

The compounds most commonly used are:

- Nootropics such as piracetam, oxiracetam, aniracetam, pramiracetam and pyroglutamate (see above).
- ACh precursors such as choline, lecithin and acetylcarnitine (see above).
- Stimulants available over the counter such as caffeine, ginseng or gingko biloba.
- Hydergine, derived from ergot, a fungus that grows on rye. It is closely related to lysergic acid diethylamide (LSD). Claims have been made that hydergine protects brain cells from damage by free radicals, increases blood supply to the brain, enhances brain cell metabolism, and increases intelligence, memory, learning and recall. Some of the above metabolic effects may be true, but whether hydergine has consistent effects on any mental abilities is not clear. It was originally marketed for dementia in the 1960s but was later used widely in the USA, with users claiming they felt more alert, attentive and lively on it. Cynics might say that, given the amounts of money spent, it would be unlikely that takers would claim anything other than clear benefits.
- Phenytoin (Dilantin/Epanutin). This drug is one of the standard treatments for epileptic convulsions. But, it has also had advocates who claim that in lower doses than those used for epilepsy it may enhance cognitive function. At present, the evidence remains anecdotal. Richard Nixon was the most famous user of phenytoin for this purpose.

- Vasopressin. This is a hormone secreted by the pituitary gland, also called antidiuretic hormone, which, as its name implies, has a role in maintaining the fluid balance of the body. It does seem to have a role in memory formation, but the precise nature of this is still unclear. Vasopressin is used widely as a smart drug, usually by nasal inhalation, with users typically claiming to feel more alert and attentive within seconds of taking it.
- Vitamins. Vitamins are used increasingly for smart drug purposes or as cerebroprotectants. Among those most commonly used are the B vitamins, B1 (thiamine), B3 (niacin), B5 (pantothenic acid), B6 (pyridoxine) and B12 (cyanocobalamin). Also used for this purpose are vitamins C and E. It is true that deficiencies of any of these compounds may cause nervous tissue damage and affect psychological performance, but there is no evidence that increasing levels of these vitamins beyond the normal enhances cognitive functioning.
- Hormones. The stress hormone cortisol leads to brain cell loss when levels are raised chronically. One of the body's antidotes to cortisol is dehydroepiandrosterone (DHEA). This enjoys considerable sales over the counter in North America as an anti-ageing agent. Another such agent is melatonin.
- Nutriceuticals. The smart drugs interface with the issue of health foods that have a cognitive benefit. Individuals enthusiastic about cognitive enhancement are also likely to spend money on vitamins or foods aimed at lowering lipid levels or otherwise boosting brain power.
- Classic stimulants. The most potent cognitive enhancers available at present are the classic stimulants, dexamphetamine, methylphenidate and modafinil (Chapter 8). These drugs are increasingly used by students and others working to deadlines who use them to maintain wakefulness and focus and restore vigour after brief sleeps. The extent of use of such drugs, often obtained on prescription by pleading adult ADHD or off prescription through Internet sources, has led to deepening concerns.[14] The concerns have to do with establishing whether the drugs actually do what it is assumed they do but also with the possible consequences of progressing down a cognitive enhancement pathway – are we facing a series of what have been called looping effects? Looping effects have been described when treatments such as an oral contraceptive or hormone replacement therapy (HRT) produce such changes in an activity from its norm or in expectations that it later becomes impossible to appreciate an earlier worldview that might have seen concerns with taking these treatments.[15]

In this case, if enough students take enhancers, it may become almost impossible for others not to – the risk of losing out competitively will drive the process. One suggestion from the compounds investigated in AAMI research has been that effective compounds there are primarily effective for older individuals who do not have dementing processes rather than for those who have begun to dement or for those under the age of 50 seeking some competitive edge. But in the case of the stimulants, there is no such clear gradient, and these smart drugs are not likely to be of any greater benefit to the socially disadvantaged than they are to those who are gifted.

REFERENCES

1. Waldmeier P. From mental illness to neurodegeneration. In: Healy D, editor. The psychopharmacologists. London: Chapman & Hall; 1996. pp. 565–86.
2. McKeith IG, Galasko D, Wilcock GK. Lewy body dementia – diagnosis and treatment. Br J Psychiatry 1995;167:708–17.
3. Black IB. The changing brain. Alzheimer's disease and advances in neuroscience. Oxford: Oxford University Press; 2001.
4. Rothman SM, Olney JW. Excitotoxicity and the NMDA receptor. Trends Neurosci 1987;10:299–302.
5. Healy D. Notes towards a future history of treatments for cognitive failure. In: Ballenger J, Whitehouse P, Lyketsos C, et al., editors. Treating dementia. Do we have a pill for that? Baltimore: Johns Hopkins University Press; 2009. pp. 25–41.
6. Caroff SN, Campbell EC, Harvey J, et al. Treatment of tardive dyskinesia with donepezil: a pilot study. J Clin Psychiatry 2001;62:772–7.
7. Chez M, Buchanan T, Becker M, et al. Donepezil hydrochloride; a double-blind study in autistic children. J Pediatr Neurol 2003;1:82–8.
8. Knoll J. The psychopharmacology of life and death. In: Healy D, editor. The psychopharmacologists, vol. 3. London: Arnold; 2000. pp. 81–110.
9. Mizuno Y, Mori H, Kondo T. Potential of neuroprotective therapy in Parkinson's disease. CNS Drugs 1994;1:45–56.
10. Graveline D. Lipitor. Thief of Memory. Infinity, Haverford PA, 2004.
11. McEntee WJ, Crook TH. Age-associated memory impairment: a role for catecholamines. Neurology 1990;40:526–30.
12. Ray O. A psychologist in American neuropsychopharmacology. In: Healy D, editor. The psychopharmacologists, vol. 2. London: Arnold; 1998. pp. 435–54.
13. Dean W, Morgenthaler J. Smart drugs and nutrients. Santa Cruz, CA: B and J Publications; 1990.
14. British Medical Association Ethics. Boost your brain power: ethical aspects of cognitive enhancement. www.bma.org.uk/ap.nsf/cognitiveenhancement2007.
15. Hacking I. The looping effect of human kinds. In: Sperber D, editor. Causal cognition. Oxford: Oxford University Press; 1995. pp. 351–83.

SECTION 8
MANAGEMENT OF SEXUAL DIFFICULTIES

SECTION CONTENTS

The range of sexual difficulties

19

CHAPTER CONTENTS

INTRODUCTION

When this book came out in 1993, it was difficult to find anything on the use of psychotropic drugs to treat sexual problems or on the sexual problems caused by psychotropic agents. Pre-Viagra, it was almost inconceivable that impotence and treatments for it would be talked about openly in both the academic and lay media. Among the things that have contributed most to this change of attitudes have been competition in the antidepressant marketplace and the advent of Viagra. Whilst almost all antidepressants were known to cause some sexual dysfunction from the start, the greater frequency of this with selective serotonin reuptake inhibitors (SSRIs), the unacceptability of this problem to people who were not used to having this happen on benzodiazepines, and the chance for non-SSRI-producing companies to highlight these problems combined to raise the profile of the area. This incoming tide was supplemented by something of a tidal wave with the advent of Viagra, which firmly put the mechanics of both male and female sexual functioning on the map.

MALE POTENCY

The sexual problem in men most likely to lead to medical input and the flagship condition of the new sexual pharmacology is impotence, now rebranded as erectile dysfunction. This refers to an inability to achieve or sustain an erection. Impotence may derive from what have traditionally been termed organic and psychogenic sources,[1] although physical and social might be better terms here.

The organic causes of impotence stem from problems with either the nervous supply to the blood vessels of the penis (neurogenic causes) or the blood vessels themselves (vasculogenic causes). The commonest vasculogenic causes involve blockage of the blood vessels by atherosclerosis, consequent on cigarette smoking, or disorders that can destroy the smooth muscle walls of the penile blood vessels, such as diabetes.

The commonest neurogenic causes stem from diseases that damage nerves such as multiple sclerosis or diabetes, or trauma to the spine or to the nerves serving the sexual organs. There are two neural pathways involved in mediating the erectile response and either can be damaged separately. One is the parasympathetic nervous system, which runs from the end of the spinal column and mediates reflex erectile responses, such as when the penis rubs up against material, etc. It also mediates the spontaneous erections that happen through the day and night in a rhythmic manner.

There is a sympathetic pathway also. This has been seen as a more 'psychogenic' pathway leading to erections at the sight of erotic material.

A number of other disorders may cause problems. There are local diseases of the penis, such as Peyronie's disease, which involves excessive curvature of the penis (few penises are entirely straight when erect). Diseases that affect the whole body, such as liver or kidney disease, may also affect sexual functioning through an accumulation of toxic metabolites or other effects. Finally, drug treatments of various sorts from antihypertensives to analgesics may cause impotence, and psychotropic drugs may either compound or minimise these problems.

EJACULATION AND ORGASM IN MEN

In men, climax usually involves an ejaculation. The extremes of pleasure – orgasm – are usually associated with this function. Ejaculation and orgasm, however, need not be tied together. There are a number of common problems affecting ejaculation and orgasm, but there is a separate set of problems that can affect orgasm, indicating that these two functions are not identical. In women, orgasm is not tied to as obvious an ejaculatory event, and the differences between the two functions are more clear-cut.

Male ejaculation depends on the production of seminal fluid from the prostate gland and the mobilisation of semen from the testes. Seminal fluid is produced before ejaculation and may be noticeable on the tip of the penis during arousal, when it appears to add to the sensitivity of the penis and to facilitate intromission.

Ejaculation involves a complexly organised set of events in which the bladder neck must be closed off, seminal fluid produced and passed down the urethra to mix with semen coming from the testes, and the whole then discharged by a coordinated 'Mexican wave' of muscle movements. At any point along this chain of events, a quite minor imbalance may compromise the whole operation.

Problems with ejaculation may involve premature, delayed or retrograde ejaculation. Premature ejaculation involves consistent ejaculation too early in sexual activity, often before entry or else within an unsatisfyingly short time of entry.

Delayed or retarded ejaculation involves an inability to ejaculate within a reasonable period of time so that no release is achieved. With time, this makes for tension and frustration.

Retrograde ejaculation involves the bulk of the seminal discharge passing back into the bladder. This gives the experience of ejaculating but not the results. Afterwards, urine may be cloudier than usual because of the seminal fluid it contains.

In women, the corresponding event is lubrication. Quite apart from the achievement of ejaculation or lubrication, most people will be aware of a certain quality to their orgasms, which varies, so that some may be more pleasurable than others. This quality of orgasm may be affected by drugs so that, although ejaculation or lubrication takes place, orgasm may not be the pleasurable thing it once was or the quality may be altered in other ways. It is possible to ejaculate without orgasm, but as ejaculation is the usual signifier of orgasm in men, they may be more inclined to miss any disconnect between mental and physical events than women.

In this context, it is usual to talk about female orgasm being context dependent (social). However, a focus on drug side effects necessarily sheds light on the physical aspect of things, and the effects of drugs on the quality of orgasm point to the difficulties there may be in deciding what is of physical and what of social origin.

Treatment with psychotropic drugs may cause ejaculatory or orgasmic problems in both men and women, and conversely the very same drugs may be used to help manage problems triggered by other causes. In the case of the antidepressants, there are probably both central and local changes following drug treatments – thus SSRIs can slow ejaculation by acting centrally, in which case the genitalia will feel normal. However, they can also produce genital anaesthesia that quite separately can slow ejaculation/orgasm in both men and women. The only person who can work out what is happening, therefore, is likely to be the person taking the drug.

LIBIDO

A third aspect of sexual functioning is libido. This refers to the degree of interest in sexual stimuli and activities – sex drive. As with erections and orgasms, libido appears to have several components. There are the diurnal and seasonal surges of interest that appear to have no specific trigger. They come on in much the way that hunger does, as though something builds up gradually and then needs discharge. There is also the specific increase in sexual interest and the preoccupation with sexually related imagery that develops on exposure to erotic stimuli or situations. Drug treatments may impact on all these aspects of libido, increasing or decreasing either the involuntary or the voluntary components.

SEXUAL ORIENTATION, OBJECTS AND PRACTICES

Sexual orientation refers to the subject matter that an individual finds erotic. This ordinarily refers to members of the opposite sex. It may involve members of the same sex. And practice and orientation may differ: a person may be homosexual or heterosexual in their practices but have fantasies at odds with this practice. If the fantasies consistently involve members of the same sex, even though the person's usual sexual partner is of the opposite sex, then there are elements of a homosexual orientation.

A great range of individuals and materials may be used as sexual objects. Sexual intercourse or relief, for example, may be obtained with animals. The fact that this is so does not indicate that an individual is necessarily zoo-sexual in orientation, as it is most likely that, whilst engaged in such practices, the sexual fantasies driving the process are elsewhere.

Related to this is the fact that a wide variety of props and ancillary material may provide a stimulus to the sexual act. If straightforward intercourse between a man and a woman is taken as the sexual norm, then practices other than this may be said to deviate from the norm. As there are so few reliable data on the range of activities that normal individuals engage in, pinpointing where normal behaviour ends and deviant behaviour begins is arbitrary.

It is worth noting that the first English language article on imipramine[2] and 30 years later *Listening to Prozac*[3] both describe cases of 'deviant' sexual activity apparently transformed by antidepressants into more orthodox behaviour. The serotonin system on which both drugs act seems involved in impulse management. A wide variety of automatic behaviours, such as eating, sleeping or orgasm, can be increased or decreased by drugs acting on this system.[4] This being the case, it is quite possible that the impact of drug treatments may extend to a 'normalisation' of sexual behaviours. When it happens, this normalisation is likely to be 'celebrated'. But just the opposite outcome has to be as likely to happen – with some people finding that their normal responses have become what some might term deviant.

This issue enters a very uncertain area. Multiple personality disorder shows that in some sense we all house more than one personality. Psychotropic and other drugs such as dopamine agonists can effectively flip some of us from one of these personalities into another. This might only be recognised when we stop treatment and revert back.

Of critical importance for this book is the attempt to make people aware that this could happen and that the best way to move this field forwards is if people talk about what is happening to them – especially when what is happening cannot be found in textbooks.

SEXUAL RESPONSES IN WOMEN

If there was a general silence within medicine surrounding male sexual responses until the mid-1990s, the position as regards women was much worse, compounded by disinclination to consider the mechanics of female responses that left the subject shrouded in mystery. This is also changing.[5]

Women also have an erectile response. As with men, there may be two components to this: a spontaneous rhythmic one and a psychogenic one that arises in response to the presentation of erotic material. Whether or not both are differentially affected is unknown. The extent to which diabetes, multiple sclerosis, trauma or other disorders affect these functions is also unknown, almost certainly because, to a greater extent than with men, female sexual activity can proceed even though aspects of functioning may have become deranged.

Women have a wider distribution of erectile tissue than men; a large area of skin may become sensitised to touch in women in a way that it may not happen as clearly in men.

As with men, there is also in women a twin-component ejaculatory response. The first component involves the release of fluid from the walls of the vagina, which derives from an increasing congestion of the blood vessels to the vagina leading to transudation. This fluid helps to lubricate sexual conjunction. Its absence may produce dyspareunia – uncomfortable or painful intercourse. A further amount of fluid is released on orgasm proper. An increase in vaginal lubrication is probably the single most reliably observable component of the female response. It is not clear to what extent drug treatments inhibit or enhance either or both components of this response. This issue can be even more difficult to determine in the presence of the vaginal analgesia that antidepressants cause.

In women, orgasm is not as clearly tied to an ejaculatory event as it is in men. Because there is a less clear-cut ejaculatory event, in women there has traditionally been a broader focusing on the quality of sexual arousal than on the specifics of an event. This leads to some questioning as to whether orgasm is normal or necessary in women.[6] In fact, this may be true for both men and women. In men the 'triumph' of ejaculation may be confused with the boundary dissolving pleasure of orgasm, and orgasm in fact may be less common in men and indeed less necessary than is commonly thought.

Perhaps more obviously than in men, the quality of orgasmic episodes in women may vary considerably. It is important here to distinguish between the actual physical quality of an orgasmic event and its pleasurable significance. An event may be amongst the most significant sexual encounters but yet have a lesser orgasmic intensity. Conversely, a meaningless encounter may involve an intense orgasmic outcome. It is not clear what specific factors make for intensity of orgasmic outcome or how psychotropic drug intake impacts on this.

In women, as with men, there is also sexual libido. When in full flood, libido in either sex is easy to recognise in that it leads to a mental state dominated by thoughts and fantasies of sexual activity and heightened awareness of others as potential sexual partners. However, while such mental states happen to all of us on occasion, in the normal course of events attempting to judge the state of our libido is more difficult. A person's libido is intact if they are noticing as sexual objects members of whichever sex they have been used to noticing as sexual objects in the past. Libido is intact if, when someone walks down the street, they find themselves aware of others as men and women rather than just as people. Libido is low if there is little or no spontaneous sexual fantasising.

All of these factors – libido, orgasm and female potency – come together in the case of sexual fantasies, orgasmic dreaming and masturbation, when the various elements of the sexual response may be more readily disentangled than in conjugal situations. Orgasmic dreaming corresponds to the male wet dream or nocturnal emission. It consists of a semi-awakening to find oneself aroused and on the verge of or immediately post-orgasm. If it is happening more or less frequently than before whilst on a particular drug, the question arises as to whether the drug may be playing some part in the change. Very much the same thing is true of sexual fantasising. Masturbation offers a chance for an individual to become aware of the various components of her sexual response and to determine in the event of a change which element is most affected.

Effects of drugs on aspects of sexual functioning

20

CHAPTER CONTENTS

DRUG EFFECTS ON SEXUAL FUNCTION: MALES (SEE APPENDIX 20.1)

POTENCY

The central factors that determine potency are blood supply to the relevant tissues and sensitivity. In general, blood supply increases during sexual activity, leading to tumescence in men and in women. Anything that interferes with this will compromise performance. Anything that improves this will enhance performance in men. Viagra, which has become the leading treatment for male potency problems, acts on just this issue.

Anything that diminishes sensitivity of skin in the genital area risks diminishing potency – and selective serotonin reuptake inhibitors (SSRIs) do exactly this.

One of the main controls on blood flow is the sympathetic system, and increases or decreases in blood flow can be brought about by stimulating or blocking a variety of receptors on which noradrenaline acts, either in the penis and vagina or in the brain.[7,8]

Many tricyclic antidepressants, as well as the selective noradrenaline reuptake inhibitor reboxetine and a number of antipsychotics, produce erectile problems by this means. These effects on potency need to be distinguished from the effects on libido that antipsychotics and antidepressants can also produce. Many of these drugs can produce what was once termed brewer's droop. This appears to come about because of an action on α1 receptors, which reduces blood supply to the sexual vasculature. The incidence of this problem with antipsychotics in general is uncertain, although it was regarded as common on thioridazine when it was in wider use. A further problem possibly caused in the same way is retrograde ejaculation.

Noradrenergic inputs to sexual functioning are mediated through the sympathetic system. This system handles 'psychogenic' responses – lubrication or tumescence in response to sexual stimuli. There is also a parasympathetic system input, mediated by acetylcholine, which handles the rhythmic inputs to sexuality – the rhythmic increase and decrease in tumescence that takes place, usually unobtrusively, throughout the day and night. Tricyclic antidepressants and antipsychotics, with their anticholinergic effects, may affect either of these.

Many blood pressure treatments reduce noradrenaline output making it difficult to vasodilate the sexual blood vessels. These include clonidine, guanethidine and methyldopa (Aldomet).

Agonists of α-adrenergic receptors are generally antagonised by β-adrenergic antagonists. So one might expect beta-blockers, such as propranolol, to interfere with sexual potency, and there are some reports of this, although it is unlikely to be a common effect as there are few β-receptors in the sexual tissues.

The role of the cholinergic system in erectile and sexual functioning is less certain than that of the monoamine systems. A series of cases has been reported of sexual dysfunction precipitated by a range of different agents that has proved to be responsive to the addition of bethanechol (Myotonine), a cholinergic agonist. Bethanechol also appears to have a place in impotence or erectile failure stemming from back injuries. This may have something to do with the fact that the parasympathetic nerves to the sexual areas start from the sacral area of the spine. Bethanechol has also been reported in some cases to reverse problems produced by antidepressants or neuroleptics.

The role of the cholinergic system may come into greater focus with the increasing use of cholinesterase inhibitors for cognitive dysfunction. Whilst these agents are primarily used for dementia, in a group of patients unlikely to report on the effects of these drugs on them, a number of other people can expect to be given them on a more experimental basis, to treat the effects of head injuries for instance, and these individuals are the ones who may be best placed to report on the effects. There are some reports from groups such as these that donepezil, rivastigmine and galantamine may be treatments for erectile dysfunction in men.

EJACULATORY AND ORGASMIC EFFECTS

Whilst erectile responses depend critically on the action of noradrenaline on its receptors, the dopamine and serotonergic systems appear to affect the threshold for ejaculatory or orgasmic responses. Whilst not actually responsible for erections, effects on these systems may, however, make erectile and ejaculatory/orgasmic responses more or less likely.

Awareness of the changes in sexual functioning associated with SSRIs has triggered interest in this area and increased understanding of the mechanisms involved. In practice, S1 agonists, such as buspirone, and S2 antagonists, such as cyproheptadine and yohimbine, bring orgasm forwards, whereas S1 antagonists and S2 agonists, such as lysergic acid diethylamide (LSD), delay it. There is an interplay between the sexual hormones and serotonin, such that the sexual hormones mediate their effects by leading to increases or decreases in serotonin synthesis, whilst serotonin in turn does not act other than in the presence of a normal hormonal milieu.[4]

It is now estimated that SSRI drugs, and many other antidepressants with effects on serotonin reuptake such as imipramine and clomipramine, will lead to ejaculatory/orgasmic dysfunction in up to 80% of people taking them.

However, according to company marketing estimates up to one-third of men suffer from premature ejaculation. The short-acting SSRI, dapoxetine, was marketed for just this. Cases of premature ejaculation may also be treated with paroxetine 10 mg or clomipramine 10 mg taken 1–2 hours before sexual relations. The risks of longer-term sexual dysfunction however should be considered before embarking on this.

A further related effect of SSRIs is to produce penile or vaginal anaesthesia. This will be experienced as loss of normal sensation, which can be linked to an inhibition of ejaculatory or orgasmic function or to a change in the quality of any orgasm experienced.

LIBIDO AND AROUSAL EFFECTS

SSRIs can lead to a profound loss of libido. It can be difficult to tease apart libido and arousal from potency and orgasmic functioning. A change in one will tend to affect the others. Initial research with these neurotransmitters suggested serotonin was involved in ejaculation and orgasm, and noradrenaline and acetylcholine in potency, whilst dopamine was more linked to libido, but these considerations seem simplistic now.

The role of dopamine in libido underpins the libido increasing effects of cocaine and stimulants. More recently the dopamine agonists used for Parkinson's disease and other conditions like restless leg syndrome such as L-dopa, apomorphine, amantadine, pergolide, ropinirole and bromocriptine have been reported to bring about serious increases in libido in up to 15% of those taking them, sometimes producing compulsive promiscuity. There are elements of increased libido and impaired judgement combined here that neither clinical care nor medico-legal system have yet got to grips with.

Drugs that antagonise dopamine, such as the antipsychotics, antagonise sexual functioning and decrease libido. Over 50% of individuals taking antipsychotics have impaired sexual functioning and a loss of libido. The loss of libido appears to be dose related, so that the higher the dose of an antipsychotic, the more likely the sexual problem. One antipsychotic, benperidol, was in fact marketed for the management of hypersexuality, although there is little evidence to suggest that it has any more marked effects on libido and potency than any of other antipsychotic.

Dopamine antagonists may act directly through the dopamine system, but dopamine blockade also increases prolactin levels and this can produce amenorrhoea and gynaecomastia and can reduce libido.

The role of dopamine in libido underpins an older use of apomorphine. This dopamine partial agonist in higher doses leads to vomiting. In the 1960s it was used in an effort to 'cure' homosexuality; treatment involved exposing men to pictures with homosexual content and using apomorphine to produce vomiting in the hope that this would turn these men away from same-sex to heterosexual desire. The treatment failed, perhaps because in low doses it enhances libido and probably produced arousal at the sight of the homosexual material. The treatment wheel has now swung full circle and low-dose apomorphine (Uprima) is being used as a treatment to enhance potency and libido.

SEX HORMONES

The sex hormones have clear effects on libido, particularly testosterone. Testosterone can increase libido in both men and women, and, indeed, in women androgens (male sex hormones) appear to be primarily responsible for libido.[5] Some takers of contraceptive pills report a decrease in libido, which may stem from an alteration in the ratio of androgen to oestrogen so that there are proportionately fewer androgens. The ratio of androgen to oestrogen, in both men and women, is likely to be the main determinant of the incidence of side effects from hormonal preparations. These can include excessive sexual interest and drive or 'masculinisation' – an increase in male secondary sexual characteristics, such as facial hair. There has been a clear use of testosterone for male potency and libido problems for some decades now, but in recent years this has been supplemented by the use of testosterone in women.

Finally, the opiates, heroin, morphine, pethidine, etc., have been associated with a decrease in libido. However, the acute use of opiates such as papaverine is associated with enhanced sexual performance and there are opiate receptors in the sexual tissues. The apparent contradiction can probably be explained in terms of the reduction in libido that occurs as a consequence of long-term opiate use, leading to a more general impairment of health and nutritional status. It may also be partly a secondary impairment of libido rather than a primary impairment, in that the consuming focus of appetitive interest has become the getting and taking of opiate drugs, and this displaces sexual libido from its usual place in the emotional economy.

DRUG EFFECTS ON SEXUAL FUNCTION: FEMALES (SEE APPENDIX 20.2)

The traditional headings under which female sexual functioning has been considered were dyspareunia and anorgasmia. These terms have been replaced by hypoactive sexual desire disorder, sexual arousal disorder, female orgasmic disorder and painful intercourse, which parallel classifications of male sexual disorders.[5] Women and men are supposedly the same.

However the medicalisation of what is now commonly referred to as female sexual dysfunction, or FSD, has been the subject of a vigorous and growing critique.[9–12] Pharmaceutical companies, in combination with experts interested in the medicalisation of this area, have been active in convening consensus conferences that represent one point of view exclusively and in forming patient and other groups to lobby for the investigation of and the promotion of awareness of FSD. It is now possible to find sexual advice columns where young women with three young children who complain of loss of interest in sex are advised that they need their testosterone levels checked. The opposition to this has come from feminists and sexologists. Whilst one drug has been approved for FSD in Europe, Intrinsa (low-dose testosterone), FSD has more generally become the pharmaceutical industry's Vietnam/Iraq.

Just as in men, in women there is a complex set of functions involved in ejaculation and orgasm. Whilst ejaculation itself is a peripheral act in both men and women, it is linked intimately to a central event, orgasm, so that disruption of one set of functions tends to compromise the other. It is also difficult to disentangle this complex from general questions of libido. Drugs that reduce libido and tumescent responses can also be expected to interfere with orgasm and ejaculatory responses.[7,8]

Whilst there are areas of overlap, there are also clear differences between erectile and orgasmic functions and these differences have become more apparent with the widespread use of the SSRIs. The commonest effect of the SSRIs on sexual functioning in both women and men is a delay of ejaculation/orgasm. There is a separate but less often commented on change in the quality of orgasms. There are varying estimates of the frequency with which these effects happen, but the data sheets for the agents involved suggest that up to 80% of individuals taking an SSRI or clomipramine may experience changes in sexual function.

In cases of drug-induced anorgasmia, a number of serotonergic antagonists such as cyproheptadine or trazodone may help, as may buspirone, which is a serotonergic agonist. Premature orgasm is something that may afflict women also, although the extent of the problem is unknown. It is a possible side effect of some treatments like cyproheptadine.

Discontinuing SSRIs may also lead to problems, with complaints of anorgasmia, for example, being replaced by problems with uncontrollable spontaneous orgasms. This has been reported primarily in women rather than men although whether it is commoner in women is not known.

Spontaneous orgasm also appears to be a side effect of SSRIs in a small proportion of takers. This seems to happen because we are all 'wired up' slightly differently. Thus a few people given a beta-blocker, which slows heart rate in over 90% of cases, will find an increase in their heart rate. Again this increase in spontaneous orgasms on SSRIs has been reported in women rather than men although what this means is less clear.

As regards loss of desire in women, there is an increasing resort to the use of either testosterone or apomorphine, and Intrinsa, a testosterone patch, is now licensed in Europe for hypoactive sexual desire disorder in post-menopausal women. The choice of testosterone may sound odd, but endogenous testosterone has a role in mediating sexual desire in women. It is increasingly common now to have blood tests of testosterone in women, even though at present normal ranges for testosterone in women remain uncertain. Treatment is sometimes instituted against a background of apparently low levels. It is not clear if the risks of masculinisation are dependent on what the original testosterone levels were.

But there are ambiguities in using testosterone in women that go beyond the issue of female endocrinology and the risk of masculinisation. Testosterone appears to increase desire in men, but whilst desiring a man may be an issue for women, desiring to be desired is also a component of female libido, and it is not clear what effect testosterone or altering the balance of oestrogens to androgen is likely to have on this.

Before proceeding to aphrodisiacs in general and phosphodiesterase inhibitors in particular, it is worth making one further point. The marketing of Viagra and its congeners brought in its wake vigorous efforts to 'sort out women', who it was suggested essentially have the same mechanics as men, leading to the differentiation into the four types of sexual dysfunction outlined above. Efforts to develop a pink Viagra have however failed, casting doubt on this mechanical exercise, with suggestions women are more complex than men.[13] Another option however may be that even men are less simple that previously thought and that for instance there are distinctions between ejaculation and orgasm that warrant further investigation.

APHRODISIACS

For millennia there has been a search for agents to enhance sexual functioning.[14] This has tended to mean agents that increase male potency, although some agents such as cocaine may increase sexual interest quite separately from any effect on potency (see below). Among the agents quoted most consistently as being aphrodisiac is powdered ginseng root, which probably acts to increase noradrenaline release.

Another widely cited aphrodisiac is cantharides, also called Spanish Fly, which is composed of the dried and ground parts of the *Cantharis vesicatoria* beetle. Sprinkled on the penis this leads to erections by virtue of being an irritant. It can also be taken orally and, when excreted through the kidneys, leads to irritation of the genitourinary passages, which in turn makes erections more likely or prolonged. As it is a frank irritant, the effects are unpleasant.

Other herbs and vegetables have been cited as aphrodisiac, including garlic, leeks, khat (quat; Abyssinian tea), liquorice and sea-foods, especially oysters. In Japan, the puffer fish or fugu is used. Shark fin is sought after in the Orient, whilst eels enjoyed the same reputation in the Occident and the conch in the West Indies. This large variety of agents has been rapidly supplanted by Viagra; it remains to be seen which of the traditional methods may contain traces of phosphodiesterase inhibitors, the active ingredient in Viagra.

YOHIMBINE, TRAZODONE AND CYPROHEPTADINE

Before the advent of the SSRIs and Viagra, the most evidence-based treatment was yohimbine. This is derived from the bark of the Yohimbe tree.[15,16] The theoretical side effects are an increase in blood pressure or in anxiety. These can happen, but appear to be infrequent. The response seems better in cases where there is a psychogenic component to the problem but is not absent in straightforward cases of organic impairment.

In the case of yohimbine, it seems likely that benefits are brought about by a combination of actions on receptors for noradrenaline and serotonin. It is both an α2-adrenergic antagonist and an S2 antagonist. Both of these systems appear to affect the threshold for erectile and ejaculatory responses so that, whilst not actually responsible for erections, effects on these systems may make erectile responses more or less likely.

The antidepressant trazodone has a very similar receptor profile to yohimbine. One of its notable side effects is priapism (sustained erections). Whilst this side effect has been widely publicised, what has been less touted is the fact that a great number of people, male and female, show an enhancement of sexual interest whilst taking trazodone.

Priapism involves erections that fail to reduce over several hours. Any erections lasting longer than 8–12 hours warrant medical attention. If such erections are not reduced, there is a risk of damage to the penis. The reduction of priapism involves aspirating blood from the penis by syringe, usually accompanied by the injection of drugs, which leads to vasoconstriction (closing down) of the blood vessels in the area.

Another agent with a similar profile is cyproheptadine, a tricyclic which was first developed in the 1950s. Cyproheptadine increases appetite and improves sleep, but failed to find a marketing niche in the 1960s – other than as a tonic. It now seems that, along with trazodone and yohimbine, it facilitates orgasm and enhances libido.

Many antipsychotics can also cause priapism but in this case usually against a background of reduced libido.

INTRAPENILE TREATMENTS

Some drugs like dosulepin can have effects if rubbed into the skin of the penis – but absorption is patchy. One way to get over the problem of absorption is to inject compounds into the body of the penis. This is done by plunging a needle into the side of the penis about an inch back from the tip. Surprisingly, it is relatively painless. The method was first described in 1982.

The initial compounds administered in this way were papaverine, a smooth muscle dilator, or a combination of papaverine and phentolamine, which increase noradrenaline release from sympathetic nerve endings. More recently prostaglandin E1, which is found naturally in the sexual tissues and whose levels are increased during sexual activity, has been used. This appears to lead to a lower incidence of priapism. The preparation that has displaced most others is intracavernosal alprostadil (Caverject). Alprostadil is a prostaglandin E1 analogue that inhibits α1-adrenergic receptors in the penis.

Apart from priapism, the side effects of intracavernosal injections include bruising, discomfort and, more seriously, the production of plaques or nodules. Essentially these are scar tissue at the site of injection. The exuberant growth of scar tissue is something that can occur after a wound or a burn. If it happens on the penis, it can lead to distortion of its shape. This, however, seems to be relatively rare.[17]

Alprostadil has also been developed in a form that allows insertion of a slim stick containing the drug into the urethra (Muse). The side effects of this are penile irritation or burning, bleeding from the penis, or swelling of the groin or legs. Faintness or dizziness may also occur.

The use of prostaglandins to stimulate erectile function in this manner raises the possibility that many analgesics, such as aspirin or other drugs used to treat arthritic conditions, which act to inhibit prostaglandin synthesis, might lead to impairment of performance. Any screening of people with difficulties should therefore check for this possibility.

PHOSPHODIESTERASE INHIBITORS

Viagra has joined Valium and Prozac as a brand name that defines an epoch. In this case the epoch is one in which the treatment of sexual dysfunction became more successful but also an era in which it became possible to talk about sexual functioning. Viagra is sildenafil, one of a series of phosphodiesterase inhibitors, the others beings tadalafil (Cialis) and vardenafil (Levitra).

In the penis, the neurotransmitter nitric oxide increases the activity of cyclic guanosine monophosphate (cGMP), which dilates the smooth muscles of the penile blood vessels. Sildenafil inhibits phosphodiesterase type 5 (PDE-5), which breaks down cGMP. This means that nitric oxide release must take place for phosphodiesterase inhibitors to work, that is, sexual stimulation must take place and must take effect. This is different, for instance, to alprostadil, which causes erections regardless of whether there is sexual stimulation.

The phosphodiesterase inhibitors were licensed for use for impotence in men. This does not mean that they only have effects in impotence or in men. Viagra was originally discovered as part of a series of clinical trials aimed at seeing whether its vasodilating effects might be useful in angina, following the successful use of nitrates such as glyceryl trinitrate (GTN) for this purpose. Its sexual effects were noticeable by normal people (i.e. people in trials of Viagra for heart conditions who had nothing wrong with their sexual functioning). It follows that Viagra may potentially have effects in most of us, and perhaps in women, and that it would seem to have some aphrodisiac or enhancement properties rather than just an ability to treat a biological disorder.

However, trials in sexual dysfunction in women have to date not demonstrated significant effects.[13] This may say as much about the heterogeneous nature of sexual functioning in women as it does about the effects of phosphodiesterase inhibitors. In men, the primary clinical effects of phosphodiesterase inhibitors involve the reversal of what may be termed ageing effects. In women there has been something of a tendency to try the drug even in quite young women with sexual dysfunction that may stem from the trauma of childbirth or pelvic surgery or as a consequence of sexual abuse. This is a different set of problems to those that respond to phosphodiesterase inhibitors in men.

Having made this point, with the advent of these drugs sexual pharmacology burst through its medical banks, and companies began to market the drugs to younger men with the usual variations in normal functioning as something that would make all sexual events perfect.[18]

PHOSPHODIESTERASE INHIBITOR SIDE EFFECTS

The less serious side effects of phosphodiesterase inhibitors include headaches, migraine, flushing, indigestion, gastritis, abdominal pain and distension, diarrhoea, alopecia, nasal congestion, rhinitis, sinusitis and backache.

The serious problems include reports of people going blind or a range of other disturbances of vision. There are reports of optic nerve damage and retinal haemorrhage. Others have a disturbance of colour vision, with everything a different colour – most often tinged with blue.

There are many reports of people going deaf, having hearing loss, or ending up with tinnitus.

There are reports of chest pain, heart attacks, cardiac failure, arrhythmias, strokes and other cardiovascular problems. Evaluating these is difficult given that erectile dysfunction may be more common in people with cardiovascular system problems to begin with.

There are reports of pain in the extremities, burning sensations, feeling hot, hot flushes and paraesthesiae in general. There can be altered sensation in the penis or genital area, anorgasmia, priapism and penile problems including curvature and fracture.

Finally, there are significant respiratory problems. The drugs cause pulmonary hypertension, and can cause respiratory failure, pulmonary fibrosis, pulmonary embolism or complaints that may present as bronchitis or pneumonia.

These drugs need to be taken on an empty stomach and without alcohol, and should not be combined with any other nitrate drugs. The effects of sildenafil and vardenafil last for up to 5 hours, whilst tadalafil lasts for closer to 24 hours.

ANTI-APHRODISIACS

As outlined, oestrogens antagonise the effects of androgens on libido. Accordingly they are sometimes given to suppress sexual libido. Ordinarily this is likely to happen only if an individual's sex drive is such that it has been getting them into trouble. Clinically, one occasionally meets men who in the past have been given oestrogens for nothing more than worries about masturbation, with shocking consequences such as a development of breast tissue. There was also a not uncommon use of antipsychotics such as benperidol in the 1960s and 1970s to kerb what was seen as sexual promiscuity in younger women.

Two agents are sometimes given for serious sexual problems: cyproterone and medroxyprogesterone. These are synthetic anti-androgens that block brain androgen receptors. They produce a decrease in libido, a reduction in sperm count, an impairment of erectile capacity and a decreased ability to achieve orgasm. It is claimed they do not produce overt feminisation, but in fact they may do so. Their use is restricted to men convicted of sexual crimes. Cyproterone though has also been reported to lead to a resolution of erotic delusions in women, an intriguing finding for anyone considering just what is physical and what is social in the sexual area. Other drugs may have comparable effects on libido. These include drugs used to treat prostate problems such finasteride.

The steroid hormones are closely related to the sex hormones, especially to oestrogen. A not infrequent side effect of steroid therapy, therefore, may be a loss of libido along with breast development or milk production.

A number of diuretics (agents that assist in the excretion of body fluid, which are often used in cardiac failure or hypertension) are also closely related to the steroid hormones. The use of some of these, especially spironolactone and aldactone, may also lead to loss of libido. All diuretics may lead to sexual problems in about 5% of users. Given that other antihypertensive agents, such as propranolol and centrally acting agents such as clonidine or α-methyldopa, may also cause sexual problems, impairments of sexual functioning are potential complications of most treatments for hypertension.

Antihistamines have also been reported to have an inhibitory effect on sexual functioning. The anti-ulcer treatments, cimetidine (Tagamet) and ranitidine (Zantac), have been reported to reduce vaginal lubrication, to cause increased breast size in both men and women and to reduce libido generally. This may be because many antihistamines are quite potent serotonin reuptake inhibitors and have all of the effects of an SSRI from delayed ejaculation to libido suppression, irritability and suicidality.

PERSISTENT SSRI-INDUCED SEXUAL DYSFUNCTION (PSSD)

If a new openness about sexual pharmacology has been one of the biggest changes since the first edition of this book, the most recent development has been the emergence of persistent SSRI-induced sexual dysfunction (PSSD), about which pharmaceutical companies are not very open. The features of PSSD include loss of libido, genital anaesthesia, and loss of functionality that may include failure to ejaculate or have an orgasm or altered orgasmic quality, or almost any other changes in sexual functioning.

This syndrome can begin in the first weeks of treatment, where it blends with the sexual dysfunction these drugs cause any way. Or, like tardive dyskinesia, it may only appear once treatment is stopped. It affects both men and women, and it may persist for a decade or more after treatment stops. Whilst some people show some recovery, there is at present no known cure. Many people who are affected also describe depersonalisation, derealisation, emotional numbing, disconnection and despair.[19]

The problem is most common with serotonin reuptake inhibitors, but an almost identical picture can present after finasteride (Propecia) used for male hair loss, isotretinoin (Accutane) used for acne and tetracycline antibiotics like doxycycline used chronically for skin conditions.

On the Internet, PSSD forums propose all sorts of remedies based on hypotheses as to which neurotransmitters have got out of balance. This approach would never have led to the discovery that benzodiazepines are the best treatment for neuroleptic malignant syndrome (NMS) (Chapter 3) and it is unlikely to be helpful here.

For some strange reason, Wikipedia seems to have made it its mission to obliterate all information about PSSD, post-finasteride syndrome or post-isotretinoin difficulties.

It is not known what causes PSSD. Of some note is the fact that early animal work on fluoxetine demonstrated that it could shrink gonadal tissue.[20] If this happens in humans, it might account for the problem. If so, the implications for pre-pubertal or adolescent use of SSRIs are worrying.

Other possibilities include an effect on sodium channels. Local anaesthetics like lidocaine produce a genital numbing very like that found with

SSRIs and SSRIs acting through the S3 receptor affect sodium ion flow into nerves.

There is also on the Internet a growing community of people who describe themselves as asexual. The emergence of this phenomenon parallels the increased use of antidepressants in pregnancy or for children. It is likely we have always had asexual people, but it is also possible that treatment is contributing to a real increase.

APPENDIX 20.1

MALE SEXUAL FUNCTIONING QUESTIONNAIRE

Drugs being taken

1 2 3 4

Circle any options that apply to you.

1. **Have you had any change in sex drive lately?**
   An increase A decrease No change to normal
   If there has been a change lately, does this bother you?
   Not at all A little Definitely bothered Extremely bothered
   If there has been a change, do you think it is related to the drugs you are on?
   No Possibly Probably Definitely
2. **Lately, have you been fantasising about sexual matters?**
   More often than before
   Less often than before
   About the same as before
   If there has been a change lately, does this bother you?
   Not at all A little Definitely bothered Extremely bothered
   If there has been a change, do you think it is related to the drugs you are on?
   No Possibly Probably Definitely
3. **How likely has sexually explicit material been to cause you to become sexually excited lately?**
   More likely Less likely About as often as before
   If there has been a change lately, does this bother you?
   Not at all A little Definitely bothered Extremely bothered
   If there has been a change, do you think it is related to the drugs you are on?
   No Possibly Probably Definitely
4. **Erections may be more or less vigorous and sustained. How have your erections been lately?**
   Better and longer lasting than before
   Weaker and more short lived than before
   About the same as before
   If there has been a change lately, does this bother you?
   Not at all A little Definitely bothered Extremely bothered
   If there has been a change, do you think it is related to the drugs you are on?
   No Possibly Probably Definitely

5. **Spontaneous erections happen regularly during the night. Has this been happening to you lately?**
   More frequently
   Less frequently
   About as often as before
   Don't know
   If there has been a change lately, does this bother you?
   Not at all A little Definitely bothered Extremely bothered
   If there has been a change, do you think it is related to the drugs you are on?
   No Possibly Probably Definitely
6. **The commonest difficulty with an orgasm is 'coming' too quickly. Has this been happening to you lately?**
   More frequently
   Less frequently
   About the same as before
   If there has been a change lately, does this bother you?
   Not at all A little Definitely bothered Extremely bothered
   If there has been a change, do you think it is related to the drugs you are on?
   No Possibly Probably Definitely
7. **Another problem with orgasms can be difficulty in 'coming'. Have you noticed this happening to you lately?**
   More frequently than before
   Less frequently than before
   About the same as before
   If there has been a change lately, does this bother you?
   Not at all A little Definitely bothered Extremely bothered
   If there has been a change, do you think it is related to the drugs you are on?
   No Possibly Probably Definitely
8. **Sometimes you may have what feels like a normal orgasm, but nothing comes out. You may notice that your urine is cloudier than usual. Has this happened to you lately?**
   More frequently than before
   Less frequently than before
   As often as before
   Don't know
   If there has been a change lately, does this bother you?
   Not at all A little Definitely bothered Extremely bothered
   If there has been a change, do you think it is related to the drugs you are on?
   No Possibly Probably Definitely
9. **How often have you been masturbating lately?**
   Less often than before
   More often than before
   About the same as before
   If there has been a change lately, does this bother you?
   Not at all A little Definitely bothered Extremely bothered

If there has been a change, do you think it is related to the drugs you are on?
No Possibly Probably Definitely

10. **What amount of pleasure do you get from orgasms lately?**
More pleasurable than before
Less pleasurable than before
Unchanged
If there has been a change lately, does this bother you?
Not at all A little Definitely bothered Extremely bothered
If there has been a change, do you think it is related to the drugs you are on?
No Possibly Probably Definitely

11. **Orgasms may happen spontaneously (for no obvious reason). Has this been happening to you lately?**
No More often than before
For the first time ever
If there has been a change lately, does this bother you?
Not at all A little Definitely bothered Extremely bothered
If there has been a change, do you think that it is related to the drugs you are on?
No Possibly Probably Definitely

12. **How would you describe your sex drive compared to that of other people?**
A stronger than average sex drive
A weaker than average sex drive
An average sex drive

13. **How would you describe your interest in sex compared to that of other people?**
Like sex more
Dislike it more
Like it about the same as others

14. **If there have been changes in your sex life caused by drug treatment, have you considered stopping the drugs?**
Yes No

APPENDIX 20.2

FEMALE SEXUAL FUNCTIONING QUESTIONNAIRE

Drugs being taken
1 2 3 4
Circle options that apply to you.

1. **Have you noticed any change in your sex drive lately?**
An increase
A decrease
No change to normal
If there has been a change lately, does this bother you?
Not at all A little Definitely bothered Extremely bothered

If there has been a change, do you think it is related to the drugs you are on?

No Possibly Probably Definitely

2. **How often have you been fantasising about sexual matters lately?**

   More often than before

   Less often than before

   About the same as before

   If there has been a change lately, does this bother you?

   Not at all A little Definitely bothered Extremely bothered

   If there has been a change, do you think it is related to the drugs you are on?

   No Possibly Probably Definitely

3. **How likely has sexually explicit material been to cause you to become sexually excited lately?**

   More likely than usual

   Less likely than usual

   About the same as before

   If there has been a change lately, does this bother you?

   Not at all A little Definitely bothered Extremely bothered

   If there has been a change, do you think it is related to the drugs you are on?

   No Possibly Probably Definitely

4. **Moistening of the vagina (lubrication) is a common sign of sexual interest. How often has this been happening to you lately?**

   More frequently than before

   Less frequently than before

   About the same as before

   If there has been a change lately, does this bother you?

   Not at all A little Definitely bothered Extremely bothered

   If there has been a change, do you think it is related to the drugs you are on?

   No Possibly Probably Definitely

5. **Sex can sometimes be painful. How painful has it been lately?**

   More painful than before

   Less painful than before

   About normal for me

   If there has been a change lately, does this bother you?

   Not at all A little Definitely bothered Extremely bothered

   If there has been a change, do you think it is related to the drugs you are on?

   No Possibly Probably Definitely

6. **It can be difficult to have an orgasm. Have you had this problem lately?**

   More frequently than before

   Less frequently than before

   About the same as before

   If there has been a change lately, does this bother you?

   Not at all A little Definitely bothered Extremely bothered

If there has been a change, do you think it is related to the drugs you are on?
No Possibly Probably Definitely

7. **Orgasms are normally pleasurable. The pleasure, however, is not always quite the same. How pleasurable have your orgasms been lately?**
   More pleasurable than before
   Less pleasurable than before
   Unchanged
   If there has been a change lately, does this bother you?
   Not at all A little Definitely bothered Extremely bothered
   If there has been a change, do you think it is related to the drugs you are on?
   No Possibly Probably Definitely
8. **Orgasms may happen spontaneously (for no obvious reason). Has this happening to you lately?**
   No More often than before For the first time ever
   If there has been a change lately, does this bother you?
   Not at all A little Definitely bothered Extremely bothered
   If there has been a change, do you think it is related to the drugs you are on?
   No Possibly Probably Definitely
9. **How often have you been masturbating lately?**
   More often than before
   Less often than before
   About the same as before
   If there has been a change lately, does this bother you?
   Not at all A little Definitely bothered Extremely bothered
   If there has been a change, do you think it is related to the drugs you are on?
   No Possibly Probably Definitely
10. **Have you noticed any change in breast size or tenderness recently, other than the kind of changes you normally get with your periods?**
    Increased size
    Increased tenderness
    Decreased size
    Decreased tenderness
    No change in size
    No change in tenderness
    If there has been a change lately, does this bother you?
    Not at all A little Definitely bothered Extremely bothered
    If there has been a change, do you think it is related to the drugs you are on?
    No Possibly Probably Definitely
11. **How regular have your periods been lately compared to normal?**
    Less regular
    Less frequent
    More frequent
    No change to before

If there has been a change lately, does this bother you?
Not at all A little Definitely bothered Extremely bothered
If there has been a change, do you think it is related to the drugs you are on?
No Possibly Probably Definitely

12. **Compared with normal, how painful have your periods been lately?**
Increased Decreased Unchanged
If there has been a change lately, does this bother you?
Not at all A little Definitely bothered Extremely bothered
If there has been a change, do you think it is related to the drugs you are on?
No Possibly Probably Definitely
13. **How would you describe your sex drive compared to that of other people?**
A stronger than average sex drive
A weaker than average sex drive
An average sex drive
14. **How much do you like sex compared to other people?**
Like sex more
Dislike it more
Like it about the same as others
15. **If there has been a change in your sex life lately that you think has been caused by your drugs, have you considered halting your drugs?**
Yes No

REFERENCES

1. Kolodny RC, Masters WH, Johnson VE. Textbook of sexual medicine. Boston, MA: Little Brown; 1979.
2. Kuhn R. The treatment of depressive states with G22355 (imipramine hydrochloride). Am J Psychiatry 1958;115:455–64.
3. Kramer P. Listening to Prozac. New York: Viking; 1993.
4. Kafka MS. Sexual impulsivity. In: Hollander E, Stein D, editors. Impulsivity and aggression. Chichester: John Wiley; 1995. p. 201–28.
5. Berman J, Berman L. For women only. New York: Henry Holt; 2000.
6. Lloyd E. The case of the female orgasm. Bias in the science of evolution. Cambridge, MA: Harvard University Press; 2005.
7. Segraves RT. Effects of psychotropic drugs on human erection and ejaculation. Arch Gen Psychiatry 1989;46:275–84.
8. Sullivan G, Lukoff D. Sexual side effects of antipsychotic medication: evaluation and interventions. Hosp Community Psychiatry 1990;41:1238–41.
9. Tiefer L. Sexology and the pharmaceutical industry: the threat of co-optation. J Sex Res 2000;37: 273–83.
10. Tiefer L. The 'consensus' conference on female sexual dysfunction: conflicts of interest and hidden agendas. J Sex Marital Ther 2001;27: 227–36.
11. Tiefer L. Female sexual dysfunction: a case study of disease mongering and activist resistance. PLoS Med 3:e170. doi: 10.1371/journal.pmed.0030178.
12. Moynihan R. The making of a disease: female sexual dysfunction. BMJ 2003;326:45–7.
13. Loe M. The rise of Viagra. How the little blue pill changed sex in America. New York: New York University Press; 2004.
14. Meyer C. Herbal aphrodisiacs from world sources. Glenwood, IL: Meyerbooks; 1986.

15. Reid K, Surridge D, Morales A, et al. Double-blind trial of yohimbine in treatment of psychogenic impotence. Lancet 1987;i:421–2.
16. Riley AJ, Goodman RE, Kellett JM, et al. Double blind trial of yohimbine hydrochloride in the treatment of erection inadequacy. Sex Marital Ther 1989;4:17–26.
17. Kirby RS. Impotence: diagnosis and management of male erectile dysfunction. BMJ 1994;308:957–61.
18. Lexchin J. Bigger and better: how Pfizer redefined erectile dysfunction. PLoS Med 3:e170. doi: 10.1371/journal.pmed.0030132.
19. Hogan C, Le Noury J, Healy D, et al. One hundred and twenty cases of enduring sexual dysfunction following treatment. Int J Risk Saf Med 2014;26:109–16.
20. Hines RN, Adams J, Buck GM, et al. NTP-CERHR Expert panel report on the reproductive and developmental toxicity of fluoxetine. NIH publication No.05–4471. <Cehr.niehs.nih.gov/chemicals/fluoxetine/fluoxetine_monograph.pdf>; 2004.

SECTION 9

MANAGEMENT OF DEPENDENCE AND WITHDRAWAL

SECTION CONTENTS

Dependence and withdrawal

21

CHAPTER CONTENTS

INTRODUCTION

Dependence and withdrawal are a huge concern of any taker of psychoactive medication. We all want to be able to stop a treatment when the right time comes. Telling us we are like a diabetic who needs insulin might be 'a noble lie' occasionally, but it risks being an insult.

It has been traditional to distinguish between physical and psychological dependence. Physical dependence is the state that produces withdrawal syndromes like alcohol-induced delirium tremens (DTs) and opiate-induced cold turkey. These are intensely physical states with shakes, palpitations, sweating and other problems up to convulsions and death.

Psychological dependence, in the past, was thought not to involve anything physical in the brain. It gives rise to the craving that leads addicted individuals to start taking a substance again, after they have gone through the horrors of a withdrawal that should have scared any reasonable person off going back to their drug. This view has changed – see Chapter 22.

REBOUND SYMPTOMS

Many drugs cause rebound symptoms when stopped. Receptors blocked by an antagonist become hypersensitive. When the blocking drug is then removed, these receptors are flooded with the normal neurotransmitter, and they respond vigorously. It may take 48–72 hours for them to settle back to normal.

Examples are the rebound phenomena with beta-blockers, such as propranolol, leading to palpitations, sweating and flushing, or cholinergic rebound after stopping anticholinergics which may produce poor sleep and nausea or vomiting. These syndromes usually clear quickly.

The term rebound syndrome suggests a mild problem as distinct from a withdrawal reaction. Drug companies are allergic to the idea of withdrawal and have marketed the term discontinuation syndrome following stopping antidepressants. In part the hope is that most people will see the difficulties stopping antidepressants as more like rebound problems than withdrawal reactions.

WITHDRAWAL SYNDROMES

Withdrawal syndromes are dangerous and can kill. Alcohol, opiates, barbiturates and benzodiazepines are thought to come with withdrawal problems. The most dangerous is alcohol withdrawal, which in its full-blown form, DTs, can be fatal. The least serious is probably opiate withdrawal, which has a fearsome reputation but historically has usually only been fatal where medical zeal has intervened.[1] In between lie benzodiazepine and barbiturate withdrawal. These may lead to delirium and fits, but death is rare.

In Chapter 23, it will become clear that antidepressants and antipsychotics (and benzodiazepines) introduce a new problem – protracted withdrawal. Rebound lasts for a few days. Withdrawal for a few weeks. Antidepressant and antipsychotic discontinuation problems can last for much longer.

BRAIN PHYSIOLOGY

In 1954, Marthe Vogt discovered noradrenaline in brain cells. This was a first demonstration there were neurotransmitters in the brain, which had until then been thought to operate electrically rather than chemically. In 1964, it was shown that neurones containing noradrenaline formed a system within the brain that has its roots in primitive parts of the brain, the pons and the medulla oblongata, responsible for vital functions such as breathing, cardiac activity and arousal. As cell bodies that contain noradrenaline stain blue, the 'nucleus' of noradrenaline-containing cells came to be known as the locus coeruleus (the blue spot).

This system extends up through other areas of the old brain into the cortex. It is paralleled as it goes by another system, termed the raphe system, which uses serotonin (5HT) as its neurotransmitter. In general, these two systems act in a complementary fashion. Where the noradrenergic system arouses, the serotonin system sedates. In addition to its role in sleep, breathing and cardiac functioning, the locus coeruleus has a role in vigilance, alerting us to things going on around us (or within us, such as a full bladder) that may be of interest or a potential threat. It is in this role that it plays a part in anxiety, which is a state of hypervigilance in which we get ready to fight, flee or freeze as in catatonia.

Interference with these systems produces the withdrawal reactions noted above for opiates and, to a greater or lesser extent alcohol, and barbiturates. They also produce tolerance.

TOLERANCE

For a number of drugs, over time it becomes necessary to take more of the substance to induce the same effects. For example, 100 mg morphine given to someone unaccustomed to taking it would be a large amount, sufficient to cause death through respiratory depression. But for a chronic opiate user doses of 4000 mg can be tolerated.[2,3]

This phenomenon, not surprisingly, is called tolerance. This is what happens when the sedative effects of benzodiazepines or alcohol wear off. It happens with some of the side effects of antidepressants and antipsychotics so that they produce less dry mouth after a while.

Early attempts to explain tolerance focused on an aspect of the metabolism of barbiturates. Like morphine, barbiturates can be taken in ever-increasing doses, with the subject becoming progressively more tolerant as the dose rises. It was discovered that the level of a liver enzyme responsible for the breakdown of barbiturates increases with exposure to these drugs. More of the drug has to be taken simply to achieve the initial level that was obtained.

Comparable factors, it was once thought, must be involved in opiate, alcohol and benzodiazepine tolerance and withdrawal reactions. However, it is now accepted that this is not the case. It has also become clear that, far from being a purely physical matter, tolerance may involve a considerable amount of learning.

Living on a busy street or beside a train line produces a comparable phenomenon. When first exposed to the noise, it may be deafening, but after a few days the sounds are hardly heard – unless a particularly large truck roars past the window or the train driver sounds the horn while going past. The person has become tolerant to the noise. No changes in enzyme levels or brain receptors are needed to explain what is going on. The brain has simply learnt not to pay any heed to this particular event.

What seems to be involved here relates to survival. Organisms pay heed to novel events until they have assessed the threat that such events pose. When they are judged to be harmless, less heed is paid to them. If the organism remains uncertain about what is going on, attention is maintained. This means that the event remains in awareness and is subjected to all the processing capacities that can be brought to bear on what is happening. Drugs are one such event. Like loud noise or unusual visual events, they bring about change in the internal milieu. While the change is novel and its significance uncertain, animals and humans react sensitively to it. If repeated administration proves harmless, reactions will be increasingly blunted.

The event being reacted to is rarely something as simple as a noise but is rather the situation in which this noise occurs. In the wild, animals faced with novel sounds, sights or smells react not just to those stimuli, but to an entire environment. The issue is not simply one of deciding whether the beast that makes that strange noise is dangerous or not, but rather whether the environment in which such beasts occur is a safe one. Or alternatively: 'I thought I knew what was going on around here, but it seems that I don't'.

This is also the case with drugs. Work on animals reveals that the animal assesses the environment in which drugs are being taken. For example, while morphine has an analgesic effect, there are striking interactions between the environment in which analgesia is being tested and the amount of analgesia produced. If analgesia is tested for daily in the same experimental situation, more and more morphine is required to bring about a constant level of analgesia.

However, if the environment is changed, less morphine may be needed. Tolerance to higher doses can be rolled back by a change of environment – at least partly. The change of environment, it seems, makes the animal less certain that the drug-induced changes are something that can be safely ignored.

Drinkers or drug takers are all aware of similar phenomena associated with the usage of alcohol and other drugs. Typically, drinking in a particular environment at one point of the day, such as one's local in the evening, can lead to the development of an ability to handle quite large amounts of alcohol without becoming inordinately discoordinated or slurred of speech. However, having a drink over a business lunch or in the morning may go to one's head much quicker.

WITHDRAWAL SYNDROME

This account of the development of tolerance does not explain why some drugs should lead to withdrawal effects. Not hearing a train go past my window is not something that is likely to plunge me into a delirious state, but tolerance does play some part, in that the drugs that cause physical symptoms of withdrawal all produce tolerance also. This means that subjects taking them chronically often ended up on very large amounts.

In the case of alcohol and the opiates, these drugs in large amounts compromise locus coeruleus function. Locus coeruleus functioning, however, cannot be compromised without death ensuing. This system is crucially concerned with maintaining vital functions such as breathing, temperature and blood pressure. Accordingly, the effects of drugs that would tend to turn such functions off must be counteracted. This is achieved by the locus coeruleus adapting to the threat by increasing its activity.

If the depressing stimulus of morphine or alcohol is then removed, the locus coeruleus is left hyperactive, and it is this overactivity that constitutes the core of the withdrawal syndrome, with the subject overbreathing, becoming hyperthermic and having raised blood pressure. In the face of these internal events, happenings in the external environment are not as likely to be processed accurately, if at all. This is what constitutes delirium.

Whether a drug interferes with the activity of the locus coeruleus or not is, however, a matter of accident rather than a question of the perversity of personal dispositions or any intrinsic evil in the compound. For example, the hallucinogens, cocaine and the amphetamines do not cause withdrawal syndromes of this type. In the case of the antidepressants and benzodiazepines we get a comparable withdrawal problem, but we do not know what the locus coeruleus equivalent is in this case.

User issues

Detoxification from alcohol

The management of alcohol withdrawal involves the use of diazepam or chlordiazepoxide to suppress the manifestations of withdrawal. Locus coeruleus function will usually return to normal some 1–2 weeks after withdrawal from alcohol. There have been reports indicating that clonidine and calcium channel blockers may also be useful, but as management with minor tranquillisers is safe and established, it seems unlikely that these other agents will find much place.

There have now been a number of studies in which alcohol-dependent subjects were detoxified and put on a regimen of naltrexone, nalmefene or placebo, in which those on naltrexone or nalmefene were less likely to relapse.[4,5] The reason for this is at present uncertain, and it is not clear whether this effect holds for all types of alcohol dependencies or for a particular subset. Another agent, acamprosate, has also been shown to reduce relapse rates.

User issues

Detoxification from opiates

The opiates suppress locus coeruleus function more directly than does alcohol or the benzodiazepines. Based on this, it was predicted that clonidine, which reduces locus coeruleus activity, would suppress the effects of opiate withdrawal. This has proved to be the case. The use of clonidine has been replaced in recent years by lofexidine, a related agent. These drugs offer significant benefit but do not completely abolish withdrawal symptoms from opiates.

Some years ago, there was a trend to combine clonidine with the opiate antagonists naloxone or naltrexone,[6,7] which push opiate users into withdrawal more rapidly than would otherwise be the case. Using them, it is possible to shorten the length of time detoxification takes. The whole procedure only takes a matter of hours, although residual symptoms may persist for some days, but the approach is not used as much now as before as the management of craving after detoxification is now seen as a more important issue than simple detoxification.

User issues

Detoxification from barbiturates and benzodiazepines

In the case of barbiturate withdrawal, individuals are switched to benzodiazepines and withdrawn according to the schedule outlined in Chapter 10.

Where the benzodiazepines are concerned, the schedule in Chapter 10 is standard practice at present despite the development of the benzodiazepine antagonist flumazenil, which can precipitate a more rapid withdrawal.

Benzodiazepines can also lead to protracted withdrawal issues – see Chapter 23.

User issues

Detoxification from antidepressants and antipsychotics

First, in the case of either antipsychotics or antidepressants, problems that arise within hours, or days and even weeks, of discontinuing treatment should lead to suspicion that this is a dependence syndrome rather than a new illness episode. If the person has discontinued treatment whilst seemingly well, it should be several months before a new psychotic or affective episode appears.

Second, if, on the emergence of problems, re-instituting treatment leads to the problems clearing up quickly, this indicates a dependence syndrome until proven otherwise. New illness episodes that emerge months after treatment has been discontinued commonly respond slowly and often poorly to the treatment that helped the person to get well previously.

Finally, if the pattern of symptoms shown by the person is different to the initial pattern of symptoms, this is good evidence for a withdrawal syndrome.

Antidepressant withdrawal

We do not know what is going on in antidepressant withdrawal, so there is no drug like clonidine that can be given to intervene and damp things down. The key element therefore has to be a slow taper. This probably helps the withdrawal syndrome, which compromises electric zaps, dizziness, nausea and vomiting as well as anxiety and depression, but it may not help the disturbances that underpin protracted withdrawal.

1A. Tapering is easier on a liquid. Convert the treatment to a liquid formulation – every drug can be made up as a liquid, but doctors or providers may quibble at the price if the drug does not already come as a liquid.
An alternative is to convert to an equivalent dose of fluoxetine liquid. Paroxetine 20 mg, venlafaxine 75 mg, citalopram 20 mg, escitalopram 10 mg, sertraline 50 mg are equivalent to 20 mg of fluoxetine liquid. The rationale for this is that fluoxetine has a longer half-life, which may minimise withdrawal problems. Rather than switch straight from one to the other, however, it would be better to lower the dose of selective serotonin reuptake inhibitor (SSRI) slowly over a week or two, as fluoxetine takes time to build up in the system, whilst paroxetine, for example, is removed rapidly from the system.

Some people become agitated on switching from paroxetine to fluoxetine, for instance, in which cases one option is take a short course of diazepam until this settles down.

1B. An alternative is to change to clomipramine or imipramine 100 mg per day. These come in 25 mg and 10 mg capsules and as liquids, permitting a more gradual dose reduction than with other SSRIs.

Imipramine, in particular, is a less potent serotonin reuptake inhibitor, and reducing potency at the reuptake site can be useful in its own right.

A related option is to switch to St John's wort. This also inhibits serotonin reuptake and does so less potently.

2. In all cases, stabilise on one of these options for up to 4 weeks before proceeding further.
3. The standard approach is now to reduce the dose in 10% steps. The rate at which these steps are taken, however, varies from person to person. It can be weekly or monthly.

User issues—cont'd

Rigid adherence to 10% steps or a fixed interval is not a good idea. There may be a need to stay longer at certain shelves in the withdrawal process and reduce by even less at some points.

4. If there are difficulties at any particular stage the answer is to wait at that stage for a longer period of time before reducing further.

Some people are extremely sensitive to withdrawal effects. If there are problems at any point, return to the original dose and from there reduce as tolerated.

Withdrawal and dependence are physical phenomena. But if the experience is literally shocking, it is possible to become phobic. Input from a clinical psychologist or nurse therapist may help manage the phobic problem, but it is important to ensure that someone who knows little about antidepressant withdrawal does not convert the difficulties of withdrawal into a psychological issue.

Self-help support groups can be invaluable. Join one. If there are none nearby, consider setting one up. There will be lots of others with a similar problem.

Whether it is or is not possible to withdraw, it is important to note ongoing problems (legacy effects – see Chapter 23) and to get a physician or someone to report them to the appropriate bodies. New health problems such as diabetes or raised blood lipid levels may have a link to prior or ongoing treatment.

The SSRIs have clear effects on the heart and may lead to cardiac problems during withdrawal. Such problems should be noted and recorded.

SSRIs impair sexual functioning. The conventional view has been that once the drug is stopped, functioning returns to normal. This is not be true for everyone. If sexual functioning remains abnormal, it should be brought to the attention of a physician (see Section 8).

Withdrawal may reveal other legacy effects, similar to the ongoing sexual dysfunction problem, such as memory or other problems. It is important to report these. The best way to find a remedy is to bring the problem to the attention of as many people as possible.

Antipsychotic withdrawal

There are at present no antipsychotics recognised as being the best treatments to switch to for withdrawal purposes, but haloperidol, trifluoperazine and clozapine are harder to withdraw from. The best agents to use are likely to be low-potency agents with longer half-lives. Sulpiride, quetiapine and levomepromazine fit this bill.

As with SSRI withdrawal, there is a need to taper slowly. Against a background of prior difficulties when attempting to stop, a taper may need to take 1 year or more.

All other steps should be carried out as for antidepressant withdrawal but with these additional possibilities. On theoretical grounds, there are some reasons to think that calcium channel blockers may ease some aspects of the withdrawal syndrome. Other agents proposed include S2 antagonists such as mirtazapine or cyproheptadine, but these should be used with caution given that part of the problem lies in the individual's susceptibility to psychotropic drugs.

Dependence and craving

22

CHAPTER CONTENTS

INTRODUCTION

In 1954, Olds and Milner discovered that there appeared to be pleasure spots in the brain.[8] Implanting electrodes in certain areas of the brain and enabling a rat to stimulate that area by pressing on a lever that activated an electric current produced in most brain areas nothing of note. In some brain areas, however, the rats seemed keen on the effects of self-stimulation; in some cases, if left to their own devices, they would self-stimulate to the exclusion of all else – this was most likely to happen in a degraded environment devoid of stimulation.

As mentioned in Chapter 21, noradrenaline was discovered in the brain in 1954. In 1959, dopamine was identified. This was shown to be deficient in Parkinson's disease, and replacement with the dopamine precursor L-dopa brought about substantial benefits.

Mapping dopamine neurones showed that they originated in the ventral tegmentum. Some of these neurones run to motor areas of the brain and constitute the nigrostriatal system. It is the loss of nerve cells in this pathway that leads to Parkinson's disease.

Other dopamine neurones run to higher areas of the midbrain and to cortical areas. These are involved in incentive learning – the kind of learning that occurs when an animal encounters a biologically important stimulus such as food or a potential sexual partner.

The ventral tegmental system is closely associated with the systems discovered by Olds and Milner.[8] These are not simple pleasure hot spots but rather areas that respond to familiar signals pleasurably and unfamiliar signals with displeasure. The 'pleasure' may be a function of the familiarity of the message being relayed through the system. Or the compulsive behaviour may be a stereotypy. Dopamine agonists cause stereotyped behaviour.

CRAVING

Why do so many alcohol or opiate users return to their addiction after detoxification? If the terrors of withdrawal were such a significant factor in producing chronic abuse, it might be expected that anyone with the least bit of wit would keep well clear of further involvement. What perversity or self-destructive impulse is it that leads to further abuse?

The traditional response to this problem was to distinguish between physical dependence and psychological dependence. It is usually argued that the latter is a state of mind, one that may stem from deep-seated psychological difficulties. It is this state of mind that some people see as the real problem with the addictions. Whilst it is relatively easy now to take in drug addicts and 'dry them out', it is a much more difficult problem to ensure they remain drug free.

When asked why they return to their habits, sufferers often mention cravings. The notion of cravings seems to suggest a depravity or perversity in keeping with the social opprobrium accorded to addicts. It suggests some weakness on their part that fits in with the idea they have psychological difficulties. Current research suggests that this picture is quite wrong.[9]

It seems, increasingly, that cravings are a very tangible physical reality rather than something psychological. Not all drugs of abuse cause cravings. Cocaine, the amphetamines, nicotine, alcohol and the opiates notably do, but lysergic acid diethylamide (LSD), phencyclidine, the psychedelic drugs generally and the benzodiazepines, antidepressants and antipsychotics do not.

BEHAVIOURAL SENSITISATION

Experimental work on drug effects on the brain has revealed that continued administration of certain drugs, far from leading to tolerance, appears to produce just the opposite effect, even when the environment is held constant. Indeed, in a mirror image of the production of tolerance, the holding of the environment constant, in these experiments, appears to facilitate the production of increasingly enhanced effects in response to certain drugs.

This phenomenon is called behavioural sensitisation.[3,10] Certain drugs induce it, others do not. Morphine is capable of inducing both sensitisation and tolerance within the one animal: the animal develops tolerance to some of the effects of morphine, such as analgesia, and sensitisation to others – one of which is the fact that continued intake becomes increasingly pleasurable.

Initial experiments suggested that morphine produced behavioural inactivity and was somewhat unpleasant. Animals who were linked to electrodes connected to the so-called pleasure spots in the brain were less likely to self-stimulate themselves when given morphine. This ran contrary to the popular belief that opiates are pleasurable but fits the experience of many people trying opiates for the first time.

Subsequent experiments demonstrated that morphine becomes increasingly pleasant to take. Chronic exposure to morphine in experimental animals gradually brings about increases in activity and self-stimulation. There is an odd aspect to this, which is that such increases are at their height some 3 hours after morphine administration, in contrast to analgesia which is at a maximum 1 hour after administration. Maximal brain levels of the drug also occur 1 hour, and not 3 hours, after administration. Furthermore, analgesia and the respiratory depression brought about by morphine can be antagonised by morphine antagonists, such as naloxone, but the pleasurable effects of the drug are not antagonised by these agents.

APPETITES

What is happening? It appears that morphine, alcohol, cocaine and the amphetamines feed into the brain systems responsible for the generation of appetites, of which the ventral tegmental system outlined above is a component. The last thing an appetitive system could do with is tolerance to the sight of food, drink or sex – rather, just the opposite. In contrast to the effect of environmental cues in helping to bring about tolerance because they signal the non-threatening, or insignificant, nature of what is happening, environmental cues might be expected to lead to increased effects where appetites are concerned. That is, we become increasingly sensitive to aspects of an environment that indicate the possibility of food or sex or drink. Such cues lead to increased rather than decreased interest. Typically, however, we do not notice the accumulation of environmental prompts pushing us towards the consummation of an appetite, unless we have been removed from the environment artificially for a while. Try dieting, seriously, and you will become aware of all the prompts to eat in the environment – advertisements in magazines, smells of food, cooking, etc.

The effect of public houses and the cultures surrounding both drink and drugs provide a host of small prompts, each of which prime an appetite that has already been created. This can even extend to having one's appetite aroused by the sight of needles.

Once stimulated, appetites, whilst not imperative, have a way of grabbing attention. It is natural to bend our minds to the satisfaction of our appetites when they require satisfying. As the weight of cues to indulgence builds up, we typically come closer and closer to behaving on automatic pilot. We less and less regard alternative cues in the environment. Thus the hacking cough is not registered as we light up another cigarette, or the amount of food we take are not realised as we sit down for a little soothing snack, and the children's Christmas presents get forgotten until the drink runs out.

The establishment of appetites can be blocked by giving morphine accompanied by dopamine-blocking drugs (antipsychotics) or naloxone. However, once appetites have been established, they cannot easily be extirpated. Neither opiate antagonists nor antipsychotics abolish cravings for opiates once they have become established.

It does not make sense that appetites could be abolished – controlled, perhaps, but not abolished. It is possible to manage one's appetite. For example, the amount of food habitually taken bears some relation to the amount of food felt to be needed. Thus eating a lot creates a big appetite. Decreasing one's intake can lead to reduced cravings. Similarly sexual appetites are to some extent set by the frequency of indulgence. The notion that some of us are born with greater sex drives than others has little solid evidence in its favour. However, even in the case of total abstinence, we would not expect our sexual appetite to vanish entirely.

However, while appetites may not readily be abolished, the notion of craving should not be taken to imply that something has been created that is insatiable and beyond human resources to combat. For example, opiate-induced craving, while a real phenomenon, does not appear to be uncontrollable. Rather, as the experience of American GIs returning home from Vietnam suggests, the vast majority of regularly indulging individuals can put aside the habit when they are removed from social situations conducive to it. Once removed from the cues that prompt cravings, only a minority of individuals have overwhelming difficulties.

Current therapeutic strategies lean towards the management of cravings on the model of managing appetites for food when these are disordered as in bulimia or anorexia nervosa. The issue is often one of helping the individual set a reasonable management strategy rather than having them insist on complete self-control. For example, subjects with bulimia will often plan to eat only one meal a day. This leaves them liable to be overcome by hunger pangs on some other occasion, leading to rushed unsatisfying snacks that in turn lead to eating more food and feeling guilty afterwards. Management aims at recognising when an appetite has been stimulated and how to handle it in a manner that allows the individual to bring into play the usual controls we all have where appetites are concerned.

PHARMACOLOGICAL MANAGEMENT OF APPETITES

DISULFIRAM

The first treatment for alcohol problems was disulfiram (Antabuse). This operates on a behavioural principle and aims to abolish an appetite or help with its control. Alcohol in the body breaks down to an aldehyde compound and then to an acid. Disulfiram blocks the conversion of the aldehyde to the acid. This leads to an unpleasant increase in the amount of the aldehyde in the bloodstream so that after a drink or two subjects taking disulfiram may feel extremely nauseated and/or have a severe headache. This experience is supposed to deter them from taking any more alcohol. In practice, if individuals want to drink, they simply do not take their disulfiram that morning.

NALTREXONE AND NALMEFENE

A similar approach has been taken with opiate users, putting them on maintenance naltrexone. This is supposed to block the pleasure that they would get from their drugs. There is debate about how well it does this, but there is some evidence it can help.[5] Naltrexone can cause dysphoria, which, in the case of an opiate user, might make them liable to seek out relief. In all cases the use of naltrexone should be delayed until the user has been opiate free for at least 5 days because of the risk of precipitating withdrawal effects. The initial dose of naltrexone is 10 mg per day, increasing to 150 mg over 2 weeks. The effects of naltrexone last up to 3 days, and therefore dosing needs to be only every 3 days thereafter.

However, another use for naltrexone has emerged recently, which stems from the role of brain opioid systems in the genesis of appetites. A number of trials have now indicated that the use of naltrexone after alcohol detoxification reduces the risk of relapse, probably by reducing craving.[4] This has led to it and nalmefene being licensed for this purpose.

ACAMPROSATE AND BACLOFEN

Another drug licensed for the management of relapse in alcoholism is acamprosate.[11] This acts on the γ-aminobutyric acid (GABA) system on which the benzodiazepines act. Whether it produces a direct anticraving effect or reduces cravings by being in some way anxiolytic is less clear. Naltrexone and acamprosate seem to work best for different patient groups. There is, however, very little clinical work aimed at mapping out which groups of patients will respond to which agent. This is not the kind of work that drug companies are likely to be inclined to do, as it would mean settling for a restricted segment of the market.

Another drug used widely to manage alcohol craving is baclofen. This also acts on the GABA system. Acamprosate has some clinical trial support but baclofen at present does not. However, on the ground many clinicians claim to see dramatic benefits with it not seen with other treatments.

BUPROPION AND VARENICLINE

There are two further drugs marketed for cravings. Bupropion, a dopamine and noradrenaline reuptake inhibitor, with antagonist effects at nicotinic receptors, marketed as an antidepressant in the USA (Wellbutrin), is also marketed as Zyban for smoking cessation. In so far as this works it seems to do so, in part at least, by minimising cravings for nicotine and cigarettes. Another agent, varenicline (Chantix), also acts on nicotinic receptors among other sites and has been licensed for smoking cessation. It supposedly reduces the pleasure in smoking and alleviates cravings.

Bupropion and varenicline induce suicidality. The respective companies blame smoking cessation for the suicidality, but the degree of suicidality on treatment seems out of all proportion to naturally occurring difficulties on withdrawal. There is also a very significant rate of aggression, anger, agitation and violence on varenicline in particular.

Varenicline can also cause convulsions, hallucinations, psychosis, labile affect, depressive mood, nightmares and insomnia along with marked abdominal discomfort and altered taste and smell.

There is every reason for believing that each of these agents may in fact work for particular individuals rather than for different conditions such as alcohol, opiate or nicotine dependency. Judicious clinical trials of each, even in the conditions for which they are not licensed, are appropriate. The rationality with which these drugs are used would be further enhanced by studies that pay heed to how takers who find the drugs effective say they are working.

PSYCHOLOGICAL FACTORS IN SUBSTANCE ABUSE

The induction of appetites and cravings used to be seen as psychological dependence. If it is, in fact, just as physical as the dependence and tolerance that underpin withdrawal, is there any other psychology involved?

There almost certainly is.[1] For example, LSD, phencyclidine and many of the new designer drugs do not cause either physical dependence or craving, yet they are abused – and increasingly so. Despite evidence that phencyclidine, for example, led to a considerable number of deaths and despite the fact that it did not lead to any obvious euphoria, during the 1980s it became for a period the second most common drug of abuse in the USA. Why?

Common to many of these drugs is the fact that they alter consciousness. As a result, they are interesting to take. They permit an escape from reality. This suggests that two factors in their use will be a certain amount of playful activity and a need to escape reality.

As regards playfulness, there are two aspects to this. First, there is the notion that people will try something new simply because it is there, just as they will climb mountains or run across continents. Allied to these things 'simply being there', there is the matter of our innate curiosity. The other aspect to playfulness is that it is a means to handle boredom. For want of something better to do, humans will turn to virtually anything, no matter how dangerous it may be. Even Russian roulette, as Graham Greene confessed, may be tried as a way of livening things up or structuring them. Indeed, it can often seem that everything that happens is just a game to counteract boredom, from intrepid mountain climbing to scientific endeavours, the writing of books or the taking of the most recently designed drugs.

When we are bored, we do things: we eat or shop. New clothes, books or records often seem to restore a sense of purpose to things. One of the central problems of treating alcohol and opiate dependence, aside from physical dependence of both types, is the question of what will the individual now do to structure their time. Frequently, it turns out that keeping an alcohol-dependent individual away from pubs also means abolishing their entire social life at a stroke. What are they to do with the yawning hole that opens up where their social life used to be?

From this perspective, the question of drug abuse becomes, to a large extent, a matter of accident, which stems from the fact that, at various points in life, some of the activities available to be sampled cause physical dependence and others produce cravings – just as it is an accident that some of the pursuits available to be taken up, such as motorcycling, have a high fatality rate.

Just as with motorbikes, it seems that if one can get through an experimental stage between the ages of 15 and 25 years without having been too involved in high-risk pursuits or in taking of drugs with a high dependence potential, then one is not likely to be killed accidentally or to become substance dependent accidentally. It is not that playfulness diminishes after this age, so much as the burden of commitments and responsibilities restricts for most of us the opportunities to participate.

One more factor should be mentioned. LSD was used widely in clinical practice in the 1950s for what were perceived to be problems from homosexuality to frigidity, neuroses, personality disorders and substance dependence problems. This use is discredited now except for a use in chronic alcoholism or other substance dependence states, where the original reports were quite convincing.

There is also a growing clinical literature on the use of psychedelic agents to manage the anxiety linked to terminal cancers or other end-of-life issues. It appears that psilocybin and ketamine given as a one-off treatment in the appropriate setting can produce a degree of equanimity in the face of death that no other treatments can offer. Ketamine is also being used for severe mood disorders.

It is therefore possible that some psychedelic use is of benefit rather than just play.

DISINHIBITION

Along with the fear that drugs may cause dependence, there is a fear that they may change personalities by either abolishing the normal personality of an individual or by liberating demons from the unconscious. The adage *in vino veritas* is often taken to mean something like this. Both alcohol and benzodiazepines are supposed to disinhibit people. What is happening?

One thing that may happen, but which is relatively rare, is that these compounds, like almost any other drug that gets into the brain, may cause dissociative reactions. These are outlined in Chapter 3 and Chapter 5.

The more usual disinhibition on alcohol is socially disinhibited behaviour, from inappropriate pinching of bottoms to violence towards a partner. In such cases, it is argued that alcohol is a general depressant that depresses brain inhibitory pathways first. Accordingly, with an inhibition of inhibitions, there is a brief period of disinhibition before increasing levels of alcohol blot out all behaviour in a general stupor. The supposed inhibitory tracts that are especially sensitive to the effects of alcohol, benzodiazepines or barbiturates are rarely specified. There is little evidence to support this idea other than the popular presumption that something like this must be the case. But must it?

There is no question that alcohol discoordinates and slurs speech. This can be demonstrated reliably in experimental situations and can be correlated precisely with the actions of alcohol on coordination centres, such as the cerebellum. Alcohol and benzodiazepines also reverse the inhibition that fear may cause, enabling someone to go on stage and give a lecture, for instance. However, in the case of someone behaving outrageously in a public situation, who then gets some troubling news such as their house is on fire, they are liable to 'sober up' instantly – although they may still remain less than perfectly coordinated as they set about getting home. Or the social disinhibition that I show one evening may be quite different to the disinhibition I show the following evening, in contrast to the discoordination, which will be approximately the same.

An alternative account of what is happening is that, misled by the very real effects of alcohol on gait, coherence and anxiety, we also put other changes in behaviours down to the drug that are more properly seen as a function of the social situation in which it is taken. In general, there is a gap between our knowledge of what drugs reliably do and our difficulties in explaining the complexities of social interactions that can be exploited by both substance abusers and those who would put down societal ills to such abuses.

There are a number of factors that almost compel such an identification. There is, first, our tendency to seek an explanation for what is happening to us. This shows up well in placebo-controlled studies of drugs generally. It is the common experience of many investigators that a not inconsiderable number of subjects have to be withdrawn from such studies because of intolerable side effects from what turns out to be placebo.

A probable explanation for this is that, of 100 subjects who enter a study, a number of them are bound to get obscure aches or physical complaints of some sort, on at least one occasion anyway. Such discomforts are borne none too happily in the normal course of events. We put up with them because it is not clear what the cause is, and accordingly we have little option. If they occur during a week when we are taking some new pill, it may be very difficult to believe that the pill is not responsible.

Applied to alcohol, such arguments yield the following picture. That alcohol itself does not disinhibit. That alcohol is commonly consumed in situations where the usual rules of restraint are altered. That alcohol, by altering the physical state, provides a cue that a certain state has been entered in which the subject has learnt that the usual rules of accountability do not apply. Thus, if after drinking I go home and beat my wife, I know that my friends, who know me for a basically decent sort, will not attribute what has happened to me but rather to the drink they saw me having. This, it should be noted, is not an *in vino veritas* argument.

These issues also play a considerable part in the abuse of other drugs. In the case of cannabis, it is quite clear that takers have to 'learn' to get stoned. Initial taking of the drug produces the effects on perception that are typical of cannabis but not 'stoned' behaviour. It is subsequent smoking in the company of others who are 'stoned' that brings about stoned behaviour.

When it comes to the abuse of street drugs, generally, the analysis of urine samples indicates that users are often taking mixtures that contain a wide variety of white powders – and perhaps none of the particular white powder they think they are getting. Some of these extras may be other stimulants, such as strychnine, but the behaviour the users display will be behaviour appropriate to the culture surrounding the drug they think they are on.

Dependence and protracted withdrawal

23

CHAPTER CONTENTS

HISTORICAL PERSPECTIVE

Until the 1940s, the main theories of addiction focused on the personality of the addict. Addiction was a matter of addictive and sociopathic personalities – low-lifes. This began to change only with a proposal by Abe Wikler that alcohol dependence was maintained by fear of withdrawal. This idea was then applied to opiate and barbiturate dependence. Wikler's ideas revolutionised treatment of the addictions.[12]

The next breakthrough came in the 1960s following the work of Olds and Milner (see Chapter 22). This gave rise to the concept that certain drugs had an addictive potential. Animals might crave them. The concept of drug dependence in 1969 emerged to explain why people became addicted to drugs that did not cause withdrawal such as cocaine and amphetamine. Neither the antidepressants nor the antipsychotics cause drug dependence of this type, but neither do the benzodiazepines cause this problem. As the selective serotonin reuptake inhibitors (SSRIs) are currently sold as not causing the dependence that the benzodiazepines can cause, this marketing involves a profoundly misleading message to anyone who might have to be put on either set of these drugs.

ANTIPSYCHOTIC AND ANTIDEPRESSANT DEPENDENCE

While all this was happening, in 1957 Leo Hollister conducted a placebo-controlled randomised controlled trial of chlorpromazine in tuberculosis. On discontinuing treatment 6 months later, it became clear that up to one-third of those on chlorpromazine had a significant physical dependence and great difficulty in stopping the drug.[13,14] By the mid-1960s, a large number of research groups had reported marked and severe physical dependence on antipsychotics. At an international meeting in 1966 the concept of therapeutic drug dependence was recognised.[15]

The kind of problem that was recognised was as follows. People, commonly women, who take 1 mg per day trifluoperazine (Stelazine) for several months might be unable to get off this, ever again.[16,17] Another problem in the frame was tardive dyskinesia, which was first recognised on discontinuing antipsychotics. This set of disfiguring facial and sometimes truncal movements could last for years after the discontinuation of treatment (see Chapter 2 and Chapter 3).

Therapeutic drug dependence was recognised with both antipsychotics and antidepressants, but this recognition vanished almost immediately after it was born. It was 30 years before another article on dependence on antipsychotics appeared. What had happened?

In the late 1960s the Western world was in upheaval, and student revolutions from the USA through Europe across to Japan were closely associated with antipsychiatry. Departments of psychiatry were occupied, and research was brought to a halt. The new psychotropic drugs were a central part of what was happening. From the same laboratories that had produced the antipsychotics came lysergic acid diethylamide (LSD), benzodiazepines and oral contraceptives, all of which were transforming society. Previously drug treatment was a matter of treating diseases to restore a person to their place in the social order. These new drugs threatened the social order. They gave women freedom from men, and they threatened to liberate the young from the social hierarchies imposed by their parents.

The establishment responded with a war on drugs. LSD, cocaine, amphetamine and a range of other drugs were scheduled. The supposed characteristic of the bad drugs was that they caused dependence, even though LSD, for instance, appears to produce neither physical dependence nor craving. If dependence was a characteristic of bad drugs, good drugs, therefore, could not cause it. The idea of therapeutic dependence could not survive in such a climate.[12]

The problem returned to haunt us in the 1980s when benzodiazepine dependence was recognised. The initial response from medical bodies was that there was no such problem. Then the establishment argued that it was necessary to distinguish between dependence and addiction. The benzodiazepines did not lead individuals to mortgage their houses and souls to get a supply of these drugs. They didn't make people junkies. However, this subtle distinction was lost on the public for whom being hooked was the definition of addiction. The new benzodiazepine 'addicts' were seen as victims of a medicopharmaceutical complex (see Chapter 10).

The consequences are with us still. Buspirone, the first serotonergic drug, was initially marketed as a non-dependence-producing anxiolytic (see Chapter 11). It never took off because, besieged by legal actions about the benzodiazepines, physicians were sceptical of the idea that there could be a non-dependence-producing tranquillizer.

As a result of benzodiazepine crisis, when the SSRIs came on stream they had to be marketed as antidepressants rather than anxiolytics, even though they are not very effective for depression. Patients who, in the 1980s, had been seen as cases of anxiety to be treated with an anxiolytic were, under the marketing weight of the pharmaceutical companies, transformed in the 1990s into cases of depression to be treated with antidepressants.

In Japan the problem with benzodiazepine dependence never happened and, as a consequence, Prozac (fluoxetine) for instance never became available on the Japanese market as an antidepressant. In Japan for a long time the antidepressant market remained a small one compared with the market in the West. In contrast, anxiolytics remained widely prescribed. In other words, the age of depression in the West, with depression being touted as one of the greatest causes of disability in the world today, stems from the conflicts about dependence on therapeutic drugs. When any SSRIs finally reached Japan, it was for the treatment of obsessive–compulsive disorder and social phobia rather than depression.

STRESS SYNDROMES

The concept of therapeutic drug dependence runs smack up against current concepts of addiction and dependence. Tardive dyskinesia is an example of dependence on antipsychotics or SSRI antidepressants. It is manifest not only when treatment is halted, but it can also emerge during the course of treatment. In other words, it is a consequence of a drug acting as a stressor on the brain. For individuals vulnerable to this kind of stress, some brain systems get 'pushed out of shape' and simply do not revert to normal on discontinuation of treatment.[17]

When dependence on antipsychotics was described in the 1960s, neurological problems such as tardive dyskinesia were the most obvious manifestations. But neurological problems accounted for only about one-third of the presentations. In other cases, patients had dysthymic syndromes, heat and pain dysregulation syndromes and stress insensitivity.

One of the consequences of these syndromes is that it can become almost impossible after the first few months of treatment with an antipsychotic to know where the treatment begins and ends and where the disease begins and ends. This is not an argument against treatment. It is simply to state that the act of therapy changes people forever, and that both the therapist and the patient need to be aware of this and to work together to manage the situation for the best. Starting and stopping treatment is not the same as not starting.

With the SSRIs dependence on antidepressants has come into focus. This is a problem that happens with all serotonin reuptake inhibitors such as paroxetine and venlafaxine but also serotonin reuptake inhibiting tricyclics such as imipramine and serotonin reuptake inhibiting antihistamines such as chlorphenamine. Initially, SSRI companies termed the problem discontinuation syndromes in an attempt to avoid the word withdrawal with all its connotations. More recently they have switched to using terms like symptoms on stopping (SoS).

SoS appears to happen in over one-quarter and perhaps up to one-half of individuals who take SSRIs. The commonest symptoms are anxiety and depression, followed by nausea, vomiting, dizziness, fatigue, poor concentration, vivid dreams, suicidality, electric shock-like or other strange sensations in almost any part of the body, but often in particular linked to the head, temperature dysregulation so that the subject may be blazingly hot and sweating or chilly.

Clearly in the case of anxiety and depressive symptoms both taker and carer may wonder if this is the original problem returning. But if the problem emerges on missing or lowering a dose or a few days of treatment, when the taker was quite well then it is likely to be withdrawal as once well new illness episodes should not appear for months or years. If the problem clears on reinstituting treatment it is likely to be withdrawal as a new illness episode or a breakthrough episode should take weeks to respond. Finally, if the disturbance has features not found in the original disorder, such as shock like sensations, dizziness or nausea, it is more likely to be withdrawal. The problem is that anxiety and depression are among the commonest withdrawal symptoms – in healthy volunteers.

As with antipsychotic and benzodiazepine dependence, the common response of physicians to difficulties on discontinuing SSRIs has been that these are a manifestation of the illness for which treatment was being given and that treatment should simply be restarted – you are like a diabetic who needs insulin.

The antipsychotics and antidepressants can also lead to 'poop-out', a term that refers to the loss of potency that can happen on SSRIs in the course of treatment. The fact that this happens has been supported from clinical trial results.[18] It has also been clear for some time that treatment with SSRIs may set up a series of dyskinesias that persist for months or years after treatment halts.[19]

The consequences of therapeutic drug dependence (stress syndromes) are far reaching. Essentially, the recognition that significant dependence and withdrawal can occur on these drugs punctures a hole in current theories of addiction and dependence:

- Tolerance is not required for therapeutic drug dependence to happen.
- The drugs do not have to be pleasurable or craved.
- The personality of the taker appears to play little part in what has happened.

Current biological theories of addiction stress the enduring brain changes that happen following intake of illicit drugs, but these enduring brain changes are no greater and certainly no longer lasting than the enduring changes brought about by antipsychotics or antidepressants. A disease model of addiction based on the idea that enduring brain changes after illicit drug use mean that this is a disease does not hold up unless applied to antipsychotics and antidepressants also.

Addiction is a social concept in two senses. It is social in the sense that drugs of addiction are ones that society has deemed to be addictive. Some factors can create an appetite for the drug, but it is social laws that restrict availability and lead to criminal behaviour to fund a habit.[20] Drugs of addiction are social also in the sense that there is an exquisite interplay between environmental and biological factors. Addictions, while having clear biological components, arise in degraded environments. Tackling these latter problems is not a matter of treatment with a further drug.

PROTRACTED WITHDRAWAL OR LEGACY EFFECTS?

Withdrawal from antipsychotics can lead to tardive dyskinesia. This is rarely thought of as drug dependence even though it appears on treatment withdrawal and demonstrates tolerance – in some cases it can be managed by raising the dose of treatment. Tardive dyskinesia may be better seen as a legacy effect rather than protracted withdrawal – but it could be either.

Legacy effects are ones that arise in the course of treatment and endure after a treatment has stopped. This means they can become confounded with withdrawal, making it difficult to be certain what's a withdrawal effect and how long withdrawal lasts.

In the case of the SSRIs, post-SSRI sexual dysfunction (PSSD) (Chapter 20) just like tardive dyskinesia arises in the course of treatment where it is confused with the sexual dysfunction that affects up to 90% of patients taking SSRIs or it can appear for the first time on withdrawal. PSSD can endure after treatment stops for 10 years or more. At present there is no known treatment. The symptoms involve genital numbing, which suggests an element of neuropathy, just as tardive dyskinesia involves some neuropathy.

Poorly understood symptoms like these are often dismissed as 'neurotic'. There is a growing divide between those who have difficulties getting off antidepressants, or have enduring problems after withdrawal, who refer to protracted withdrawal syndrome, and doctors who deny that these complaints fit any known model of dependence or withdrawal.

The first point to make is that withdrawal syndromes from antidepressants are real and in many instances more severe than many concede. Healthy volunteer studies on paroxetine in the mid-1980s found that up to 66% of subjects had withdrawal problems after 2 weeks of exposure to treatment. This happened in both young and old, in males and in females. The withdrawal syndrome included anxiety, depression, malaise, dizziness, agitation, insomnia and nightmares, essentially most of the features of major depressive disorder even though these individuals had not begun with any affective disorder.

It is now clear that all SSRIs cause significant dependence and withdrawal problems with many SSRI users who have also used opiates, cocaine or other drugs of abuse saying that it can be more difficult to get off an SSRI than these other drugs. The company line remains that studies show any problems are transient. But the studies typically cited have looked at symptoms that emerge shortly after the discontinuation of treatment in people who have had short-term treatment. These studies have not taken legacy effects into account or attempted to recruit from the large pool of people who find it difficult to stop.

In most Western countries, there is now one antidepressant prescription per year for every member of the population. Of these, upwards of 90% are for people on treatment chronically. This should not happen if there is no problem stopping. There have in fact been more reports to regulators about dependence on SSRIs than there have been for any other psychotropic drugs.

C-FIBRE NEUROPATHIES

Patients with a peripheral sensory neuropathy present with problems for which they often cannot find words. The complaints may seem bizarre – pain for instance triggered by heat or touch (tactile allodynia), paraesthesia, or complaints of tight band-like sensations that do not map onto standard dermatomes, hot, or burning or numb sensations in feet or hands that present in stocking or glove distributions. Where pain is involved, the conditions respond poorly to standard treatments for pain.

These conditions are linked to C-fibres rather than the larger fibres that mediate discriminative touch. There are links to drug treatment. Burning hands and feet are termed causalgia, and this has long been linked to alcohol use, even though it is reported more often in women than men. Triptan use for migraine is linked to tactile allodynia. PSSD and persistent genital arousal disorder (PGAD), which commonly entails vulvodynia, are linked to serotonin reuptake inhibitors, isotretinoin and finasteride.

C-fibres have input from histamine and serotonin through S3 receptors and transient receptor potential (TRP) receptors of which there are now eight superfamilies and efforts are underway to map the functional roles of each.[21] TRP receptors are linked to a series of channels that mediate calcium and sodium ion transport across membranes. They are present on all types of nerves but especially on C-fibres mediating tactile sensitivity, pain, itch, smell and taste.

There are new distinctions between C-fibres mediating touch and fibres mediating affective tactile sensitivity.[22] There is a growing body of evidence that this component of the peripheral sensory system and its mediation of maternal touch in early life is an important determinant of the development of the social brain in the first instance and later abilities to regulate mood states.

These developments fit the James-Lange Theory of the Emotions: this theory suggests our emotions may lie primarily in our bodies and are only interpreted centrally. There is much more of ourselves outside our brains and in our body than we usually think. In this case, nurturing touch sets affective tone, and if the fibres mediating this are disturbed, affective tone is likely to be also. Similarly, while there may be central input also, peripheral genital sensations may drive libido so that when genital numbness happens as in PSSD, libido falls off as a consequence.

There is little information on C-fibre input to memory processes, but there are a great number of patients taking drugs from statins to fluoroquinolones to antidepressants complain about 'Chemo Brain' or 'Brain Fog' but have normal results on cognitive function tests. Complaints like this, against a background of normal results, are consistent with a disturbance in C-fibre function.

It is worth noting that there are smell and taste receptors in the gut, where 90% of the body's serotonin lies, and in general a substantial proportion of the nerves in the gut wall are C-fibres. A disturbance here would give rise to food and drug intolerances.

Finally, TRP channels play a significant role in cardiac functioning. Through mechanisms not clearly understood, as groups of drugs, antidepressants and antipsychotics have significantly more effects on aspects of cardiac functioning expressed in QT intervals and rhythm abnormalities than other groups of drugs.

Consider now the classic symptoms linked by sufferers to protracted withdrawal difficulties with antidepressants, benzodiazepines and antipsychotics:

1. Heart palpitations.
2. Increased anxiety.
3. Restless legs.
4. A pain syndrome.
5. Muscle tightness.
6. Food and drug sensitivities or intolerance.
7. Muscle twitches.
8. Feeling very flat.
9. Taste or smell changes.
10. Sensitivity to sound and light.
11. Heat sensitivities.

These differ significantly from the electric zaps, dizziness, nausea, vomiting and nightmares that are prominent features of acute withdrawal, but these acute withdrawal features do seem to clear up after several weeks or 1 month or two.

Case A: Waldinger and colleagues have reported a case that might point a way ahead.[23] Their patient was referred for paroxetine-induced penile anaesthesia. The gentlemen lost his sense of smell and taste whilst taking an SSRI in addition to having diminished skin sensitivity over large parts of his body including the genital area. Smell and taste returned whilst on treatment, and after he stopped paroxetine, his skin sensitivity returned to normal, but his genital numbness persisted. He could apply Tiger Balm without sensation to his genital area.

This led to treatment with LPLI (low-power laser irradiation) to the penile area, which produced a degree of restoration to the ability to distinguish between warm and cold stimulation and about a 40% recovery in touch sensation. The researchers speculate that the action of LPLI treatment is mediated through TRP channels.

Case B: A 60 year old woman who had 20 years' successful treatment with dosulepin until following a parathyroidectomy the benefit of treatment failed. Having previously been unable to stop treatment, she was now able to stop successfully.

One year later her mood slipped. She was given a series of serotonin reuptake inhibiting drugs but found herself intolerant to all of them, with disturbances of vision, smell, touch, heart rhythms, and an aggravation in terms of intensity and extent of a previously mild degree of numbness and muscle stiffness in her feet. She developed food and drug intolerances she did not have before.

Her current situation is that most antidepressants cause problems in ever lower doses while stopping them also causes problem. There appears to be an instability of some system.

'My hearing is a lot worse; I have vertigo and balance problems. I feel unsteady on my feet. My ears are ringing. They are also supersensitive to sounds. I feel like I am only 50 percent here – kind of like a bad head cold feeling or living in a dream state. I feel shaky and out of sorts and panicky. I feel weird and feel like I am going to pass out. I can be fine one minute, and then BAM – all of a sudden I feel this odd feeling coming on as if my hearing gets very quiet. I feel as if I am chilled. I get a tingly feeling in my head, and then I feel a sort of darkness and closed-in feeling about to happen. I start to shake and sweat, and I just feel as if I am drifting away'.

LEGACY OR PROTRACTED WITHDRAWAL?

SSRI and related antidepressants have effects on peripheral sensory systems, especially on C-fibres. If this underpins protracted withdrawal effects, as with tardive dyskinesia, we would expect these effects occasionally to appear within weeks of starting treatment but to be more likely to arise later in the course of treatment and to endure after treatment stops.

It would support the standard understanding of the basic withdrawal process, which is that this is time-limited. So we would expect some individuals to have a straightforward withdrawal process, lasting a number of weeks. This might in some instances be more severe than is often conceded. There is substantial evidence that this process, for instance, doubles the rates of suicidal and aggressive acts within 30 days of stopping. These effects may be so severe than in some instances the process of withdrawing may be impossible.

We would expect a number of clinically disturbing features to emerge on treatment or its discontinuation that persist relatively indefinitely after treatment stops. The evidence from PSSD suggests strongly that neuropathic disturbances do happen – so the question is how far beyond PSSD they extend. Such enduring post-withdrawal outcomes, however, are legacy rather than withdrawal effects.

These peripheral sensory neuropathies should create some instability of affective tone especially as anyone suffering from them would run into a dismissal from their prescriber. They would also create a variety of dysphoric and other conditions. Just as tardive dyskinesia can be alleviated in some temporarily by re-instituting treatment, so the same might be expected with SSRIs (or benzodiazepines), but overall the contribution from the neuropathy is to lead to a situation of instability so that neither increasing nor decreasing dosage brings relief. Against this background, adding the effects of withdrawal to an already uncomfortable situation can only make the discomfort worse, sometimes making withdrawal itself impossible – think antipsychotic withdrawal compounded by the emergence of tardive dyskinesia.

In the face of clinical difficulties such as this, the history of tardive dyskinesia shows that many clinicians are likely to attribute the difficulties to the disorder being treated. In the case of the antidepressants, this response might lead to suggestions the patient is bipolar and needs a mood-stabiliser added to an antidepressant. Drugs like pregabalin (Lyrica) may offer temporary relief but will often add to the instability.

We know genetically coded channelopathies mediate shorter or longer QT intervals, that increase or decrease the risk of an arrhythmia from treatment-induced QT changes. Similar genetic effects may predispose some subjects to the development of treatment-related peripheral sensory neuropathies

The pharmacology of channelopathies and TRP channels remains rudimentary, but there are likely many treatments out there that have potentially helpful effects. Drugs acting on calcium or sodium channels would seem to offer the best prospects.

REFERENCES

1. Bakalar JB, Grinspoon L. Drug control in a free society. Cambridge: Cambridge University Press; 1989.
2. Baker TB, Tiffany ST. Morphine tolerance as habituation. Psychol Rev 1985;92:78–108.
3. Jaffe JH. Addictions: what does biology have to tell? Int Rev Psychiatry 1989;1:51–62.
4. Srisurapanoni M, Jarusuraisin N. Opioid antagonists for alcohol dependence. Cochrane Database Syst Rev 2005;(1):CD001867.
5. Kirchmayer U, Davoli M, Verster A. Naltrexone maintenance treatment for opioid dependence (Cochrane Review). In: The Cochrane Library, Issue 4. Oxford: Update Software; 1999.
6. Preston KL, Bigelow GE. Pharmacological advances in addiction treatment. Int J Addict 1985;20:845–67.
7. Loimer N, Schmid RW, Presslich D, et al. Continuous naloxone administration suppresses opiate withdrawal symptoms in human opiate addicts during detoxification treatment. J Psychiatr Res 1989;23:81–6.
8. Olds J. Studies of neuropharmacologicals by electrical and chemical manipulation of the brain in animals with chronically implanted electrodes. In: Bradley P, Deniker P, Radouco-Thomas C, editors. Neuropsychopharmacology. Amsterdam: Elsevier; 1959. p. 20–32.
9. Pickens RW, Johanson C-E. Craving: consensus of status and agenda for future research. Drug Alcohol Depend 1992;30:127–31.
10. Hand TH, Franklin KB. Associative factors in the effects of morphine on self-stimulation. Psychopharmacology (Berl) 1986;88:472–9.
11. Mann K, Lehert P, Morgan MY. The efficacy of acamprosate in the maintenance of abstinence in alcohol-dependent individuals: results of a meta-analysis. Alcohol Clin Exp Res 2004;28:51–63.
12. Healy D. The creation of psychopharmacology. Cambridge, MA: Harvard University Press; 2002.
13. Hollister LE. From hypertension to psychopharmacology: a serendipitous career. In: Healy D, editor. The psychopharmacologists, vol. 2. London: Arnold; 1998. p. 215–35.
14. Hollister LE, Eikenberry DT, Raffel S. Chlorpromazine in nonpsychotic patients with pulmonary tuberculosis. Am Rev Respir Dis 1960;81:562–6.
15. Battegay R. Forty-four years in psychiatry and psychopharmacology. In: Healy D, editor. The psychopharmacologists, vol. 3. London: Arnold; 2000. p. 371–93.
16. Tranter R, Healy D. Neuroleptic discontinuation syndromes. J Psychopharmacol 1998;12:306–11.
17. Healy D, Tranter R. Pharmacopsychiatric stress syndromes. J Psychopharmacol 1999;13:287–90.
18. Baldessarini RJ, Ghaemi SN, Viguera AC. Tolerance in antidepressant treatment. Psychother Psychosom 2002;71:177–9.
19. Fitzgerald K, Healy D. Dystonias and dyskinesias of the jaw associated with the use of SSRIs. Hum Psychopharmacology 1995;10:215–20.
20. DeGrandpre R. The cult of pharmacology. Chapel Hill: Duke University Press; 2007.
21. Nilius B, Owsianik G, Voets T, et al. Transient receptor potential cation channels in disease. Physiol Rev 2007;87:165–217.
22. McGlone F, Wessberg J, Olausson H. Discriminative and affective touch: sensing and feeling. Neuron 2014;82:737–56.
23. Waldinger MD, van Coevorden R, Schweitzer D, et al. Penile anesthesia in Post SSRI Sexual Dysfunction (PSSD) responds to low-power laser irradiation: a case study and hypothesis about the role of transient receptor potential (TRP) ion channels. Eur J Pharmacol 2015;753:263–8.

SECTION 10
CONSENT, ABUSE AND LIABILITY

SECTION CONTENTS

Consent

24

CHAPTER CONTENTS

INTRODUCTION

Over the past two decades, there has been a shift within health care from an expectation that patients should entrust themselves passively to the care of physicians to an expectation that they should cooperate in their own care. These changes are reflected in the terms we use; for instance, the word patient, which means someone who endures, is often replaced by terms such as client or consumer, which suggest a more active participant in the medical process.

Informed consent was not an issue in medical practice before the 1970s.[1] Today, it forms a central issue. It may seem clear what informed consent is, but in a famous study where volunteers were given varying amounts of information about the drug's expected side effects, the more information the volunteers were given, the less likely they were to take the drug, despite being offered money.[2] But when they found out that the drug being investigated was aspirin, most subjects said that what they now knew would not change their attitude to aspirin.

Despite its name, therefore, there seems to be a sense in which informed consent cannot be about being fully informed. Both too much and too little information can prejudice valid consent. Rather than meaning fully informed consent, informed consent must mean something more like valid or voluntary consent.

VOLUNTARY CONSENT

When an individual attends for a consultation, although this is changing, the assumption has been they will take the advice offered by the healthcare professional. A prescription often seems to function in two ways: as a treatment and as a symbol of the advice being offered.

Arguably, however, informed consent is such a contested issue now because we expect more negotiation than formerly. There are problems in that a surgery or outpatient setting is not one that is conducive to any of us being able to articulate our concerns. We may be worried by the condition that has led us to seek help. We may be anxious when faced with the doctor, nurse, psychologist or whoever. We may be aware of the queue of others after us, who need to be seen, and of the prescriber who seems to be wondering whether they are likely to get to lunch if all consultations are going to take as long. Not the best arrangements for considering whether it's a good idea to commit to 'a poison' or not.

For these and other reasons, we often take the prescription. However, evidence suggests that most people given antidepressants, for instance, do not take them for longer than 4 weeks. One reason for this may be that the pill prescribed does not suit them, but another may be that once away from the pressures generated in clinical settings, people withdraw consent.

The lack of consent involved here probably does not reflect an opposition to drug treatment so much as an opposition to a style of treatment delivery, in which an authoritarian doctor decides what is best and issues instructions. Implicit in this authoritarian approach is the idea that medical science has developed to such an extent that there is something approaching certainty regarding the proper management of most conditions.

In contrast, many have argued that care should involve a greater acknowledgement of uncertainty on the part of the practitioner and an invitation to collaboration.[3–5] According to this approach, treatment would be a matter of negotiation rather than one of instruction: a negotiation that would recognise that an illness is one event within the drama of someone's life and that, for a variety of reasons, rigid adherence to a treatment regimen, with all the side effects that may be entailed, may not be that person's top priority.

From this perspective, voluntary consent is key to good clinical practice. This is not something that can be properly defined at law. Even signed consent forms, in certain circumstances, may not be interpreted by a court as indicating valid consent, whilst on the other hand the lack of a signed consent will not necessarily be taken to indicate a lack of consent should someone apply for legal redress for a claimed injury.

The law is only a blunt instrument. Ideally a profession should give some indications about what it thinks on certain key issues. The possession of a book such as this or access to a website like RxISK.org can perhaps help by offering a clear set of statements with which a therapist may agree or disagree and in the process reveal something of their approach to therapy.

A clinical style that is more likely to result in valid consent to taking the risks involved in any act of health care hinges on an ability of healthcare professionals to live with explicit ignorance about the likely outcome of their interventions in the circumstances of their patient's life. The sharing of knowledge and power that such an approach advocates is not one that all healthcare professionals accept or one that all can live with easily, even in limited circumstances. Indeed, it is not the approach that all patients want – sometimes we just want someone who knows what they are doing to take over responsibility for us.

Until things go wrong, that is. When things go wrong and people want to stop taking an antidepressant or antipsychotic because the trade-off is no longer acceptable to them, the system often regards them as 'mad'. Taking medication has come to be seen as evidence we are handling our problems. Today we get stigmatised instead if we are not taking our meds – people wonder about our capacity.

INFORMATION AND COMPREHENSION

How much information do people need about the risks and benefits of treatments? Most commentators come down in favour of informing the taker of a drug of the significant risks associated with treatment rather than making them aware of every possible risk. There are a number of issues here.

One is the question of being able to make an informed judgement of whether to consent to treatment or not. A bald list of side effects or complications is unlikely to help any of us to make up our minds. In contrast, meeting someone who is taking the drug or who has undergone the treatment in question and had problems is more likely to offer a tangible example of the issues involved.

We are often very isolated in making decisions. It is not an easy matter for anyone to be faced with 'facts' in clinical settings; these facts often bring with them implicit requests to make our minds up soon. Where psychotropic drug taking is concerned, this isolation and the disempowerment that it brings about could be managed by encouraging prospective drug takers to visit local user groups or 'Mind' branches, by having advocates on wards or with access to first person accounts of treatment.

Groups such as 'Mind' have sometimes been seen as hostile to medical practice in the past. But those giving treatments need to realise the role of the community at large in accepting medical practices. This is a message pharmaceutical companies understand all too well as they get ever more active in setting up patient special interest groups. Many doctors still live in a world of medical authoritarianism, but 50 years ago doctors were thought to be on their patients' sides. The relentless progress of technical developments since and pharmaceuticalisation of medicine has led to a disintegration of this community of understanding. This became very clear with the benzodiazepine crisis, in which doctors and pharmaceutical companies rather than the addicted patient were regarded as the problem by the wider community.

A further important point is whether the information that is given comes with implicit or explicit permission to return with further concerns and queries at a later date, or even the permission to consult a third party. In this case, the privileges of the wealthy, who think nothing of seeking further advice elsewhere if they are not happy with what they have paid for, contain a pointer to the state of affairs that would be desirable for all.

Finally, on the question of information, there is the issue of comprehension. Clinical settings are often very stressful, and there is a good deal of research to suggest that only half of the information imparted in a consultation is retained afterwards. One way to overcome this would be to copy letters sent to the patient's general practitioner to the patient also. This would give people an opportunity to remind themselves of the recommendations that were made and a chance to review these recommendations in a less stressful setting.[6,7]

The language in which recommendations are made may pose its own problems. The practice of medicine, as with the practice of anything else, involves the comprehension of a jargon. This jargon becomes so commonplace to practitioners that they often forget that the terms they use may be meaningless to the person they are seeing. The term schizophrenia, for example, is likely to suggest something akin to a split personality disorder to most lay people – a condition that would not, on the face of it, appear to be appropriately treated with drug therapy.

In clinical trials, for example, despite what appear to be clear instructions, a patient may simply not grasp that of the two pills they are taking only one is active, whilst the other is a placebo. Again and again in clinics it becomes clear that many patients do not appreciate that an anticholinergic drug (see Chapter 3) may be an antidote to side effects their antipsychotic is causing.

CLINICAL TRIALS AND LEGAL JEOPARDY

There is another issue. What are we being asked to consent to? Every medicine is comprised of two things – a chemical and the information a prescriber has from clinical trials.

In clinical studies before launch, the selective serotonin reuptake inhibitors (SSRIs) were associated with akathisia and agitation, occurring with sufficient frequency and intensity to lead to recommendations that benzodiazepines be co-prescribed in clinical trials.[8] Leading textbooks on the clinical profile of psychotropic agents mention SSRI's well-known propensity to cause akathisia. Akathisia has been implicated as a mechanism whereby SSRIs may lead to violence and suicide (see Chapter 5). Yet the clinical trials database for these drugs contains almost no mention of akathisia. We are now in a world where prominent effects can go 'missing' for 10 to 20 years.

Emotional flatness or blunting is a not infrequent side effect of treatment reported by patients on SSRIs. Arguably, this effect is the key thing these drugs do. Most patients mention it either as a useful or as an unhelpful thing. It has been linked to a range of harmful behaviours, yet nothing resembling emotional blunting appears in the clinical trials side-effect database for SSRIs.

These examples point to problems with the side-effect data from clinical trials. One is the failure of systems to cope with 'new' problems. Another is a dependence on self-reporting methods for the collection of data on side effects. In the case of the SSRIs, these methods detect only one in six of the side effects detected by systematic checklist methods.[9]

If the side-effect profile of a drug drawn from clinical trials was used just for marketing purposes, there might be little problem with this state of affairs. We could all take them with a grain of salt. After all, although clinical trials indicated that sexual dysfunction on SSRIs occurred at a 5% rate, no-one believed this. These side-effect profiles have, however, also been used in marketing and for legal purposes to deny that claimed adverse effects are happening.

This means that anyone entering into any clinical trials where side-effect data are collected by spontaneous reporting methods and there is no access to the data are putting any patient who suffers a drug-induced adverse event into a state of legal jeopardy. When you become suicidal, the data from trials in which I may have become suicidal are hidden from your doctor and the hiding is used to deny that this drug could cause anyone to become suicidal.

Clinical trials these days are an industry, and even the government encourages people to participate in trials, arguing that it is almost a civic duty to do so – the doctors doing the persuading are much less likely to participate themselves in trials or to encourage their own family members to do so. But given the lack of access to trial data it may be time to stop participating in these trials that often yield thousands of pounds per patient for the clinician running the study, but only increased legal jeopardy for the rest of us.

Another way forwards might be for ethics committees and patient advocacy groups or others to transform the informed consent form into a contract between patients and investigators and companies giving rights of access to the raw data. This is not an issue just to leave to patient groups within mental health. It applies across medicine and applies as much to those who are not at present patients as it does to those at present in treatment. This is a matter for lawyers and politicians to consider closely as it is their friends and families who are being put in a state of legal jeopardy should treatment lead to drug-induced injury.

COMPLIANCE

There is an overlap between consent and compliance. Those who do not consent to treatment are unlikely to comply with it afterwards. Many people, when they consent, do so only provisionally. For instance, a consent to antidepressant treatment will often involve an agreement to take the medication only until some improvement appears; it will not mean an agreement to go on taking it forever.

Playing on concerns about poor compliance with antidepressants, companies provided many SSRIs in one pill a day form. This, however, was largely a marketing exercise and should not be thought of as the answer to problems with compliance. The issues involved in non-compliance hinge on relationships and education, rather than whether the pills come in a once-a-day formulation. Current research suggests that the greatest single determinant of compliance is the quality of the relationship between the patient and their keyworker or prescriber.[10]

Another important element in the equation is an individual's personal situation. Becoming a patient is just one more episode in personal dramas that involve getting or holding down jobs, sexual relations, driving safely and so much more.[4] Nursing staff and other mental-health staff may be much more aware of this than their medical colleagues and could probably do a great deal to minimise confrontation by bringing out how much treatment is getting in the way of a person getting on with their life. This happens more often areas of healthcare such as the management of diabetes than it happens in mental health.[11]

One of the weapons a patient or their keyworker can use in the face of medical power is the weapon of data. Filling up rating scales such as the LUNSERS (Liverpool University Side Effect Rating Scale)[12] is a way to face a physician with data; if the physician is being as scientific as they claim, this tests how they will respond to data.

A more specific version of the same would be to create rating scales specially designed for each problem being faced by the patient – this is easily done (see Fig. 24.1). Using scales such as this, the individual (perhaps helped by a keyworker) would rate how much difficulty they were having from voices, for instance, and how much from a side effect such as weight gain, stiffness or sexual dysfunction. The progress of problems stemming from both the illness and the treatment could be charted over the course of several weeks in this fashion and then presented to the prescriber (Figs. 24.2–24.4).

If a prescriber refuses to respond to these data, or if their behaviour is not manipulable by feedback of this sort, it may be time to change prescriber.

PRESCRIBING

One of the most significant changes since the first edition of this book has been the appearance of nurse prescribing. This is one more step in a history that now spans a century.

A prescription, initially, was an order to a pharmacist to dispense a particular medication, but until the 1950s it was not the only way a patient could obtain medication. Most drugs, including thalidomide, for example, were sold over the counter (OTC). Alternatively, based on an earlier prescription, a patient could go back to the pharmacist for virtually endless repeats. The idea of prescription only medicines (POM) was introduced in 1914 for heroin and cocaine – it was a system to control addicts.

This situation changed in 1951 when the US regulators made new drugs available on prescription-only.[13] Extending a system designed for addicts to restrict the availability of the first really effective agents, the new antibiotics, seemed odd to many. The thalidomide disaster of 1962 copper-fastened the new system in place, and since then all of us have been forced to hand over control of our health care to professionals in a way that we did not have to do before.

In recent years, some of the new 'wonder' drugs have become available OTC – the histamine H2 blockers such as cimetidine and ranitidine, for instance. Is there any reason why the SSRIs or antipsychotics could not also be available OTC? The SSRIs are at least as safe as H2 blockers – or the serotonin reuptake inhibiting antihistamines that have always been OTC. The problem with SSRIs often lies in the fact that patients unwilling to make their doctor unhappy continue taking a drug that makes them feel bad in a way they would never continue with something bought OTC.

If chlorpromazine had been available OTC, it seems a safe bet that it would never have been self-prescribed by users in the megadoses given during the 1970s and 1980s. It is more likely that users would have opted for regimens pretty close to what medical opinion 40 years later seems to be coming around to recommending as optimal.

Sold OTC, the tricyclic antidepressants would probably have been marketed as tonics rather than antidepressants: they improve sleep, appetite, energy, etc. Seen in this light, they might be far more acceptable to many people. Part of the appeal behind alternative medicine and the use of health

Self-assessment questionnaire

Usual experiences/problems (enter your own problem)

1 Today, how much have you had paranoid feelings/low mood, etc?

Not at all ☐☐☐☐☐☐☐☐☐ A great deal

2 Today, how much have you heard voices?

Not at all ☐☐☐☐☐☐☐☐☐ A great deal

Distress caused by unusual experiences/problems

1 Today, how much have you been distressed by your paranoid feelings?

Not at all ☐☐☐☐☐☐☐☐☐ A great deal

2 Today, how much have you been distressed by voices?

Not at all ☐☐☐☐☐☐☐☐☐ A great deal

Side effects (enter your own side effect)

1 Today, how much have you had agitation caused by your drugs?

Not at all ☐☐☐☐☐☐☐☐☐ A great deal

2 Today, how much have you had dry mouth/sexual dysfunction, etc?

Not at all ☐☐☐☐☐☐☐☐☐ A great deal

Attitudes to medication

1 Today, I have felt that my medication:

Has not helped at all ☐☐☐☐☐☐☐☐☐ Has helped a great deal

2 Today, I have been distressed by my side effects:

Not at all ☐☐☐☐☐☐☐☐☐ A great deal

FIGURE 24.1 Rating scales used to determine a person's experience whilst taking psychotropic medication.

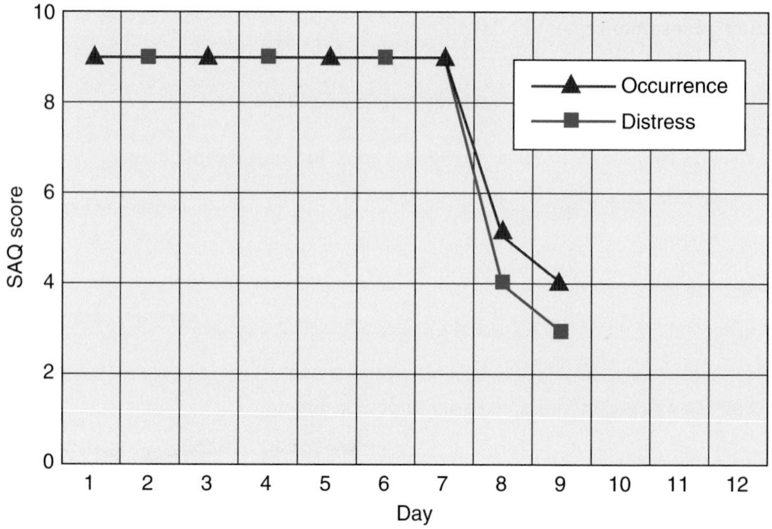

FIGURE 24.2 Occurrence and distress caused by paranoid feelings, as rated by Self-Assessment Questionnaire (SAQ).

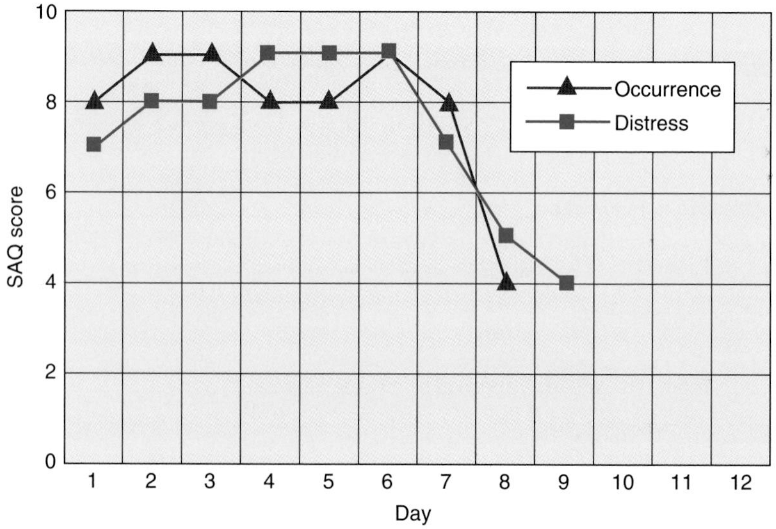

FIGURE 24.3 Occurrence and distress caused by voices, as rated by Self-Assessment Questionnaire (SAQ).

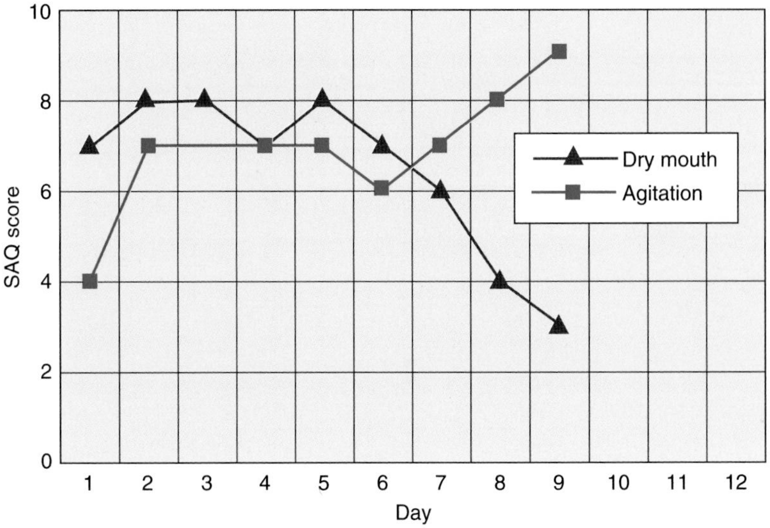

FIGURE 24.4 Dry mouth and agitation as rated by Self-Assessment Questionnaire (SAQ).

foods is that this kind of management leaves control of health in one's own hands, and there are not the same disease implications. If you are stressed or burnt out – something we all are from time to time – you can take St John's wort. To get Prozac (fluoxetine), you have to be given a mental illness first of all.

Prescriptions are also bound up intimately with the question of disease. In 1962, the US Food and Drug Administration (FDA) attempted to minimise the risks of treatment by restricting the use of drugs to people who were genuinely ill, so that any risks brought about by a drug could be weighed in the balance of clear benefits also produced. In the case of depression, it would seem that many people simply do not accept a disease model of depression: they do not consent to treatment on these premises and, as a consequence, they very often do not comply. In addition, what the regulators in 1962 failed to anticipate was the ability of pharmaceutical companies to sell diseases. Restricted to marketing pharmaceuticals for serious diseases, they have responded by making us all diseased (see Section 11). To give someone Prozac, a prescriber first has to make them depressed.

Pharmacological abuse

25

CHAPTER CONTENTS

When chlorpromazine was first introduced, doctors prescribed and patients took what they were given. The prescription of a medicine now is much more likely to be based on the assumption that a patient should understand the condition for which the prescription is given, the nature of any treatment, its duration, its chances of success, the risks of side effects and they should be free to ask for any information they want from the prescriber, who will respond genuinely.

Clearly, respect for the autonomy of the patient has to be balanced against a respect for the autonomy of others. In mental-health care it is necessary on occasion to give treatment without consent, but society has put mechanisms in place to compensate for a patient's loss of autonomy in such situations.[14,15] The issue here does not apply to these emergency situations but to situations where a paternalistic approach to patients may involve an insidious loss of autonomy that may be counter-therapeutic and ethically dubious and ultimately go close to compromising much of mental healthcare.

THE PROBLEM

Consider the following. Many patients, when first admitted to the hospital, will be started on medication regimens that they will not know exceed local or national formulary limits and greatly exceed what research has shown to be optimally effective. They are unlikely to know that there is rarely a pharmacological justification for the co-prescription of two different oral antipsychotics or for a combination of both an oral and depot antipsychotic, or for cocktails of anticonvulsants and antipsychotics. If given an anticholinergic agent, they may not know that this has been given as an antidote to the side effects of the primary medication. If they do know this, they are unlikely to know that, quite commonly, it would be possible to avoid the need for an anticholinergic agent. If they are on a combination of antidepressants and antipsychotics, they almost certainly will not know that their 'depression' may be a consequence of treatment with antipsychotics and, if so, will not be responsive to antidepressant medication.

On a broader front, the worry is that patients admitted to hospital will have their treatment discontinued abruptly with a new treatment started immediately with little or no consideration being given to the possibility of withdrawal from the earlier treatment. In practice antidepressants and antipsychotics are treated as though switching from one to another involved no more than switching between vitamins. This, however, is not the case. Putting patients on psychotropic drugs should be regarded as giving people a pharmacological life event.

Against this background, it seems certain that in clinical practice betrayals of trust occur and that situations may arise that are 'abusive'. Let us consider therefore to what extent dynamics that are familiar from the sexual abuse arena might also apply in this domain.

THE DYNAMICS OF ABUSE

As in other forms of abuse, a 'victim' of 'abusive prescribing' may be dependent on the 'abuser'.[16] This dependence may be brought about by virtue of an unavailability of psychiatric services in the victim's area other than through the prescriber and by virtue of the unavailability of psychotropic compounds other than by prescription. The victim, therefore, may have to maintain an interaction with the perpetrator and may in the process have to cope with the fact that the perpetrator at some level may show, or may be regarded as showing, concern for them. A common response to this point is that there is a difference between the intent to take advantage of children found in child abuse and the worst that clinicians can be accused of: doctors do not casually or deliberately 'violate' their patients. This probably underestimates the harm that can be done by clinicians 'who know best'.

As with other forms of abuse, there will necessarily be a low incidence of disclosure to others, for a number of reasons. First, it is necessary to disclose the illness in order to disclose the abuse, and victims may understandably be reluctant to do this. Second, there may be a legitimate fear of reprisals should complaints be made, which many suspect might take the form of an increase in the dose of the treatment being complained about. Third, in addition to being seen as ill, just as any other victim of abuse, a victim of abusive prescribing risks further stigmatisation as a 'loser'. Fourth, there are difficulties in ventilating concerns in this area as complaining about nervousness and other problems as a consequence of treatment leaves the subject open to the perception that all that has been demonstrated is the problem that led to the initial prescription.

Indeed, many may not make the connection between their treatment and the way they are feeling.[17,18] It may only be when they see someone else that they become aware of a connection between their treatment and symptoms such as anxiety, depression, demotivation, fatigue, a variety of psychosomatic symptoms, nervousness, impulsiveness, irritability, weight gain, sexual disturbances, suicidality, emotional blunting and other problems.

Finally, if a patient complains, there will often be a lack of support from significant others. This, as in other forms of abuse, may be important in its own right. Indeed, there may be considerable external pressure on the individual – from relatives and friends as well as from mental-health professionals – to accommodate to the situation and to internalise blame. This will lead to a sense of defectiveness on the patient's part or denial of the difficulties that are being experienced. This is compounded by blanket company denials that treatment could cause problems and indeed company suppression of the data indicating that there can be problems.

As with other forms of abuse, unpredictability may make things worse, as may the duration of the abuse, the extent to which the abuse pervades all aspects of the subject's life and the extent to which prescribing is seen as reactive to conflicts rather than aimed at rational and agreed therapeutic ends. Particular difficulties are raised in the case of violent incidents in clinical settings. In such circumstances mental-health staff risk assuming the role of both judge and jury.

Ongoing abuse has also traditionally found justification from evidence that the discontinuation of treatment leads to serious problems. This is invariably interpreted as a re-emergence of the illness, a situation that, ethically all but demands the resumption of treatment. However, there is a considerable body of evidence to indicate that what is typically taken as a new illness episode following a reduction or discontinuation of medication may in a large number of cases be evidence of a dependence syndrome (see Chapter 3 and Chapter 23).[19] It is known that clinicians routinely fail to warn patients about the risk of tardive dyskinesia owing to their own emotional discomfort at raising this possibility. Probably for similar reasons, they appear to have managed to ignore evidence indicating the existence of tardive dysthymias and other drug-induced stress syndromes. Clinicians seem in practice all but unable to inform their patients of these significant risks.

PRESCRIPTION 'RIGHTS'

Some of this potential for abuse may arise from the prescription-only status of psychotropic medicines (See Chapter 24). One consequence of prescription-only status is that it is not only when a patient has been formally detained that a prescriber is given more than the usual amount of power in determining the outcome of a clinical condition. Every writing of a prescription involves a potential deferral to a medical opinion in a manner that does not happen when people manage their own conditions by non-pharmacotherapeutic means or by means of over-the-counter medications or health food supplements. The potential for abuse in prescription-only arrangements was recognised when it was put in place in 1962 when it was noted that the person who prescribed consumed by putting something into the mouth of another – 'he who orders does not buy and he who buys does not order'. This is consumption without side effects – for the prescriber.

Potentially abusive prescribing of the type outlined probably applies in the case of all medications, given indicators from 1996 that drug-induced conditions were the fourth leading cause of death and may have led to up to one-third of admissions to hospital.[20] The issue, however, probably applies with extra force in the case of the psychotropic agents, in that the problematic effects of medication are most pernicious in this domain. However, where the women's movement has been able to lobby effectively for a consideration of sexual abuse and harassment both on a legal level and in terms of raising consciousness in society, mental-health patients have fewer levers available to them and would seem to be even more vulnerable.

A vignette may bring some of the issues home. MC is a 65-year-old well-educated articulate woman who became depressed for the first time in her life. She had concomitant osteoporosis that restricted the choice of antidepressant medication that might have suited her. She was accordingly put on sertraline. After several weeks on this she developed chest pain, probably anginal, and breathlessness. After attendance at a clinic, I wrote to her general practitioner recommending a change from this antidepressant. He did nothing. A follow-up letter copied to the patient, suggesting that this was selective serotonin reuptake inhibitor (SSRI)-induced angina and an SSRI-induced respiratory dyskinesia, again advising a change of medication from SSRIs, also had no effect. The doctor's interpretation was that the angina was unrelated to her treatment. He interpreted her breathlessness as panic attacks and therefore as evidence that she should continue with treatment and preferably with an SSRI. The woman herself continued with treatment, afraid that if she stopped and had to call her general practitioner out in an emergency, and he were to find that she had gone against his instructions, he would refuse to treat her when she really needed it. The general practitioner was finally persuaded to change to a non-SSRI, and after several weeks MC's chest pains and breathlessness cleared up.

This vignette illustrates how dependent people can become in therapeutic situations. Children are almost certainly even less capable of maintaining their perceptions of drug-induced abnormality in the face of contradictory interpretations from both clinicians and their parents. This is not just a theoretical issue. There has been a huge increase in antidepressant and antipsychotic prescribing to children, with estimates that there are several million prescriptions per year in the USA alone.[21–23] This increase has taken place even though the randomised trials of these drugs undertaken in paediatric populations have shown no benefit of the drugs over placebo. There is an ethical issue as to whether this kind of treatment should take place at all in the face of so much negative evidence but, more to the point, the potential for abuse would seem to be huge in such situations.

As with other situations of abuse, the adverse effects of abusive prescribing will remain invisible as long as the existence of a problem remains unacknowledged.

Although not about prescribing, the question of abuse in therapy formed the heart of the Osheroff case, in which a man who was depressed was treated for 9 months with psychotherapeutic approaches that had not been shown to work. Subsequent treatment with antidepressants brought about a prompt improvement in his condition, but this was too late to save his marriage or his job. The issues were debated at length in the pages of the *American Journal of Psychiatry*.[24,25] In brief, there was no agreement that therapy should necessarily follow evidence of efficacy, but there was agreement that persistence with one therapeutic line, in the face of a lack of progress without a genuine review of other options, was indefensible. Even where the therapy being delivered has been shown to have some evidence of efficacy, a failure to review may well be abusive.

The Osheroff case makes clear that it is good practice for all therapists, prescribers or not, to specify what outcomes they are aiming at, the period of time for which they are likely to persist in a particular course of action in the face of non-response or partial response and what other treatment options they would consider should the current treatment fail to deliver the expected benefits. Exactly these recommendations were written into a 1997 British Association for Psychopharmacology consensus statement on prescribing for childhood and learning disability indications.[26]

THE RIGHT NOT TO BE DISABLED BY TREATMENT

In one of the most extraordinary books in medicine, *Dear Luise*, Dorrit Cato Christensen outlines what happened to her daughter Luise.[27] Luise did not have a mental illness. She may have had an Asperger-like syndrome. She slipped into the mental-health system owing to adverse effects stemming from anticonvulsant medication she was given for a diagnosis that was unfounded. Even though Dorrit was a passionate and articulate advocate on her behalf, Luise never managed to escape from the system. She predicted her own death, which followed.

The challenge for all of us is to work out what kind of mechanisms to put in place to avoid what now seems an inevitable fate for some patients.

Up to 1845 the scanty Mental Health Legislation was worldwide aimed preventing abuses – stopping the occasional unscrupulous relative from getting someone locked up in order to steal their money. In 1845, a new kind of asylum was created that aimed at cures. Where before people who were dangerous were locked up, after 1845 we began to detain people whose families recognised were ill rather than possessed or criminal. This was the point in history where the idea of a patient was properly born – not just within mental health, although mental health was the first to have specialist hospitals and journals.

The 1845 Lunacy Act created an entirely new framework based on therapeutic optimism. Specialist treatment would enable patients to recover. It was similar in spirit to the way we sometimes compulsorily detain patients with tuberculosis today – because we have treatments that can make a difference.

It was recognised that the bulk of caring was being undertaken by families and communities, but the hope was that a new therapeutic instrument, the asylum, might support community efforts. Treatment in the asylum depended on the consent of the family. The decision to detain was the families usually. The family could discharge the patient 'against advice' if they believed no benefits were being realised, or the patient might remain in hospital when families felt unable to cope with them after discharge.

The data for moral treatment supported the case. For the first 40 years of the asylum era, schizophrenia was rare, and the psychoses and melancholias that came into hospital were turned around within a 3- to 6-month period with good hygiene and monitoring. Detention was an evidence-based treatment.

Later in the century as admissions for chronic psychoses became more common and hospitals began to silt up, the spectre of commitment to a hospital without the prospects of a benefit began to raise concerns. The notion of a warehouse for the insane began to take shape, into which the elderly infirm and mentally handicapped found their way also.

Interventions, whether medical or legal, can have unintended consequences. Drugs with a short-term benefit can produce long-term harms. The asylum system was not intended for long-stay patients and with longer stays the problems of institutionalisation emerged.

And once a medical system and a legal process is put in place, some component of what happens next will, on a simply bureaucratic basis, involve actions by the system to perpetuate itself. This an almost inevitable consequence of any intervention in human affairs. It leaves people grappling with the 'system'.

THE DILEMMAS OF THERAPEUTIC OPTIMISM

The hope that had been extinguished by 1900 re-emerged in the late 1950s with the first effective psychotropic drugs.

Just as the 1845 Act assumed asylums would work, current mental-health legislation assumes these drugs work. The evidence certainly shows these treatments can offer a beneficial tranquilisation, but there is less evidence of cures and much evidence that a proportion of patients rather than becoming more contained become more agitated and are at greater risk of harming themselves and others than they were in the first instance. The data points to a loss of up to 20 years of life expectancy. If the stated reason for detention is on the basis of reducing risks to self, or others or to the patient's health, this raises a problem.

The problem is that justified by an expectation of benefit, we deprive people of their liberties to a greater extent in the mental-health system than in the criminal justice system.

To compensate, the patient can appeal against the loss of liberty on the basis that they were not as ill as was claimed in the first instance, that the risks to their health and safety or the health and safety of others were not as great as was claimed or that detention is disproportionate in the circumstances.

But the system makes no provision to address a problem that many patients point to, which lies in the capacity of these treatments to cause adverse effects with significant behavioural consequences. In addition to triggering danger to self and others, these treatments can cause behavioural disturbances that mimic mental states that can lead to detention. The antipsychotics in particular can cause auditory hallucinations, stereotypies, mannerisms, agitation and can produce a 'psychotic look'. Under the influence of one of these drugs, if the doctor is unaware of the situation, a normal person could be detained in the interests of their own health and safety.

If detained, although there is an appeals process with an independent doctor, who may even be good at keeping patients out of hospital, these doctors are not trained in the recognition of treatment-related adverse events. They have not seen the evolution of the problem that almost by definition in the medical records will rarely be recorded as an adverse event, or may not be recorded. Tribunal doctors lack expertise to explore this domain and are unlikely to have an inclination to recognise treatment-induced problems. It is also difficult to sanction the release of someone whose condition has deteriorated since admission.

The people who are often best placed to recognise a deterioration or a failure of the original promise of detention are members of the individual's family, people like Luise's mother, Dorrit. But their protests that treatment is not helping are likely to be viewed as a questioning of medical authority leading to efforts to displace family members as the nearest relative or to bypass them, de facto displacing them without going through a judicial process.

Families have effectively lost an historic right – the right to discharge – and the patient has lost an important protection.

The problem extends beyond mental health and is growing. New treatments in health have engendered ever greater therapeutic optimism. Clinicians want to bring these benefits to the patients that come under their care. Many will think that patients who are reluctant to engage with treatment must lack capacity.

However for pretty well all pharmacological treatments on patent within medicine today, close to the entire scientific literature that fuels the therapeutic optimism that leads to their use is ghost written, and there is a total lack of access to the data underpinning the claims doctors make. The data supporting a patient's or families' perception that the treatment is not working is sequestered. In these circumstances, to claim that the patient and family lack insight or capacity and must be forced to comply is close to psychotic.

Families are increasingly at risk of isolation as they have to swim against a tide of increasing treatment seeking in communities sold the benefits of modern treatments by the most sophisticated marketing on earth. This marketing plays on the fact that families want to do the best for their members. The most striking examples come from the mental-health domain and involve families bringing children along for treatment for attention deficit/hyperactivity disorder (ADHD), depression or variations in development that would never before have come to medical attention.

CRISIS POINT

When arrangements are born in an era of therapeutic optimism, the eagerness to bring benefits may make medical, legal and government parties to the intervention susceptible to missing the harms that can arise.

We have reached a crisis point. Families and communities have traditionally provided the overwhelming bulk of care for relatives whether they were mentally infirm, elderly and dementing, younger with learning disabilities or suffering from physical illness. The impetus to care for a relative supported the creation of modern health services to help deliver the best possible care.

While the services have sometimes been compromised by abuses on the part of a small minority of families or in the institutions set up to deliver care, and while families will often push for treatments that many doctors are reluctant to give, the tendency to regard families who question things as suspect should be the exception not the rule. Abuses involving families need to be but should never obscure the primary reality, which is that families have by far the greatest incentive to secure the best possible outcome for a family member.

At a time when many still cannot access services, when many are in prison when they should be in hospital, we now paradoxically are facing a growing need to provide an exit route from healthcare for people who are rendered mentally infirm or alienated by the effects of treatment or held hostage by services supposed to support them.

Once in healthcare systems, the voices of professionals now trump the voices of those who know the person better – a child, parent or partner. This is unprecedented. Review tribunals, advocacy and other mechanisms put in place to ensure that patients get care that is the least restrictive possible, in many instances work to support incarceration rather than to support a person in taking risks they may wish to take.

Against this background, we need to recognise that:

- eliciting consent to treatment is a more complex process than is often recognised
- a lack of capacity should never mean disagreement with a healthcare professional
- those delivering treatments should not be allowed dictate what are a person's best interests
- risk management is biased towards locating risks in the person rather the system; we need to recognise that the greatest source of risks lies in the system – in the lack of access to clinical trial data and lack of provision of services by cash strapped health providers
- people need to be supported to embrace the risks they decide to take
- patients whose 'rights' are suspended must be treated as though their most passionate advocate were present to observe all that is happening them
- independent mechanisms need to be put in place to monitor the rates at which people are being injured by current systems of care
- advance directives and named person status must mean something
- detained patients should be provided with a copy of every medical report produced on them as a matter of course
- patients and families who speak out have legitimate fears of reprisals.

REFERENCES

1. Shorter E, Healy D. Shock therapy. A history of electroconvulsive treatment in mental illness. New Brunswick: Rutgers University Press; 2007.
2. Epstein LC, Lasagna L. Obtaining informed consent: form or substance. Arch Intern Med 1969;123:682–8.
3. Bursztajn HJ, Feinbloom RI, Hamm RM, et al. Medical choices: medical chances. London: Routledge; 1990.
4. Kleinman A. The illness narratives. New York: Basic Books; 1988.
5. Seedhouse D. Liberating medicine. Chichester: John Wiley; 1991.

6. Fitzgerald F, Healy D, Williams B. Shared care. Some effects of patient access to medical communications. J Ment Health 1996;6:37–46.
7. Healy D. Involving users in mental health services in the era of the word-processor and the database. In: Crosby D, Barry M, editors. Community care: evaluation of the provision of mental health services. Aldershot: Avebury Press; 1995. pp. 209–31.
8. Healy D. Let them eat Prozac. New York: New York University Press; 2004.
9. Rosenbaum JF, Fava M, Hoog SL, et al. Selective serotonin reuptake inhibitor discontinuation syndrome: a randomised clinical study. Biol Psychiatry 1998;44:77–87.
10. Day JC, Bentall RP, Roberts D, et al. Attitudes towards antipsychotic medication. The impact of clinical variables and relationships with health professionals. Arch Gen Psychiatry 2005;62:717–24.
11. Mol AM. The logic of care. London: Routledge; 2008.
12. Day J, Wood G, Dewey M. A self rating scale for measuring neuroleptic side effects. Br J Psychiatry 1995;143: 129–50.
13. Healy D. Pharmageddon. Berkeley CA: California University Press; 2012.
14. Brabbins CA, Butler J, Bentall R. Consent to antipsychotic medication for schizophrenia: clinical, ethical and legal issues. Br J Psychiatry 1996;168:540–4.
15. Ormrod R. Therapy, battery and informed consent. Psychiatr Bull 1987;11:185–6.
16. Healy D, Savage M, Thomas P. Abusive prescribing. OpenMind 1998;September:18.
17. Healy D, Farquhar GN. Immediate effects of droperidol. Hum Psychopharmacol 1998;13:113–20.
18. Sharp HM, Healy D, Fear CF. Symptoms or side effects? Methodological hazards and therapeutic principles. Hum Psychopharmacol 1998;13:467–75.
19. Tranter R, Healy D. Antipsychotic discontinuation syndromes. J Psychopharmacol 1998;12:306–11.
20. Lazarou J, Pomeranz BH, Corey PN. Incidence of adverse drug reactions in hospitalized patients. JAMA 1999;279:1200–5.
21. Fisher R, Fisher S. Antidepressants for children. Is scientific support necessary? J Nerv Ment Dis 1996;184:99–102.
22. Sharav VH. The impact of FDA Modernization Act on the recruitment of children for research. Ethical Hum Sci Serv 2003;5:83–108.
23. Healy D, Le Noury J. Paediatric bipolar disorder. An object of study in the creation of an illness. Int J Risk Saf Med 2007;19:209–21.
24. Klerman GL. The psychiatric patient's right to effective treatment: implications of osheroff vs chestnut lodge. Am J Psychiatry 1990;147:409–18.
25. Stone AA. Law, science and psychiatric malpractice: a response to Klerman's indictment of psychoanalytic psychiatry. Am J Psychiatry 1990;147:419–27.
26. Healy D, Nutt D. British Association for Psychopharmacology consensus statement on childhood and learning disabilities psychopharmacology. J Psychopharmacol 1997;11:291–4.
27. Christensen DL. Dear Luise. Portland: Jorvik Press; 2012.

SECTION 11

THE MARKETING OF TRANQUILLITY

SECTION CONTENTS

The ethical industry

26

CHAPTER CONTENTS

INTRODUCTION

Before the second half of the 19th century, the dominant medical and popular notions of disease rested on a humoral theory of disease, dating from the Greeks. According to this, there were four humours – phlegm, choler, bile and sanguine – and diseases resulted from an imbalance of these humours or between the humoral state of the individual and conditions in the environment.[1] Masturbation and menstruation led to disease or madness because of a loss of secretions disrupting the internal balance of the humours leading to disharmony.

A version of this theory survives to this day in the notions of yin and yang and in the three dhosas of Ayurvedic medicine, both of which are popular in complementary medicine settings. These systems aim at is a state of harmony, and treatment consists of efforts to restore balance or internal equilibrium. Until the 19th century this was done by regulating diet, by bleeding, purging, inducing vomiting, raising blisters (in which noxious vapours could collect), or by giving a variety of tonics – agents that were stimulant or strengthening in some way. Diet and tonics of various sorts remain the most popular methods today.[2]

Healers aimed at mimicking the body's own reactions: sweating, bleeding, purging, vomiting, the passage of water, etc. Producing what we would now call side effects like these seemed to be the obvious thing to do and, far from suing the way patients might do nowadays, these side effects were taken as a welcome sign that the treatment was working.

Against this background, a large industry flourished, aimed at satisfying consumer needs (or profiting from their misery) through the provision of tonics, elixirs, and so on. The market was almost entirely consumer led as numerous plays, novels and operas, such as Donizetti's *L'Elixir d'Amour*, attest. It was a regular feature of village life to have the pedlar of medicines come around with a range of potions for sale. Even when quite seriously ill, it was common until the 20th century for afflicted individuals to have a go at treating themselves first.

In the 19th century, patent medicines emerged – medicines containing 'secret' remedies. These were marketed vigorously in the popular press, and a great number of the techniques underpinning modern advertising developed in an effort to sell these compounds. Their success became an increasing problem in orthodox medical circles and amongst regulators.[3] The patent medicine industry survives today in over-the-counter (OTC) medicines, in the health food industry, in internet pharmacies selling smart drugs (Chapter 18) and in nutraceuticals such as lipid-lowering spreads.

The modern pharmaceutical industry took shape in the early 20th century as a reaction to these patent medicines. The drug companies that emerged termed themselves 'ethical' companies in contrast to the patent medicine industry. These companies saw themselves as being ethical, in their willingness to purify the compounds that went into their preparations and to specify exactly what a medicine contained.

THE MAGIC BULLET

The development of specific theories of disease was the most significant factor affecting the outcome of competition between the ethical and patent pharmaceutical industries. The discovery by Pasteur of bacteria and their role in infection led to a growing belief in specific causes for specific diseases. The key breakthrough came with the development of diphtheria antitoxin in 1896, which led to the eradication of diphtheria.

Allied to this, there was during the 19th century an increasing awareness that the many natural herbs and compounds that appeared to be helpful in the treatment of disease all contained specific compounds and that it was these compounds rather than the whole herb that were the curative factors. For example, it turned out to be the morphine in the poppy rather than the entire poppy that was helpful, the digitalis in foxglove and the salicylic acid in the bark of the willow tree (*Salix alba*). The emergence of anaesthesia led to more specific surgical procedures and specific cures. The growing trend found expression in Paul Ehrlich's concept of the magic bullet. Magic bullets would enter the body and act on a disease process specifically, leaving all other metabolic processes undisturbed.[4]

The antibiotics have come closest to this ideal in practice. The idea, however, has taken hold that all modern drugs are magic bullets of some sort, and this leads many, if not all, of us who are prescribing or taking drugs to believe that we are taking something that will work specifically on just one faulty piece of the human machinery.

The reality, however, is quite different. It is not just that most drugs, particularly psychotropic drugs, may cause side effects but rather that they all act throughout the body. For instance, the calcium channel blockers have therapeutic actions on almost every system in the body. The antipsychotics may be used as anxiolytics, antipsychotics, antidepressants, antipruritic agents, antihypertensives or antiemetics. Company marketing attempts to obscure this.

The advantage of purification is that the amount of a drug given could be controlled. In the case of foxglove, for example, crushing and administering the plant may help cardiac failure if the dose is right but may be poisonous if the dose is too high. In principle, if there is an active ingredient in a natural compound, it should always be possible to purify it and make its use safer.

The next step was the manufacture of entirely synthetic compounds, such as the barbiturates. The production of chlorpromazine in the 20th century was a laboratory-based exercise of this nature that was spectacularly successful.

But despite the rhetoric of magic bullets, the last thing the pharmaceutical industry actually wants – arguably – is a series of drugs that clear up the problem. The best-selling compounds are the antihypertensives, lipid-lowering drugs, gastric acid-reducing agents and antidepressants. These drugs lower risks, whether of strokes or suicides, rather than curing diseases such as strokes. The problem is where diseases can be cured, so that treatment can stop, risks go on forever so there is always a case for keeping the person on treatment. The human body however can cope with being poisoned in the short term by a magic bullet, like an antibiotic, but it's not designed to be poisoned long-term.

THE INTERFACE BETWEEN ETHICS AND MARKETS

In 1906, in an attempt to curb the production of dangerous patent medicines, what was later to be the Food and Drug Administration (FDA) was set up in the USA. The operation of the FDA led to the removal of many patent medicines from the market and to the demise of a large number of small companies producing such compounds. This fostered the growth of the ethical industry.[3]

Over the next 50 years in response to drug disasters culminating in thalidomide, the FDA began to put in place a set of regulations aimed at forcing the manufacturers of pharmaceuticals to provide demonstrations of efficacy and safety.

When new medicines are produced, there is a prima facie case for conducting a series of open studies in clinical populations to establish their actual effects in humans as opposed to the effects proposed by current theories or by extrapolation from animal experiments. This, however, is not the way the modern pharmaceutical industry works.

Given the costs of demonstrating efficacy and safety, and the liabilities involved in selling drugs, the modern production of a drug requires a prior determination of market returns balanced against liabilities: on what basis might we be sued and how much is this likely to cost? The initial requirement of demonstrating profitability acts as a mould into which subsequent developments must fit. This leads to a number of strategies and a number of consequences.

One strategy is that drug companies attempt to determine, early in the process of a drug's development, what kind of drug it is: is it an antidepressant, antihypertensive, antipsychotic, or what? The reason is that the company must make calculations regarding potential market size and liabilities should things go wrong. This can be done only if it is known what the drug is likely to do. Accordingly, whilst new drugs could be developed in a manner that produces safe compounds, with the aim of leaving it to clinicians or consumers to establish what these compounds do by prescribing and taking them, this is not how development happens.

There is a further aspect to this. Advance information about the compounds that a company has in its pipeline may have a substantial impact on the company's share price.[5] Stockbrokers employ analysts to pore over the proceedings of pharmacology conferences for indications of what may be forthcoming. Based on this there may be considerable shifts in market capital. As a consequence, companies have a predilection for the 'rational' development of drugs. Rational development in this context means that the drugs are produced as the consequence of some established theory. Companies want you to think that all the 'science' has been done before a drug comes to the marketplace, and all that remains is for a clinical trial to confirm the predicted benefits. The belief that drug development is a rational process and that all the significant science has been done before a launch is, however, at odds with the evidence.

Most major breakthroughs, like Viagra, for instance, still come about essentially by accident. Observations that the drug is doing something that was not predicted pose serious problems for companies – they upset the balance sheet of profits and potential liabilities. Far from being grateful when new observations are pointed out and new uses indicated, drug companies are liable to be less than enthusiastic. The interesting observations of consumers or their keyworkers are a problem, even where these interesting observations might offer the prospect of increased sales. They do so, but at an uncertain cost. If these drugs are doing something we do not know about, what else might they be doing that might be a potential liability?

Added to this company disinclination to have new information come to light is the fact that they spend large sums of money understanding prescribers better than they understand themselves (currently approximately £30 000 per doctor per annum). Everyone has heard about the free conferences in exotic locations or under-the-counter gifts, but the key marketing lies in the use of randomised controlled trials (RCTs) and in being able to deny access to the data from these trials and ghostwrite the publications from the trial to the point where even negative trials are described as positive studies.[6]

The intense marketing of drugs has all the characteristics of any other marketing enterprise, from automobiles to washing powders. There is market surveillance beforehand to determine what sales pitch will work. There is a variety of post-launch strategies that have been worked out for other industries and applied equally to medical practitioners. This is an inevitable hazard of the modern way of drug development, but it seems to run against our wishes that medicine in general not be a business and that all concerned with it be motivated by a wish to relieve suffering rather than any desire for money.

There is nothing new about the unease some feel about the business side of medicine, but there are in fact some genuinely new things about current business developments. In an effort to manage the development process, it has become increasingly common for pharmaceutical companies to have all of the key articles linked to their drugs ghostwritten. Somewhere between 50% and 100% of articles on therapeutics appearing even in the most prestigious journals such as the *Lancet* or the *New England Journal of Medicine* may now be ghostwritten.[7] A general problem with this is that such articles will not deviate from the company line. A more specific problem is the evidence indicating that company articles on therapeutics often fail to refer to the data on serious hazards of treatment such as suicidal acts or indeed evidence that not only has the raw data been suppressed, but it has in some instances been significantly changed.[8] In contrast, efforts to get materials on drug hazards published may pass through the peer review process, but even the premier journals such as the *BMJ* and the *Lancet* will still not publish because they are afraid of being sued by a pharmaceutical company.[9]

What medical prescribers have failed to realise is that the clinical trial is the key marketing device of pharmaceutical companies rather than the free pens and Post-its and lunches that clinicians focus their concern on. Health professionals in general also have a great deal of difficulty grasping the concept that marketers know more about marketing than they do, and in particular they fail to see what the consequences might be for the evidence they say they rely on.

What is new about the situation is that companies are able to make claims without providing access to the data from trials underpinning these claims. This breaches both the norms and the ethics of science, and medical prescribers have let companies get away with it. This is the greatest challenge facing medicine today.

CONSEQUENCES

One of the consequences of these strategies to ensure profitability is that a fundamental observation central to this book has been overlooked. The fact is that the development of most psychotropic drugs so far has come about serendipitously and by clinical observation rather than by a process of 'rational' development, and this is likely to remain the case for some time.

There is another way to put this. Clinicians assume that the compounds they are given and have been told are anxiolytics and antidepressants are just that. They, accordingly, ask their patients the question: 'Did it improve your depression?' Psychopharmacologists assume that what is important about a compound is what receptor it acts upon and therefore they ask: where did it go in the brain? The question that is not being asked, and indeed is being obscured by current clinical practice, is: what did it do to you? What did you notice while you were taking that drug? Questions such as this, if asked more routinely, would be liable to lead to important discoveries. Questions such as these would be obviously scientific questions to ask. But the current thrust of drug development strategies make questions like these unwelcome to both drug companies and academics, even though questions such as these would lead to better clinical care.

In 1956, just after chlorpromazine was developed, there was a conference involving clinicians, basic scientists, industry personnel and all those interested in further drug development to look at how to move forwards. Most parties agreed on a need for clinical trials, rating scales and a range of screening tests for new drugs. However, Ed Evarts from the National Institutes of Mental Health in the USA pointed out that chlorpromazine would have done as much to control the behaviour of patients with dementia paralytica (tertiary syphilis) as it did for those with dementia praecox (schizophrenia). If the drug companies had gone down the same route to develop new drugs as that they were now proposing for new treatments for schizophrenia, a therapy and research establishment would have grown up around producing variations on chlorpromazine for dementia paralytica and the benefits of penicillin for this condition would never have been discovered.[10]

This is exactly the kind of blind-alley we have wandered into in the last 50 years. Drugs like chlorpromazine and imipramine were wonderful breakthroughs but rather than move on to better medicines and better care, we have stymied ourselves. Clinical trials are in part to blame.

Evidence-biased care

27

CHAPTER CONTENTS

ACCESS TO DATA

The biggest issue in medicine today hinges on the question of access to clinical trial data. The controversies surrounding the risk of suicide on antidepressants did more than anything else to face medicine generally with the fact that we simply don't have access to the data from clinical trials but this is as true for the statins and drugs for asthma as it is for the antidepressants.

The evidence we have consists of a selection of trials, with industry doing the selecting. Almost all these trials are ghostwritten. In some cases negative trials have been written up as studies showing the drug worked and was safe.

The most important trigger to reform was Study 329, a trial of paroxetine in adolescents who were depressed. This completed in 1998 and was published in 2001 claiming the drug worked well and was safe.[11] In 2004, it became clear that the makers of paroxetine had published the bits of the data that suited them whilst internally conceding the trial was negative. When they became aware of this, New York State sued. As part of the settlement of the case, the company agreed to put Company Study Reports up on their website. This marks the point where the access to the data bandwagon started rolling.

Using the Company Study Reports for Avandia, Steve Nissen, a cardiologist from the Cleveland Clinic, demonstrated that this treatment for diabetes caused cardiac problems. Shortly afterwards a Cochrane group looking at Tamiflu found that with every little bit of data they were able to prise out of the company (Roche) the efficacy of the drug seemed to get slimmer and slimmer. As governments had spent billions stockpiling this drug in the event of a pandemic, this clearly revealed the cost of lack of access to data.

Study 329 has since been rewritten and the key message from the rewrite is this: Where we don't have access to the data, scientific articles apparently written by distinguished professors and appearing in journals like the *Lancet* can adopt a Biblical tone – this is the Word of God and all that is left for clinical staff to do is to ensure the patient gets the treatment.[11]

But once the data are available it becomes clear that scientific articles should be provisional in tone rather than authoritative. There are always different ways to organise the data and some of these will bring out one set of possibilities, whilst another cut will emphasise other possibilities. Trials do not offer the definitive last word.

Every practitioner must interpret the results in the light of their personal experience. The problem is that evidence-based medicine (EBM) at present encourages us to lay our personal experience aside in favour of 'the evidence'. Independent judgement is supposedly suspect. Yes, there are problems with randomised controlled trials (RCTs) their proponents concede, but this is because they are done by companies. If they were done by us, everything would be okay.

There are two arguments in this chapter. First the test of a good clinician – in any branch of healthcare – comes when they are faced with a choice between believing the patient or the experts. Second, even if done by angels, RCTs often get the wrong answer.

We need data-based medicine rather than EBM. Data based in the sense that when it comes to controlled trials, no-one should accept claims about the results of any trials if we do not have access to the underlying data. But data based also in the sense that at the end of the day the person on treatment is the data and this means being willing to go by what they say to us and being willing to trust them unless there is good evidence we should not.

THE ORIGIN OF RANDOMISED TRIALS

Ronald Fisher created the RCT in the 1920s when investigating the effect of fertilisers. Many factors can confound fertiliser studies such as differences in soil drainage, exposure to wind or sunlight and a myriad of soil elements. The known factors can be controlled for, but Fisher's insight was that he could control for unknown confounders by randomising the fertiliser to alternate soil patches.[12]

Fisher's interest was to design a good experiment. If we got the same result every time, we had designed a good experiment. Shave a bit off one side of a coin and you can expect heads to come up 19 times out of 20. Randomisation in this sense is about leaving nothing to chance. It indicates that an experimenter knows what they are doing. In contrast, most RCTs in medicine are done today when the experimenters don't know what they are doing.

Fisher also created statistical significance. If we get the same result 19 times out of 20, the findings are real world or clinically significant. They are only statistically significant in Fisher's sense if we get the same result pretty well every time. He would not have regarded the results of modern antidepressant trials as significant. He would find current distinctions between clinical and statistical significance to be bizarre.

Fisher's idea about how to design a good experiment was taken and applied to medicine, where the idea was to use RCTs to weed out the claims of hucksters that they had treatments that could help a serious illness like tuberculosis. The answer is let's see if this claim survives an RCT. This, strictly speaking, is all the trial tests.

Randomisation was first used in 1948 in Bradford Hill's trial of streptomycin for tuberculosis. Earlier clinical use had established all that is known about streptomycin for tuberculosis – that it works in the short term but that the germ becomes resistant and treatment comes with significant risks, such as ototoxicity. We did not need an RCT to tell us this. This trial showed randomisation could work rather than showing that streptomycin worked.

Whilst the hope was that trials would contain pharmaceutical company claims, by the mid-1960s Bradford Hill noted that drug company salesmen were deploying RCT evidence to encourage doctors to use their company's products. In contrast to the current enthusiasm for RCTs, Hill's own idea was that RCTs were a useful club in the golf bag but we would be mad to try to play golf with just the one club.

The fact that everyone bows to RCTs today comes not because they are more rational or logical, or coherent than other ways to evaluate treatments, but from the thalidomide crisis in 1962. Thalidomide created a political imperative to be seen to do something to make patients safer. In 1962, RCTs had just been discovered. They appeared to be a way to see if drugs worked or not. But no one knew about the problems with RCTs we know of now.

In the desperate panic to be seen to do something to make sure another thalidomide couldn't happen, in 1962 a new amendment to the American Food and Drugs Act required companies to demonstrate the 'effectiveness' of new compounds, using placebo-controlled RCTs to do so.

There is no better symbol of how little anyone knew about what they were doing than the fact that as of 1962, only one drug had demonstrated effectiveness and safety through a placebo-controlled RCT prior to marketing – thalidomide.

It was the fact that trials were built into regulations forcing companies to use them that led to the widespread adoption of RCTs, rather than any evidence RCTs worked or kept us safe.

In fact as Table 27.1 shows, most major drug groups were introduced in the 1950s without the benefit of RCTs, and the drugs that were introduced then were more effective than treatments that have come to the market since through RCTs. We don't need RCTs to get effective treatments. RCTs can, in fact, give us worse drugs.

THE PLACEBO EFFECT

RCTs of fertilisers are not controlled with placebos. The first RCTs in medicine were not placebo controlled. The first placebo-controlled trials in medicine were not RCTs.

The marriage of RCTs and placebos gives the impression that a further set of biases is being controlled. But placebos introduce a bias. An active treatment simply needs to beat placebo on some rating scale or blood test to be adjudged as working. This can be achieved for ever weaker agents by

Table 27.1 *Drug effectiveness with and without RCTs*

Drug groups introduced pre-1962	Exemplars of pre-1962 medicines	Post-1962 medicines: more effective or not
Analgesics	Morphine, paracetamol	No
Antibiotics	Penicillins, tetracyclines	No
Anticonvulsants	Barbiturates, valproate	Possible
Antidepressants	Tricyclics, monoamine oxidase inhibitors	No
Antihistamines	Chlorphenamine, diphenhydramine	No
Antihypertensives	Thiazides	No
Antipsychotics	Clozapine, haloperidol	No
Chemotherapies	Nitrogen mustard, cisplatin	Perhaps
Contraceptives	Second-generation oral contraceptives	No
Diuretics	Furosemide	No
Hypoglycaemics	Metformin	No
Steroids	Prednisone	No
Stimulants	Dexamphetamine, methylphenidate	No
Tranquilisers	Diazepam	No
Vaccines	Polio, smallpox	No

increasing the numbers of patients recruited to the trial. Manipulations of this sort mean that recent antihypertensives, hypoglycaemics and antidepressants are mostly less effective than treatments introduced without RCTs before the mid-1960s (Table 27.1).

In the 1950s, someone had to see a treatment make a real difference on an individual patient level for the drug to be developed. Now drugs can be developed on the basis of a statistical difference with no-one seeing any actual patient do better.

RCTS AND EFFICACY

The design of controlled trials in place today to establish efficacy for an antidepressant for instance involves testing active drug against placebo in trials lasting 6 weeks, using rating scales as outcome measures.

There is academic debate about whether a statistically significant finding of doubtful clinical significance constitutes efficacy or not. But in practice, regulators like the US Food and Drug Administration licence drugs for use on the basis of such data and so this debate is academic – the drugs are taken to work and are put into ever increasing use as few doctors, and no politicians want to deny treatments that supposedly work.

The problem is that, given current company abilities to hide data, to publish selected trials and to ghostwrite all publications, if the rest of us could avail of all these manoeuvres we could achieve an identical outcome as is achieved with selective serotonin reuptake inhibitors (SSRIs) by putting alcohol through these 'antidepressant' efficacy trials. Proving alcohol is an antidepressant would not be a good outcome in general.[13]

The difference between alcohol and SSRIs is that we can balance what we know about alcohol against the knowledge from RCTs. But when it comes to SSRIs, we can't do this; we don't have a reference point, and we assume that because the recommendations to take some treatment have come through an RCT that this is good-quality knowledge and a sound recommendation.

WHAT'S WRONG WITH RCTS?

Supporters of RCTs would accept many of these points but say that the problems we see are down to the use of surrogate outcomes (rating scales for antidepressants or cholesterol levels for statins), in trials of inadequate duration (6 weeks), against a regulatory background that will licence drugs on the basis of two positive RCTs even if there are 10 or more negative studies, with almost all publications stemming from these two positive studies ghostwritten and all trial data withheld.

The argument laid out here is that every time a disorder and its treatment produce a roughly similar outcome, such as antidepressants and suicidality, then RCTs in principle cannot work. People and their diseases and proving a treatment works for those diseases is not unidimensional in the way that proving a fertiliser works for crops is. Transforming a chemical into a medicine is a different matter to demonstrating a chemical is an effective fertiliser.

A fertiliser has only one action we need pay heed to, but a medicine may have 100 effects all of which need attention. We can focus on one effect of a chemical in an RCT of fertilisers and ignore the others. The fact that a small proportion of ears of corn might die prematurely because of the fertiliser is of no consequence if overall there is more corn.

But we can't do this in healthcare. The task for any of us is to look after the patient in front of us. Average effects that obscure the harm to this patient are dangerous. Clinical practice needs to manage the fact that we are different, not act as though we are clones – and RCTs do not help us with this.

ANTIDEPRESSANTS AND SUICIDE: A THOUGHT EXPERIMENT

Randomisation is supposed to control confounders. But when testing, a medicine randomisation can introduce confounders in a way that doesn't happen with fertilisers. Two examples involving antidepressants and suicide in depression help to bring the point out, but the point being made applies to all drug groups and all drug effects.

Imipramine was the first antidepressant. It was launched in 1958 without RCTs. In 1959, at a meeting convened to discuss its effects, several clinicians noted on the basis of Challenge–Dechallenge–Rechallenge (CDR) tests that wonderful though imipramine was for many patients, it could trigger suicidal and homicidal ideation in some.

Imipramine and some other tricyclic antidepressants inhibit serotonin reuptake amongst other things. They are more clinically potent than SSRIs, 'beating' SSRIs in patients with melancholia. Melancholic patients are 80 times more likely to commit suicide than mildly depressed patients. Accordingly comparing imipramine and placebo in an RCT of melancholic patients would likely show fewer suicides and suicidal acts on imipramine than on placebo. The relative risk might be as low as 0.5.

In contrast, analysing all suicides and suicidal acts in SSRI and post SSRI trials gives a relative risk that the drugs will cause suicide and suicidal acts of roughly 2.0. This outcome comes about in part because these drugs are weaker than imipramine and were tested in people who were at less risk of suicide; as a result the rate of suicidal acts on placebo falls making the risk from the drug more noticeable. Imipramine tested against less severely depressed patients would show the same excess of suicidal acts.

So in this case, a drug that causes suicide will protect against suicide on a population basis. Something similar to this can happen every time a drug and an illness cause the same thing. It is common to hear claims that RCTs demonstrate cause and effect. But this thought experiment shows that if a trial is not designed to look at an issue, it cannot show cause and effect. These RCTs tell us nothing about whether the drug causes the problem or not, except in so far in this case as there could not be an excess of suicides and suicidal acts if the drugs don't cause suicide.

Better evidence that the drugs can cause suicide in some came from the case reports from 1990 on fluoxetine and suicide that demonstrated individual patients becoming suicidal on fluoxetine with the problem clearing up when the drug was stopped and the patient able to tell the doctor they could distinguish between the effect of fluoxetine and the illness.

Similar scenarios to this unfold with cardiac rhythm problems in trials of anti-arrhythmics, with breathing difficulties in trials of anti-asthmatics, with vaccines and viral infections that cause brain or other damage. Similarly, angiotensin-converting enzyme (ACE) inhibitors improve renal function in patients with diabetes, but in some they make renal function worse. The interaction between the heart attack-producing effects of both diabetes and rosiglitazone (Avandia) obscured the adverse effects of rosiglitazone. Other hypoglycaemics like exenatide and sitagliptin produce pancreatitis, but diabetes can too.

We can expect results like this every time a treatment and an illness produce superficially similar pictures, which may apply in the case of up to half of all treatment effects.

ANTIDEPRESSANTS AND SUICIDE: ACTUAL EXPERIMENTS

In the early 1990s, SmithKline undertook a study of paroxetine (Study 106) in patients with intermittent brief depressive disorders (IBDD). The study terminated early and was never published. The rate of suicidal acts on paroxetine was three-fold higher than on placebo. SmithKline then undertook Study 057 in a similar group of patients.

In 2006, GlaxoSmithKline in a press release presented data for patients in paroxetine major depressive disorder (MDD) trials (Table 27.2).[14] The MDD patients show a significant increase in suicidal act risk on paroxetine.

The press release also contained data on the suicidal act rate in two IBDD trials.[14] Despite the fact that these studies do not support using paroxetine for IBDD, the data from these studies when added surprisingly cause the risk of a suicidal act on paroxetine in depression trials to vanish (see Table 27.3).

We can add 16 more suicidal acts to the paroxetine IBBD column in Table 27.3, increasing the relative risk of an adverse event on paroxetine to 1.4, and the combined paroxetine suicidal act number to 59, and still get the same apparently protective outcome overall.

This example points to a deep problem for all trials undertaken in mixed clinical populations – from back pain to Parkinson's disease. Just as IBDD patients can meet criteria for depression, so also can diverse sets of pain or Parkinson's disease patients meet criteria for their respective illnesses. Provided there is more than one IBDD patient entered into MDD trials randomisation will ensure these patients will hide the effect of an SSRI on suicidal acts. Similarly back pains of one type may mask what may be beneficial treatment effects on another type of pain.

This paradoxical outcome is predictable. When it comes to a medicine, unlike a fertiliser, knowing what a drug can do, makes it possible to design placebo-controlled RCTs that use a problem the drug causes to hide that same problem. The only way to overcome this problem and to get a result we can understand from an RCT is to understand the biology of the condition we are

Table 27.2 ***Suicidal acts in MDD trials***

Major depressive disorder (MDD) trials	Paroxetine	Placebo	Relative risk
Suicidal acts/patients	11/2943	0/1671	Inf (1.3, inf)

Inf, infinity.

Table 27.3 ***Suicidal acts in MDD and IBDD trials***

	Paroxetine	**Placebo**	**Relative risk**
Major depressive disorder (MDD) trials acts/patients	11/2943	0/1671	Inf (1.3, inf)
Intermittent brief depressive disorders (IBDD) trials acts/patients	32/147	35/151	0.9
Combined acts/patients	43/3090	35/1822	0.7

Inf, infinity.

treating and the genetics of the drug we are using. It is only then that the results of RCTs can be understood.

PHARMAGNOSIA

All chemicals, both fertilisers and medicines, literally have 100 or more effects. In the case of fertilisers, we don't need to pay heed to all of them but when it comes to medicines, we do need to.

When we design an RCT to manage the unknown unknowns for only one of these effects, what, in fact, we are doing is asking the doctor and patient to focus on one effect (the one a company wants them to focus on) and to ignore all the other effects. This is hypnosis, where holding a subject's attention to one focus can lead them to miss more important material out of focus, especially when for the sake of 'objectivity' patients reports are essentially ignored.

As a result, RCTs necessarily generate ignorance. There is no way they can't do this. This is a risky thing to do. If we buy into company marketing that says RCTs offer us gold-standard knowledge, we generate ignorance about ignorance regarding most of what the drug does.

In the case of the SSRIs, the choice of endpoint was dictated by business considerations. This meant powering studies to produce a statistically significant outcome on rating scales like the Hamilton Depression Rating Scale (HAMD) that measure clinical changes in a very rough fashion. But because of the focus on HAMD scores, data on sexual functioning and the other 99 effects these drugs have was poorly collected, letting companies claim afterwards that less than 5% of those taking SSRIs had a disturbance of sexual functioning, when the true figure is close to 100%.

The clinical encounter is a relationship, and good care involves close attention to the individual. Clinical trials have affected this relationship by treating individual variation as inconsequential. This has made and continues to turn clinical encounters into an industrial process, like agriculture, that aims at implementing impersonal algorithms and guidelines, leaving clinicians practising mediculture rather than medicine.

RCTS ARE RISKY

RCTs were introduced to improve the safety of drugs by forcing companies to prove their drugs worked. The move has backfired. Because no-one pays any heed to the other 99 effects of drugs, we have both compromised safety and reduced the rate of discovery of new drugs, which depend on takers and their carers coming up with 'inconvenient' observations.

The message is that just as drugs do, RCTs can have an important place in therapeutics, but even if carried out impeccably, their adverse effects may outweigh their benefits. The key contribution RCTs make to safety is when they demonstrate that claims a drug helps are bogus, as in the Women's Health Initiative study of hormone replacement therapy (HRT). With this kind of outcome, the risks inherent in RCTs of a medicine are warranted because the effect demonstrated leads to a reduced exposure to risky chemicals. It also puts the onus back on companies to find the people who are likely to benefit from taking these risks rather than leaving it up to us.

Instead, the verdict of RCTs is all too often pitted against clinical and patient judgement. This happens even though a trial may not be able to show a drug causes suicidality, but clinical judgement within a trial can do so. Clinicians and patients can usually distinguish between depression-induced and drug-induced suicidality.

People on an SSRI can make it clear for instance that the drug is producing a useful emotional numbing but that this numbing is not leading to recovery. This information is important if we want to make a decision as to whether to introduce another drug with a different mode of action into the mix or whether we want to stop the original drug and start another.

As things stand, because RCTs de facto discourage the engagement of clinicians with patients, they obscure what different drugs do. If clinicians listen to patients, they would hear that SSRIs help by producing an emotional numbing whilst noradrenaline reuptake inhibitors help by improving energy. But put through RCTs, these drugs that act on different brain systems end up looking exactly the same.

The other thing that happens is that people end up on drug cocktails because all have been shown to 'work' without any effort to match whether the kind of thing this drug might do would be helpful to this patient's needs. Going by RCTs prevents clinicians from finding the right drug for the patient in front of them.

It also blocks the possibility of the taker of a drug and their clinician wondering about what they are seeing and discovering more about the nature of the problem the person has and even something more about the constituent parts of human nature.

Marketing and risk

28

CHAPTER CONTENTS

Clinical trials do something else not often noticed – they enable the marketing of psychiatric disorders. If our drug makes a difference for post-traumatic stress disorder (PTSD) or other condition, the disorder must in fact exist. The role companies play in disease mongering of this sort has come into clearer focus in recent years.[15]

Earlier editions of this book covered the selling of obsessive–compulsive disorder (OCD), panic disorder, social phobia and other conditions to market selective serotonin reuptake inhibitors (SSRIs) or alprazolam. Section 4 covers the marketing of attention deficit/hyperactivity disorder (ADHD) to sell stimulants. This edition shows how a focus on risk management can be used to market drugs.

THE MARKETING OF DEPRESSION

In addition to mongering social phobia and panic disorder, many will be aware of company marketing of fibromyalgia to sell pregabalin and restless legs syndrome (RLS) to sell ropinirole. These examples might suggest companies have been selling disorders of lesser importance, but in just the same way there was an earlier marketing of depression.

There is, however, one difference to bear in mind with the marketing of antidepressants by marketing depression or the marketing of trigeminal neuralgia to sell carbamazepine and the modern marketing of fibromyalgia. This is that everyone could see a difference in using the first antidepressants for melancholia or carbamazepine for trigeminal neuralgia compared with the marketing of pregabalin where people are more likely to get this drug because clinical trials say so, whether or not the prescriber or the person can see a difference.

There was considerable company reluctance to market the first antidepressants in the late 1950s as no-one could see a sizeable enough market.[16] The only people who were thought to be depressed were in psychiatric hospitals, where they responded to electroconvulsive therapy (ECT). The company that took the plunge and made the market was Merck, who committed itself to selling both amitriptyline and the concept of what an 'antidepressant' might treat by distributing 50 000 copies of a book by Frank Ayd on the recognition and treatment of depression in general medical settings.[17] The company made and distributed videos on how to interview depressed patients. They sold depression. Nevertheless, the recognition of depression and the use of antidepressants remained unexciting from a marketing point of view until the 1980s and the emergence of the SSRIs.[8]

The notion that depression was conjured up by marketing departments is rather startling now, when depression has become the common cold of psychiatry. It became the common cold of psychiatry in the early 1990s, when the Royal College of Psychiatrists in the UK and the American Psychiatric Association mounted campaigns to make professionals and the public aware of depression. These campaigns were supported by companies bringing a new generation of drugs, the SSRIs, to market.[16]

The failure of buspirone, the first serotonergic drug, to make inroads into the anxiolytic marketplace made it clear that it would be very difficult to market any new tranquillisers in the post-benzodiazepine era because of concerns about the dependence potential of anxiolytics (see Section 5). The SSRIs could have followed down the buspirone route, but they became antidepressants instead, even though at the time of registration as antidepressants there were no clinical trials that showed they worked in hospitalised patients with depression.

This development did not happen in Japan where, as of 2003, there were no SSRI antidepressants on the market. Fluvoxamine was launched at the end of 1999 – as a treatment for OCD, with paroxetine launched for social phobia and depression. In Japan, the antidepressant market as of 2002 remained the same size as the antidepressant market had been in the West up to the mid-1980s. In Japan, in contrast, the anxiolytic market remained robust. The critical difference lies in the fact that benzodiazepine dependence never became a problem in Japan. This is now changing with depression and bipolar disorder being ever more heavily promoted in Japan, the consequences of which remain to be seen.

As the SSRIs are safer in overdose than the earlier tricyclic antidepressants, it became a feasible proposition to take the findings from social psychiatry and advise general practitioners that there were several times as many untreated depressives as was formerly thought; to educate them to recognise that patients with conditions presenting as anxiety, who had been given benzodiazepines up until then, often had an underlying depression; to reassure them that the publicly available evidence as of 1990 suggested that antidepressants (in contrast to anxiolytics) need to be taken chronically, to reduce the risk of relapse, and that this is a reasonable thing to do as the SSRIs are not dependence producing. From the beachhead of depression, then, raids could be launched on the hinterlands of anxiety. Whether or not the SSRIs are antidepressant rather than just anxiolytic is almost unimportant.[18]

A number of developments could lead levels of depression to sink back to the levels seen in the 1980s. First, any truly new group of drugs with a psychotropic effect, perhaps acting on substance P, neuropeptide Y or sigma receptors, is more likely to be marketed by companies as anxiolytics rather than antidepressants. The company calculation here is that few members of the public are likely to make any identification between the terms anxiolytic and tranquilliser.

A second possibility would stem from the discovery of an antidepressant effective for hospital depression – ECT in pill form, perhaps ketamine-related compounds (see Chapter 4). Such a compound would be a 'proper' antidepressant and the condition it treated would be proper depression, and it would in all probability have little effect on most cases of primary care nerves. If this happened, it would lead to a crisis in our use of the word depression. Something would have to change.

The final possibility might be if the SSRIs, which have now largely gone off-patent, were to be sold over the counter. This is much less likely now owing to concerns about suicidality and dependence, but the thought experiment is interesting. Had these drugs become available over the counter, companies would likely have marketed them in the way that St John's Wort is marketed: as agents for stress and burnout rather than for depression. A disease concept is only needed for marketing through prescription-only arrangements.

THE MARKETING OF BIPOLAR DISORDER

As the antidepressants went off-patent, bipolar disorder received the full attention of marketing departments.[19] Companies with a series of anticonvulsants from valproate through to lamotrigine, as well as newer antipsychotics, such as olanzapine, risperidone and quetiapine, collectively raised recognition of bipolar disorders (see Section 3). Lilly in particular has marketed bipolar disorder with little reference to olanzapine and in breath-taking fashion have suggested that anyone for whom antidepressants have been unhelpful may in fact have a bipolar disorder. An unprecedented number of satellite symposia have been sponsored on this topic, and everyone has been educated to recognise that ever subtler aberrations of behaviour may in fact indicate a bipolar disorder.

One of the extraordinary features of this has been the almost complete lack of clinical trial evidence that any of these agents can be considered prophylactic for bipolar disorders. The increased sales of all these agents have depended heavily on companies being able to parade a series of expert lecturers on the topic of bipolar disorders, thereby creating a linkage between the illness and their treatment with very little evidence presented that treatment is actually of benefit. The most disturbing aspect of this current trend is how children are being swept up in the process and being prescribed some of the most toxic drugs in medicine as a result.

THE MARKETING OF FEMALE SEXUAL DYSFUNCTION

Bipolar disorder has been and clearly described for 150 years. In contrast, while women may always have had sexual complaints, a new illness entity, female sexual dysfunction, has been created in recent years, largely linked to company efforts to develop and market a 'pink Viagra' (see Section 8).

This creation of female sexual dysfunction brings out a further aspect of disease marketing. Companies are not just changing the labels we might happen to use. In doing this they also change our experiences and the way we understand ourselves. Women in their 20s with three young children who have lost interest in sex are being encouraged to think they should have their testosterone levels checked rather than that their problems may stem from the circumstances in which they find themselves. While this medicalisation may be helpful in some specific cases, clearly other women will be losers in the process.

The marketing appeals to the science. In this case rating scales designed to try to show drugs like low-dose testosterone or flibanserin have effects. The items include for instance a clitoral numbness item – because this is the kind of thing that can be rated on a rating scale. But focusing on clitoral numbness risks changing the entire experience of making love. In addition to changing experience, the process creates a discontent to which a drug becomes the answer.

RATING SCALE MONGERING

As randomised controlled trials (RCTs) have been trumpeted as providing gold standard evidence, everything to do with them has taken on a reflected validity. This includes rating scales, which are increasingly being imported into clinical practice apparently on the basis that they will reduce variability in the clinical encounter and make that encounter more scientific. Healthcare practitioners are encouraged to administer depression or other behavioural rating scales when seeing patients. Thus guidelines such as the UK National institute for Health and Care Excellence (NICE) guidelines on antenatal care advocate using the Hospital Anxiety and Depression scale for all pregnant women.

Aware of this, pharmaceutical companies have for some years run symposia at major professional meetings aimed solely at introducing clinicians to rating scales. Rating scale mongering has succeeded disease mongering as the promotional instrument du jour. Pfizer at the 2007 American Psychiatric Association meeting, for example, supported a symposium 'From Clinical Skills to Clinical Scales: Practical Tools in the Management of Patients with Schizophrenia'. The practical tools were rating scales whose use would draw attention to ways in the company's antipsychotic ziprasidone was superior to some others in the field.

The hazards of taking measurement technologies like these out of clinical trial context are rarely acknowledged.[20] The first hazard is that rating scales within the behavioural domain are simply checklists. Far from being information rich, they are information poor. The advantage to companies is that their use ensures that a number of possibly irrelevant questions get asked. In time-limited clinical exchanges, if these questions are asked other more important questions are likely to be sacrificed. When applied to healthcare, this dynamic means that prescribers ask the questions for which a drug rather than something else is the answer.

Second, whilst rating scales generate data, where exclusive reliance is put on such data there is an informational reductionism that may be doing more to dehumanise clinical exchanges than the biological reductionism that is more commonly complained about. If specific measurements lead to an oversight for context or other dimensions of an individual's functioning or situation that are not open to measurement or that are simply not being measured, rather than being modestly scientific by measuring what we can, we risk being pseudoscientific.

Third, having figures for weight from a weighing scale for instance can allow us to plot norms for healthy weight. It also generates potent feedback in a weight reducing programme. But while this is the case, the figures can seduce both the person and the clinician. In the absence of figures from other areas of a person's life, against which the figures for weight can be put in context, there is a risk for the patient that the figures for weight will come to dominate their concerns, establishing a neurosis. Most of us can recognise how potent or dangerous a weighing scale is. The risk for the clinician is that she will treat the figures rather than the person. We should but we don't pathologise a clinician's figure-centredness.[20]

An older generation of clinicians would have readily made a case that even in the treatment of eating disorders weighing scales should rarely be introduced. Where in the 1970s and 1980s the treatment of anorexia differed notably from the treatment of any other condition in psychiatry by virtue of a new centrality accorded to measurement technologies, today this management style is rapidly becoming the norm, and many clinicians might be alarmed at the prospect of encountering a patient without a battery of such technologies. There is good case for getting back to seeing people without such technologies, even weighing scales, but this would involve a return to clinical discretion that is politically a problem at present.

There are two important points to note about all this. First, exactly the same is happening in other areas of medicine, for example, with the use of bone scanners to sell drugs for bone thinning (osteopenia or osteoporosis) or with blood tests for cholesterol to sell statins to lower lipid levels. None of this is unique to mental health. Second, these measurements are often about risks rather than diseases. The measurements set up a risk for which a drug is the answer.

RISK MANAGEMENT

The place where the use of rating scales becomes most problematic is in a domain that has come to the fore for everyone involved in mental health throughout the Western world – risk management.

Every day most of us are faced with forms that look like this, except for usually having far more boxes:

Areas of risk

Risk	**Y**	**N**	**N/A**
Risk to self			
Risk to others			
Risk to health			

The key point here is that risk management locates the risks in the person being assessed. It might not be as much a problem if there were boxes for ticking the risk posed to the person or the healthcare worker trying to help them from a lack of access to clinical trial data or from the lack of provision of services by a provider who is cash-strapped.

Identifying a risk leads to a push for action to eliminate it or to at least be seen to do something in the face of the identified risk. When the risks end up in the person, a drug becomes an almost impossible to resist option, whether it is covering a person with an antidepressant until their counselling appointment comes up to putting someone who is hearing voices that may be comforting and supportive on an antipsychotic to actual treatment of an actual disorder.

Mental health units that once had active occupational therapy units and social programmes are now reduced to boring sterile places where only activities that have been 'shown to work' and that address risks happen. Patients are not exercised, nor taken out on social activities, nor involved in art, music or other therapies. If they leave hospital for psychosocial reasons, it is likely to be because of boredom. Caring and absorbing risk rather than checking boxes are things that good staff used to do, but unfortunately these qualities are like placebos – undeniably but unprovably effective and as a result unsponsored.

These changes to the fabric of care might be acceptable if RCTs and risk management had done something to control the furore therapeuticus. They do the opposite. In recent years there has been a mass pharmaceuticalisation of a range of nervous and other general health conditions in primary care. This is wrong, but what is even more inappropriate is the current lack of monitoring of the therapeutic impact of intervening in these conditions. In practice, based on weak evidence of treatment effects, we have done a great deal to detect such nervous problems and to ensure people are put on drug treatments but little to monitor whether treatment has in fact delivered the desired result. Because these agents have been shown by RCTs to 'work', we have promoted a situation, virtually free of warnings, where primary-care prescribers and others, besieged by the mass of community nervous problems and all but impotent to do much for these, have been trapped by the weight of supposed scientific evidence into indiscriminately handing out psychotropic agents on a massive scale, increasing rather than reducing risks – while healthcare staff are immune provided they tick the right boxes.

THE NEW MARKETING

Pharmaceutical company marketing is seen by many people as an evil. They decry the free pens and cups and trips to meetings and meals at hotels that supposedly corrupt physicians. But these are the trinkets of the sales department, not marketing, and medical prescribers, when asked if these things influence them – say no. Asked what does influence them, they say they are primarily influenced by the evidence. Aware that evidence is the way to capture the minds of physicians and increasingly all healthcare professionals, marketing has for some time been about ensuring the evidence can only lead to one conclusion – prescribe our drug.

It has been known for a long time that only a selection of the clinical trials done get published. It was thought – incorrectly – that the regulator gets to see all the data. But of the trials that get published, it is now clear that companies have cherry-picked the data that suit them, leaving out the data that are unfavourable or pitching it in a way that minimises a hazard. Almost all trials of any importance to a company – across medicine – will these days be ghostwritten, and the writers have considerable skill in framing the issues. So suicidal acts may be coded – legitimately – under the heading of emotional lability and perhaps less legitimately under the heading of nausea or even left out of the paper entirely because there was nothing statistically significant about the finding.

When guidelines are drawn up, even by bodies completely independent of the pharmaceutical industry, they can only deal with the published evidence, and the published evidence for the most part can only lead to one conclusion. In almost all cases this is prescribe the latest drugs rather than older ones. In this way evidence-based medicine, in which many invested great hopes, becomes evidence-biased medicine and a means whereby pharmaceutical companies get a grip on healthcare.

Allied to this has been a recasting of how evidence is read so that as illustrated in Chapter 4, data that shows antidepressants may offer some benefit, but that perhaps the SSRIs at least should not be used frontline in primary care disorders, becomes evidence that the drugs 'work' and should therefore be given as quickly as possible to people. And if one drug fails to do the trick, patients should be put on cocktails of treatments.[18]

A final key element has been a misuse of the concept of statistical significance. Pharma regularly portrays the risks of treatment as insignificant – even when they may be significant in the sense of being lethal – but also when there is an excess of some hazard on a drug compared to placebo but this excess does not reach statistical significance. An excess of a hazard on a drug is an excess of a hazard, until proven otherwise. Companies however rarely conduct studies designed to look at this hazard, and as a result the figures may never become statistically significant. The figures for suicidal acts from controlled trials of antidepressants pointed to a 2.5-fold increase in the risk of suicidal acts from 1988 onwards. This should have been recognised and warned about then.[27]

Putting these elements together the world in which we all now operate is one in which pharmaceutical companies market their drugs by having articles ghostwritten with the top names in the field appearing on the authorship line and the article published in the best journals, a world in which drugs are sold by having professors talk to their colleagues at meetings and then local doctors talk to other healthcare professionals. There may be minimal evidence of pharma presence. The appeal may simply be to the evidence. And the whole operation is a lot cheaper than putting a salesforce in the field.

From healthcare to pharmageddon

29

CHAPTER CONTENTS

PERCEPTIONS OF PROGRESS IN MENTAL HEALTH

The early 20th century was a time of remarkable improvement in the health of people in the industrial democracies. The infant mortality rate fell, life expectancy increased and a number of scourges, such as tuberculosis and diphtheria, were eradicated. To a large extent technological developments in medicine – and perhaps pharmaceutical developments in particular – have been credited in the popular mind with bringing about these improvements.

The reality, as Thomas McKeown has demonstrated,[21] was more complex. The drop in mortality rate from a variety of infectious diseases antedated the development of antibiotics, vaccines or any specific drug therapies. It resulted in the main from improved nutrition, the alleviation of overcrowding and public works programmes such as the provision of better sanitation. The increasing development of 'high-tech' medicine, which has grown more spectacular with every decade since the Second World War, has done little to extend the basic improvements in healthcare brought about at the turn of the 20th century.

Public perceptions of progress in psychiatry are the same as perceptions for other medical developments. The introduction of antipsychotics and antidepressants is credited with bringing about our current programme of emptying and closing large psychiatric hospitals, by enabling the treatment of psychological disorders in the community. The reality is more complex. The closure of the large hospitals owes a great deal to administrative changes. Until the early 1950s, many of the large asylums followed a policy of lumping patients together in wards regardless of diagnosis.[22] Substantial improvements were brought about simply by separating the mentally ill from the mentally handicapped, older subjects from younger individuals, chronic patients from those with acute disturbances, and milder problems from more severe ones. This led to the development of a wider range of treatment strategies for specific problems and a change in morale within the psychiatric services, to which the advent of chlorpromazine contributed.[9] In contrast, in Japan the advent of chlorpromazine led to a quadrupling of the numbers in hospital beds indicating that there was no necessary link between chlorpromazine and de-institutionalisation.

What else of a non-specific or 'low-tech' nature can be done or needs to be done now? There is a range of issues. Among the most important are the questions of child abuse, both sexual and physical, but also mental torture, psychological cruelty and domestic violence.[23,24] It increasingly appears that programmes aimed at prevention of such abuses would lead to a reduction in morbidity in later life. It also appears that hi-tech medicine is becoming a hazard in its own right.

The process of randomised placebo-controlled trials that has been used to show that specific high-tech approaches work for certain conditions also reveals that non-specific treatments work. In trials of antidepressants, where 50% respond to the antidepressant, up to 40% respond to a placebo. What this means in practice is that, unlike the treatment of infection with an antibiotic, when it comes to the treatment of nervous conditions, neither the antipsychotics nor antidepressants are so specific that they will knock out the 'psychic infection' that an individual has regardless of the circumstances in which treatment is given. The rapport that patients have with those looking after them plays a big part in the likelihood of response to treatment and in the quality of that response.

Bamboozled by the evidence that antidepressants can be shown to add something over and above the benefits that can be obtained from a good-quality therapeutic relationship, we are at risk of forgetting that without the bedrock of a good-quality relationship they may not work at all. The psychotropic drugs should have made psychopharmacotherapy possible; the risk is that they will result in the staffing of the mental-health service with psychopharmacological technicians, who are increasingly insensitive to the dynamics of the relationships in which prescribing takes place. Physicians at least seem on their way to becoming 'pharmacologists'.

Other non-specific developments that might be as therapeutic, if not more so, than the specific benefits of drug treatment include the provision of detailed information regarding drug therapies to those who take psychotropic medicines. As this book illustrates, the harmful effects of such drugs on a person's life may entirely outweigh any benefits they could have conferred if used judiciously. Intuitively it would seem that enabling individuals to take control of their own lives in this way and to make their own decisions would be a good thing. There is considerable philosophical justification for such a position.[25] However, this runs counter to the prevailing mechanical models in medicine that underpin current drug company research and business programmes. It remains to be seen what the outcome of this potential clash will be.

HEALTHCARE VERSUS HEALTH PRODUCTS LTD

The landscape of health has been completely transformed in the past 50 years. Where once we consulted doctors and didn't dare question them, or if we did the response was likely to be that they would be prepared to discuss matters if we came back with a medical training, controlled trials put evidence on benefits and risks out into the public domain and enabled women in particular to question medical prescribers and surgeons. Medical people had to descend from a pedestal and get engaged in collaborating with their patients in a new way – as guides or experts.

This gave rise to a language of choice and rights, and terms like consumers and clients replaced the older term of patients. But these new data and processes also gave rise to what is increasingly becoming a market in health products, of which pharmaceuticals are the most obvious examples, but where entire services are in fact being packaged and managed as products. And to sell the product, the adverts for drugs and mental-health services promise what adverts for automobiles and shampoos once promised – your life will be enhanced if you purchase our product.

This is a long way from healthcare in which nurses, doctors and others tried with those of us who are suffering, often against the odds, to produce health. The term patient is a much better word for this – referring as it does to someone who endures. From a caring perspective, it makes as much sense to call a patient a client as it would for a mother to call her child a client or a teacher to call her pupils consumers. From a caring perspective, adverts for insulin that portray patients with diabetes as young and healthy and walking in the mountains are close to offensive. The reality of the illness in clinics is that this disease shortens lives, and people have to be taught to prick the side of their fingers to get blood samples because they may need the touch sensitive pulp of their fingers if they go blind.[26] Adverts for antipsychotics and antidepressants are typically equally divorced from the reality of caring, which rather than delivering cures for the most part involves a myriad of adjustments to cope with the frailties of the human body and mind.

Both those seeking help for mental problems and those whose help they seek in this sense aim at producing as much health as possible out of what are some of mankind's most debilitating illnesses. But there is an increasing problem for all of us seeking help and those of us who are trying to care in that we are being progressively alienated from any ability to care in this sense. We are encouraged to follow guidelines and protocols rather than listen to our patients and do something that may be individual. The rhetoric may be increasingly about personalised medicine, the practice is increasingly standardised and the outcomes are getting worse rather than better.

We are in a world where healthcare professionals focus on their own organs and segment risks accordingly. This means that cardiovascular physicians aim at lowering lipid levels and are happy if the drugs they prescribe do this, oblivious to the change of personality or cognitive problems the drugs may cause. Even though mortality from non-cardiovascular causes may be increased, they do not consider it necessary to inform their patients about this.[27] They are happy if they have delivered their health products even though the health of the whole person may have suffered as a consequence.

In the same way, treatments across medicine from asthma to psychosis are being standardised and patients who complain about problems are regarded as an inconvenience. Drugs from Dianette (a combination pill used for contraception and acne), to the statins, to beta-blockers can trigger an increasing burden of disability, and it can prove very difficult to rescue someone from treatments like these when they are making them worse. Acutely induced problems from suicidality to psychosis may occur on the weight loss agent rimonabant, or smoking cessation agents varenicline or bupropion, or the acne treatment Ro-accutane, and because these problems fall outside the remit of the dermatologist or whoever is doing the treatment, they seem not to see them.[6]

PHARMAGEDDON

The emergence of Viagra in the mid-1990s is significant for many reasons. The obvious one is that it marks a point where it became possible to discuss sexual issues and treatments more openly. But of longer-term significance, perhaps, was that this was a point where company executives began to talk openly about lifestyle agents rather than treatments for a disease.

It was not the focus on sex that led to talk about lifestyles. What was different about Viagra that enabled executives to begin to talk about lifestyles was the reliability of the responses it produced. Nine or 9.9 times out of 10, it produced the desired effect. This was in contrast to the antidepressants, for instance, which produce the desired response in only one out of 10 although people can be fooled into thinking it is five out of 10 (Chapter 4).

Unlike the antidepressants, Viagra produced quality outcomes. For anyone working in healthcare, quality until recently meant a situation in which the relationship between professional and patient was warm, understanding and intuitive, but this is not what the word means industrially. From the point of view of pharmaceutical companies, quality refers to reliability. Big Mac hamburgers are quality hamburgers in this sense: they are the same every time. What companies want are drugs that will be equally reliable, and once drugs become this reliable, it becomes possible to jettison talk about diseases and replace it with talk about lifestyles.

Are we about to produce a whole new generation of antidepressants or anxiolytics that are so much more reliable soon? No. There will be no great change in the drugs we have, although the use of neuroimaging to see whether drugs are working or not and pharmacogenetic testing to check for adverse effects before treatment may make a new generation of drugs more reliable. The marketing of drugs has become so sophisticated, however, that people can be persuaded of benefits that don't exist, and because of this marketing psychopharmacology is well on the way down the path plastic surgery took as it evolved into cosmetic surgery.

Plastic surgery began as a set of very unreliable procedures to repair the injuries inflicted by war. As it became more reliable, it burst out of the constraints of medicine to become cosmetic surgery.[28] In the process it changed from a discipline that restored people to their place in the social order and became a set of practices that were sold on the promise that they might help us change our place in society. Psychopharmacology, largely through the efficacy of its propaganda rather than the efficacy of its drugs, is well on its way down this route becoming increasingly less medical and more lifestyle orientated – a cosmetic psychopharmacology.

The changing scene has been caught best by Charles Medawar. 'I fear that we are heading blindly in the general direction of Pharmageddon.

Pharmageddon is a gold-standard paradox: individually we benefit from some wonderful medicines whilst, collectively, we are losing sight and sense of health. By analogy, think of the relationship between a car journey and climate change – they are inextricably linked, but probably not remotely connected in the driver's mind. Just as climate change seems inconceivable as a journey outcome, so the notion of Pharmageddon is flatly contradicted by most personal experience of medicines'.[29]

In the 1960s, my parents thought of buying a car. It was a time when people didn't need cars. My father could get to work easily on the bus or the train. The local shops were close to us so that you could walk to get all the bits and pieces that you needed. A car was a luxury. Fairly soon afterwards where we live changed, and most people began to need a car because they were living further out and work was too far away and the local shops weren't local in the way they had been before and the kinds of things you needed couldn't be bought in the local shops the way they could be before.

Everyone got cars and because of cars cities changed so that the city almost became a vehicle to sell cars. This is what the marketing departments of major companies would call a distribution channel – where everything conspires to sell the product. Cities, the way we lived, all meant we needed cars. Cars can be an unquestionably good thing. But they are also inextricably linked to a change in the world in which we live, to climate change, a change of the kind that most of us as individuals find hard to see how we could influence.

The same argument can be made for televisions through computers to the internet.

It can also be made for food. In the 1960s, it was rare for children to come home from school to a processed meal. There were no fast foods. But as the way we lived changed during the 1960s and as we didn't buy fresh food locally in the way we had before, instead using our cars to go to hypermarkets to buy food for the week, increasingly we began to buy processed foods.

But unlike the informational superhighway and climate change, it's clear to lots of people that fast foods aren't the only way to go. They can be optional, but they aren't the way we should eat routinely. It has been possible to imagine slow food, and a movement has begun to counteract fast food.

In just the same way as for food, cars and televisions, back in the 1960s drugs were not the only answer to healthcare problems. They were an option. They were a poison that it was great to have and doctors could use with care. But we have moved into a world these days where, as opposed to being regarded as poisons that could be tremendously useful if used wisely, drugs have become something closer to fertilisers to be used indiscriminately.

Controlled trials have played the same role in relation to medicines as oil has played to cars – they have turbo-charged pills compared to other elements of healthcare.

Where once it was wonderful to have mechanical vehicles to undertake arduous journeys, hoping into the car to drop down to the shop to get the paper makes us unfit and obese, as well as doing harm to the planet. In the same way it has become ever easier to convert life's vicissitudes into illnesses and market drugs like the stimulants for these, and even persuade doctors and patients that some of the most toxic drugs in medicine, the antipsychotics, should be used for minor conditions and used in minors. Whilst this is the case, there is no incentive for companies to produce drugs to overcome the real scourges of schizophrenia or proper manic-depressive insanity. Breakthroughs are only likely to emerge by accident and are as likely to come from the observations of the readers of a book like this as they are to come from the laboratories of a pharmaceutical company. But above all, between us we need to create a slow medicine.

REFERENCES

1. Vogel MJ, Rosenberg CE, editors. The therapeutic revolution. Philadelphia, PA: University of Pennsylvania Press; 1979.
2. Sneader W. The prehistory of psychotherapeutic agents. J Psychopharmacol 1990;4:115–19.
3. Liebenau J. Medical science and medical industry. Basingstoke: Macmillan; 1987.
4. Pellegrino E. The sociocultural impact of twentieth century therapeutics. In: Vogel MJ, Rosenberg CE, editors. The therapeutic revolution. Philadelphia, PA: University of Pennsylvania Press; 1979. p. 245–66.
5. Marsh P. Prescribing all the way to the bank. New Sci 1989;18(November): 50–5.
6. Healy D. Pharmageddon. Berkeley CA: California University Press; 2012.
7. Healy D, Cattell D. The interface between authorship, industry, and science in the domain of therapeutics. Br J Psychiatry 2003;182:22–7.
8. Healy D. Let them eat Prozac. New York: New York University Press; 2004.
9. Healy D. Pharmageddon. Berkeley CA: California University Press; 2012.
10. Healy D. The creation of psychopharmacology. Cambridge, MA: Harvard University Press; 2002.
11. Le Noury J, Nardo J, Jureidini J, et al. Study 329 Restored. BMJ 2015;351: h4320.
12. Healy D, Mangin D. Does my bias look big in this? In: Baylis F, Ballantyne A, editors. Clinical trials involving pregnant women. New York: Springer; 2015.
13. Healy D. Challenging the dominance of the pharmaceutical industry in psychiatry. In: Higgins A, McDaid S, editors. Mental health in Ireland. Dublin: Gill & MacMillan; 2014. p. 251–69.
14. Healy D, Bechtold K, Tolias P. Antidepressant-induced suicidality: how translational epidemiology incorporating pharmacogenetics into controlled trials can improve clinical care. Personalized Med 2014;11:79–88.
15. Moynihan R, Cassels A. Selling Sickness. Nation Books: New York 2005.
16. Healy D. The antidepressant era. Cambridge MA: Harvard University Press; 1998.
17. Ayd FJ. Recognition and treatment of the depressed patient. New York: Grune and Stratton; 1961.
18. Healy D. Serotonin and depression. The marketing of a myth. BMJ 2015;350:h1771.
19. Healy D. Mania. Baltimore MD: Johns Hopkins University Press; 2008.
20. Walsh D, Charlton B. The association between the development of weighing technology, possession and use of weighing scales, and self-reported severity of disordered eating. Ir J Med Sci 2014;183:471–75.
21. McKeown T. The role of medicine. Oxford: Basil Blackwell; 1979.
22. Valenstein ES. Great and desperate cures. New York: Basic Books; 1986.
23. Healy D. Images of trauma. London: Faber and Faber; 1993.
24. McGhee RA, Wolfe DA. Psychological maltreatment: toward an operational definition. Dev Psychopathol 1991;3:3–18.
25. Bursztajn HJ, Feinbloom RI, Hamm RM, et al. Medical choices, medical chances; how patients, families and physicians can cope with uncertainty. London: Routledge; 1980.
26. Mol A. The logic of care. London: Routledge; 2008.
27. Mangin D, Sweeney K, Heath I. Preventive healthcare in elderly people needs rethinking. BMJ 2007;335:285–7.
28. Haikan E. Venus envy. A history of cosmetic surgery. Baltimore, MD: Johns Hopkins University Press; 1998.
29. http://www.socialaudit.org.uk/6070225.htm.

INDEX

Page numbers followed by '*f*' indicate figures, '*t*' indicate tables, and '*b*' indicate boxes.

A

B

C

D

E

F

G

H

INDEX

M

N

O

P

T

U

V

W

X

Y

Z